Mario Glowik, Sławomir Smyczek (Eds.)
Healthcare

Healthcare

Market Dynamics, Policies and Strategies in Europe

Edited by
Mario Glowik, Sławomir Smyczek

DE GRUYTER
OLDENBOURG

ISBN 978-3-11-055388-8
e-ISBN (PDF) 978-3-11-041484-4
e-ISBN (EPUB) 978-3-11-041491-2

Library of Congress Cataloging-in-Publication Data
A CIP catalogue record for this book has been applied for at the Library of Congress.

Bibliographic information published by the Deutsche Nationalbibliothek
The Deutsche Nationalbibliothek lists this publication in the Deutsche Nationalbibliografie;
detailed bibliographic data are available on the Internet at http://dnb.dnb.de.

© 2017 Walter de Gruyter GmbH, Berlin/Boston
This volume is text- and page-identical with the hardback published in 2015.
Cover illustration: Monkeybusinessimages/iStock/thinkstock
Typesetting: PTP-Berlin Protago-TEX-Production GmbH, Berlin
Printing and binding: CPI books GmbH, Leck
♾ Printed on acid-free paper
Printed in Germany

www.degruyter.com

Preface

This publication discusses emerging challenges related to healthcare in the European Union (EU). The complex subject of healthcare is illuminated from the perspective of different stakeholders, such as hospital staff, political-legal decision makers, and academics, as well as medical device and pharmaceutical practitioners. This multi-level approach makes the book novel and unique and differentiates it from books currently available on the market.

Moreover, this publication is not narrowly focused on healthcare-related challenges in just one country; instead, the authors develop a multi-country perspective. Research outcomes concentrate on five leading markets: Germany, Sweden, Belgium, the United Kingdom, and Poland. These countries were selected because they represent the most important, but different, healthcare systems in the EU. Poland, the largest economy among the new EU member states, serves as an excellent case of a healthcare system that was completely revised after the fall of the Iron Curtain in 1989. This publication contributes information relevant to the necessity for increasingly integrated and harmonized healthcare systems, which is as one of the major challenges in Europe.

The *first chapter* of the book provides an introduction to the European healthcare environment. The countries of the EU have adopted different approaches to the organization of health systems in their countries. These systems have different forms of financing and also have different levels of efficiency. The characteristics of the major health systems in the EU are described; and the sources of financing for these systems, including voluntary forms of insurance, are introduced. *Chapter two* provides an analysis of the investment attractiveness of leading European healthcare markets. Because investment in healthcare is one of the most complex areas of investment, its attractiveness depends on many factors, such as the country's macro and micro characteristics. These characteristics are introduced to the reader.

Chapter three is concerned with a fine-grained identification of healthcare consumers. Several variables influence consumption of medication and the behavior of consumers who use medication. The aim of the authors is to compare these parameters based on various insurance models. The results come from medication sales from pharmaceutical wholesalers to community pharmacies and hospitals. Liberalized global trade patterns and general technological advances have led to various changes in consumer behavior in the European healthcare market. The main goal of *chapter four* is to present how these changes have resulted in new consumer behavior trends. Relationships between medical facilities and patients present a very dynamic, yet not entirely recognized, category. As a result, the literature lacks a complex and clear picture of this phenomenon, which could aid the assessment of activities related to relationship marketing. *Chapter five* seeks to fill this gap by evaluating the effectiveness of relationship marketing, describing the dimensions and strength of relationships between medical facilities and patients, and presenting a model showing the performance of medical facilities acting in the European market. *Chapter six* describes the actors and their roles in a modern hospital buying center and the corresponding network configurations with external stakeholders, such as group purchasing organizations (GPO) and medical device manufacturers.

Chapter seven focusses on the characteristics, cases, and recommendations that pertain to the integrated marketing communication of healthcare service providers in the five European countries being analyzed. In *chapter eight*, based on an in-depth analysis of all sixty-eight orphan drugs that have received designation and marketing authorization in the EU for the treatment of rare diseases since 2000, the authors demonstrate the effects of the regulatory framework for orphan drugs on company strategy.

The effectiveness of healthcare organizations is of vital importance and can be ensured through the use of performance control mechanisms. The objective of *chapter nine* is to present performance measurement control mechanisms applied to healthcare. The importance of the Internet in the European health sector has increased continuously over the last years. Various European national healthcare services and e-health infrastructures and systems are now viewed as central to the future provision of safe, efficient, high-quality, and citizen-centered healthcare. Consequently, *chapter ten* discusses the concept of e-services in the healthcare sector and the main assumptions of suitable e-health strategies as currently being implemented in the EU. Social media have become a central part of social life for many people all around the globe. Organizations use social media tools more and more frequently for their customer-targeted marketing communication. Due to the fact that the significance of social networking services has also been growing in the healthcare sector, *chapter eleven* presents the results of the author's research regarding the activity of selected hospitals that operate in the five EU countries and use social media. Particular attention is paid to Facebook. Customer attitudes concerning e-medical services depend, to a large extent, on the value expected by patients. *Chapter twelve* describes the value that patients expect from medical facilities and from the services offered by them in the virtual environment in Europe. Finally, *chapter thirteen* is devoted to efficiency control mechanisms for building relationships using social media in healthcare.

We sincerely thank Margie Dyer for her tremendous efforts proofreading our manuscript. We also wish to thank all reviewers and project supporters, particularly Professor Dr. Jochen Breinlinger-O'Reilly, for their valuable recommendations and comments. Last but not least, we would like to thank Mrs. Anja Cheong from the publishing house De Gruyter Oldenbourg for her outstanding support and very professional expertise realizing this publication.

January 2015

Mario Glowik
Sławomir Smyczek

Contents

Justyna Matysiewicz

1 Introduction to the European Healthcare Market

Abstract: The Member States of the European Union have adopted different approaches to the organization of health systems in their countries. These systems have different forms of financing and also have different levels of efficiency. This chapter presents detailed characteristics of the major health systems in the European Union and discusses the sources of financing for these systems, including the additional, voluntary forms of insurance. In particular, the chapter describes and characterizes Belgian, German, Polish, Swedish, and UK systems. The chapter also presents the results of patient surveys used in the health systems.

Keywords: Healthcare system, Financing healthcare, European market

1.1 Introduction

Every **healthcare system** is focused on meeting the health needs of a particular population. The real level and degree of meeting these needs is determined by a number of elements, in particular by the means at the disposal of the system. The result of system activities should be improvement of the health status of the population, or at least should keep health outcomes at a constant level. The particular healthcare systems in the European Union countries are related to the history, tradition, and culture of the given country. Nevertheless, there are a few main healthcare models, which differ from one another in methods of financing, organization, and efficiency. This chapter describes the main types of healthcare models in the EU, discusses expenditures on health by the individual countries and the role of private health insurance, and presents opinions of patients regarding the health systems.

1.2 Concept of the healthcare system

Equality in access to health services is one of the main rights of people, and its assurance should be the primary objective of the healthcare system. The **health policy** of each country[1] and the WHO[2] should aim, therefore, to achieve this objective through an appropriate regulatory system that takes into account financial and structural needs and promotes the principles of bioethics (equality in access to healthcare for people with identical health needs, ensuring the same quality of med-

---

1 Article 129.1 of the Maastricht Treaty of 1993.
2 The WHO strategy "Health for All", adopted in 1978.

ical services and the same use of resources and effort in pursuit of patient health) (Suchocka 2008).

Health protection refers to a wide range of social activities undertaken by public health departments and government agencies, whose aim is to prevent and treat diseases, improve mental and physical health, extend human life, and ensure the healthy development of the next generation (Encyclopedia 1999). In contrast, healthcare can be defined as a system of healthcare facilities and the services provided by them. The aim is to strengthen and improve the health of individuals and society through disease prevention, early detection, treatment, and rehabilitation (Encyclopedia 1999). The purposes of this system are the following (Poznański et al. 2000, Wlodarczyk 1996):

- providing the entire population the full range of required medical services without regard to their economic, social, cultural, and geographical status (access to care);
- providing services and benefits, preventive treatment, and rehabilitation at the highest possible level, given the level of knowledge and art of medicine and the principles of good practice (quality of medical care in accordance with the principles of its continuity and a global approach);
- organization of care in the best possible way, so as to ensure optimum use of resources – financial, personal, and technological such as health databases (effectiveness of healthcare – productivity, rationality, efficiency);
- systematic implementation of activities that improve the system; and employment of appropriate personnel prepared to work in healthcare.

The health system differs from other social systems, such as education, and from the markets for most consumer goods and services in two ways, which make the goals of fair financing and responsiveness particularly significant. One difference is that healthcare can be very costly. Much of the need for care is unpredictable, so it is vital for people to be protected from having to choose between financial ruin and loss of health. Mechanisms for sharing risk and providing financial protection are more important than in other situations where people buy insurance, as for physical assets like homes or vehicles or the financial risk to a family of a breadwinner dying young. The other peculiarity of health is that illness and medical care as well can threaten people's dignity and their ability to control what happens to them more than most other events to which they are exposed. Among other things, responsiveness means reducing the damage to one's dignity and autonomy and reducing the fear and shame that sickness often brings with it (The World Health Report 2000).

Therefore, it is assumed that the basic objectives of the healthcare system include eliminating health inequalities by ensuring equal opportunities for development and health; strengthening health; preventing disease, death and disability; and organizing the treatment to be provided so as to ensure both care for the patient and the preservation of patient dignity.

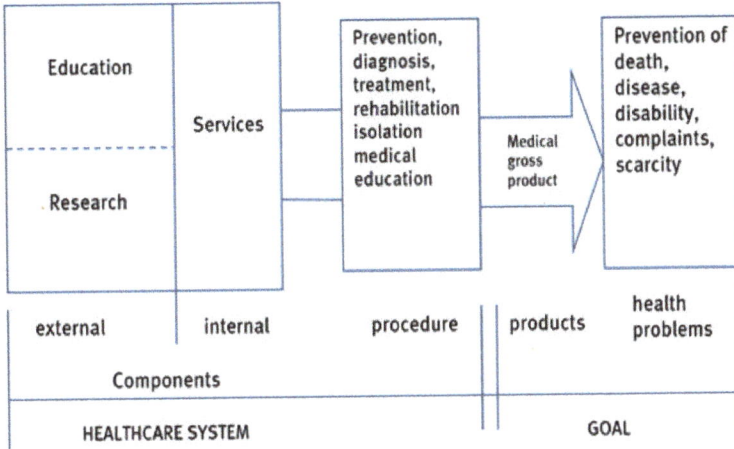

Fig. 1.1: Relationship between the functions of the health system and its goal
Source: Adapted from The World Health Report, Health Systems. Improving Performance, WHO 2000p. 25

1.3 Healthcare systems in the EU

European societies recognize that a good healthcare system should be accessible to everyone, regardless of their income. Free choice and equal access to health services for all (or the vast majority of the population) is the primary goal of each system. Due to limited resources and their nature (public), and in particular the existing disparity between resources and the needs of society, the healthcare system should use tools that enable maximum efficiency in both micro- and macro-scales. The tools used to achieve this efficiency are the different forms of organization and ownership of healthcare units, sources and methods of financing healthcare services, and methods of payment for medical services – from public funds or the private funds of patients (Jasinski 2002).

The systems chosen by European countries are different. This difference relates primarily to the method of financing healthcare in the country and the forms of its organization (Siwinska 2008).

Traditional **models of healthcare systems** are treated as patterns that describe the desired or the ideal shape of the system. The models constitute a set of possible solutions, from which countries can choose those that are thought to be the best given their circumstances. Individual countries adapt the model to their own circumstances on an individual basis, i.e. they decide to apply only certain elements that are appropriate to the situation in their country. The most common European models of health systems are

- Bismarck's model (insurance model of healthcare financing);
- Beveridge's model (supply model of healthcare financing);

- Residual model, called the X model; and
- Siemaszko's model (after the collapse of the communist system, this model is not present in any European country).

These models have a universal character because of the possibility of their use in the analysis of the health policies and systems of different countries. At the same time, they show some specifics related to the development of systems that proceeded differently in the UK, Germany, the countries of Central and Eastern Europe, and Scandinavia. Other countries, utilizing one of these models to a greater or lesser extent, proceeded in their own way, a process in which tradition and history played a very important role (Klos et al. 2005).

Finance and organization of healthcare in the EU Member States is based on national political and socio-economic traditions. These traditions translate into certain social objectives in healthcare finance and delivery, such as equity, efficiency, and affordable cost. There is considerable variation both among healthcare systems in the EU and in healthcare and other policy sectors within each country in the relative value assigned to each objective.

To finance a healthcare system, money has to be transferred from the population or patient, the first party, to the service provider, the second party. All systems in the European Union employ a third party to pay for or to insure health expenses for beneficiaries for the times when they are patients. The aim is to share the costs for medical care between the sick and the well and to adjust for different levels of ability to pay. This mechanism of solidarity reflects consensus in the European Union that healthcare should not be left to a free market alone (European Parlament 1998).

Discussing more particularly the healthcare systems implemented in Europe requires starting with Bismarck's model, which was introduced by Prince Otto Eduard Leopold von Bismarck in 1883. This model became the template for creating insurance in almost all European countries in the early twentieth century. Healthcare services are financed from premiums (paid by the employee and the employer), which are most often obligatory. The process of making decisions is decentralized, and the state creates precise legal frames of functioning for the entire system. The important thing is that funding medical care costs may be provided in full or may include some share of financing by the insured.

After World War II, in 1948, the master system of the English national healthcare services was introduced in the United Kingdom, based on the project by Lord William Beveridge. This model is called the Beveridge model. It excludes medical care from the social insurance system and calls for a special fund, financed from general taxes. The leading idea of this model is guaranteeing social security to all citizens, the so-called principle of equality of citizens. The state controls execution of healthcare services by healthcare facilities. Healthcare services are free. Hospitals are financed mostly from the central budget or are assigned funds. The above model also includes voluntary supplementary insurance facilities dedicated to increasing the standard of medical care and expanding its scope.

A residual model, called the X model, rejects or seriously limits public responsibility for providing citizen access to healthcare. In the X model, healthcare services are financed with voluntary individual premiums; thus the private sector has the dominant role. The area of public health is thus separate from individual healthcare, and the healthcare sector is regarded as an open field for economic activity. Financing of services is based on private insurance or on individual direct financing. The residual model includes the public sector, which covers only persons in special need, including very poor or old people.

In Central and Eastern Europe, Siemaszko's model (or the budget model) has been functioning since the early twentieth century. Its principles were developed by Mikołaj Siemaszko, the healthcare commissar in the Soviet Union in the 1930s. The basic premises of this model are financing healthcare services from taxes through the budget, providing a free and complete range of services except for some medicines, providing equal access to services for everyone, and having a monopoly by the state healthcare service. This model proved to be fiction – pure theory. It is now regarded as a historical form, and the states in which this model was functioning are restoring their insurance systems (Rutkowska-Podolowska et al. 2011).

Analyzing table 1.1 shows the loss of the original assumptions of the models. In these systems, we deal with the coexistence of different systems: the creation of mixed system.

Tab. 1.1: Methods of financing healthcare in the Member States of the EU
Source: Adapted from Healthcare Systems In Europe. A Comparative Study, European Parliament, Luxembourg 1998p. 18

Country	Dominant financial system	Additional financial system
Finland, Greece, Ireland, Italy, Sweden, Spain, United Kingdom	Public: Taxes	Private voluntary insurance, direct payments
Denmark, Portugal	Public: Taxes	Direct payments
Austria, Belgium, France, Germany	Public: compulsory insurance	Private voluntary insurance, direct payments, public taxation
The Netherlands	Mixed: compulsory social insurance and private voluntary insurance	Public: taxes, direct fees
New EU Member States	Public: compulsory insurance	Public: taxes, direct fees, private voluntary insurance

With reference to the earlier discussion, the EU Member States employ different methods for cost-sharing. **Co-payments** for services, which are to be paid by patients, are most frequently applied to prescribed pharmaceuticals either at a flat rate or at a percentage of the price of the product. Co-payments for prescribed pharmaceuticals have in principle been deployed in all Member States. Some Member States (Austria, Belgium, Denmark, Finland, France, Italy, Ireland, and Portugal) also apply a co-payment system for specialist physician care; whereas co-payments for services provided by general practitioners are less frequently required (Austria, Belgium, France). Co-payments for inpatient hospital care are in operation in Austria, Belgium, Germany, France, Luxembourg, Portugal, and Sweden. Co-payments for dental services can amount to 100% in a number of EU countries (European Parliament 1998).

Co-insurance is another form of cost-sharing, whereby the insured person has to pay for a set proportion of all services delivered (France). In most Member States, there is a provision to exclude low-income groups and other disadvantaged population groups from cost-sharing.

Compulsory and **voluntary insurance** is administered by insurance funds – autonomous organizations that collect a share of work-related income and in turn provide payment for healthcare either at the time of use or by repayment afterwards (European Parliament 1998).

Most of the tax-based systems operate with a national health service, where services are provided through a central public institution. However, it does not necessarily follow that government funding leads to services that are owned by the government or that all staff working in the health services are salaried staff. Only in Greece and Portugal is a salaried staff the predominate arrangement for doctors working in ambulatory care. Alternative payment systems in office-based care are fee-for-service (payments according to fixed service charges) and capitation (where the provider receives a fixed amount per enrolled person). More recently developed forms of payment to primary care providers include payment of a lump sum (budget), within which services have to be managed. Under study are payment systems based on a certain diagnosis or on achieved medical outcomes. In general practice and specialist care, out-of-hospital, fee-for-service arrangements tend to be the predominant payment type in social insurance systems in the EU (Belgium, France, Germany, and Luxembourg). There is currently a substantial effort to reform fee-for-service arrangements (European Parlament 1998). In the CEE countries, the main source of funding for health spending is social insurance. Due to insufficiency in the healthcare systems, continuously increasing sales of private insurance are being observed (Poland) as well as direct payments.

1.4 Healthcare expenditure

Health systems in Europe are at the core of the high level of social protection, and they are a cornerstone of the European social market economy. The healthcare sector accounts for 8% of the total European workforce and for 10% of the EU's GDP.[3] The large share of healthcare costs in the EU raises the issue of cost-effectiveness and the financial sustainability of the health systems. The problems caused by the economic crisis are coupled with more structural changes in demography and the types of diseases affecting populations in Europe. Clearly, health is an important part of public budgets. It represents almost a third of social policy budgets. Public expenditure accounts for almost 80% of healthcare budgets. In 2010, public spending on healthcare accounted for almost 15% of all government expenditures. In the decade before the crisis, healthcare was one of the fastest growing spending items for governments in almost all Member States, considerably outpacing GDP growth. Public expenditure on healthcare and long-term care is expected to increase by one-third by 2060. This growth is due to a number of factors. On the demand side, it is chiefly due to population size and structure, health status, individual and national incomes, and provisions regulating access to healthcare goods and services. On the supply side, the increase is driven by the availability of and distance from health services, technological progress, and the framework regulating the provision of goods and services. The relatively large share of public healthcare spending in total government expenditures, combined with the need to consolidate government budget balances across the EU, underscores the need to improve the sustainability of current health system models (*Investing in Health* 2013).

The Netherlands had the highest share of its GDP allocated to health in 2010 (12%), followed by France and Germany (both at 11.6%). The lowest share of GDP allocated to health spending was in Romania and Turkey, at around 6% (figure 1.2.). With the exception of Cyprus, public funding remains the main source of financing of health expenditure in all EU Member States, with close to three-quarters of all spending being paid by public sources. The ranking of countries in terms of public expenditure on health as a share of GDP is not very different from total expenditure on health. For a more complete understanding of the level of health spending, the health spending to GDP ratio should be considered along with health spending *per capita*. Countries having a relatively high health spending to GDP ratio might have relatively low health expenditure *per capita*, and the converse also holds. For example, Belgium and Portugal both spent around 10.5% of their GDP on health in 2010; however, *per capita* spending (adjusted to EUR PPP) was nearly 50% higher in Belgium.

---

[3] The size of the healthcare sector varies widely among Member States: above 11% of GDP in Austria, Denmark, France, Germany and the Netherlands; below 7% of GDP in Estonia, Latvia, and Romania.

% GDP

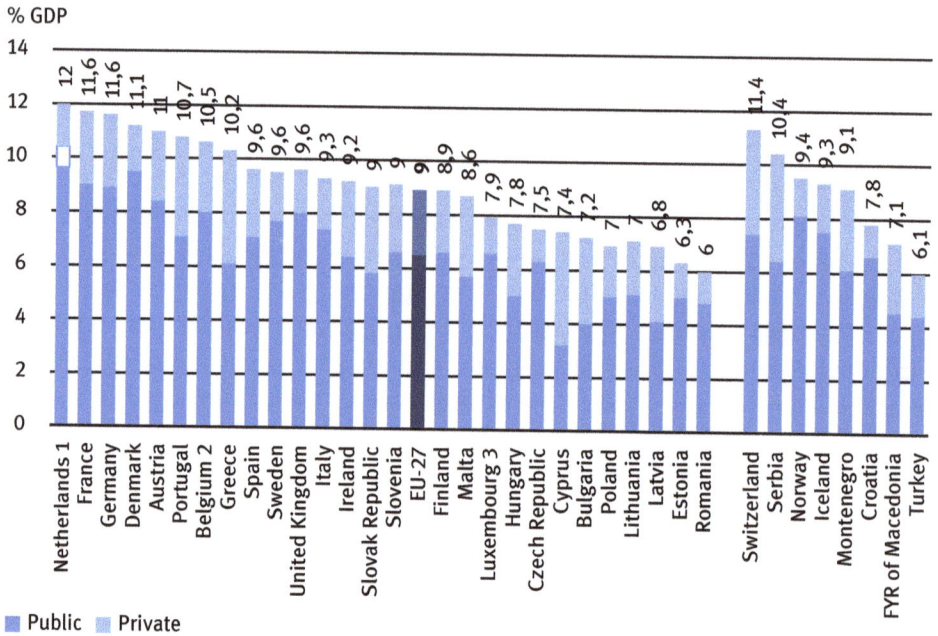

Fig. 1.2: Total health expenditure as a share of GDP, 2010 (or nearest year)
Source: Adapted from Health at a Glance: Europe 2012, OECDiLibrary, http://www.oecd-ilibrary.org/

1 In the Netherlands, it is not possible to clearly distinguish the public and private share related to investments.

2 Public and private expenditures are current expenditures (excluding investments).

3 Health expenditure is for the insured population rather than resident population.

Changes in the ratio of health spending to GDP are the result of the combined effect of growth in both GDP and health expenditures. Between 2000 and 2010, the annual average growth in health expenditure *per capita* in real terms was about 4% on average in EU member states, nearly two times greater than the growth rate in GDP *per capita*. With the exception of Bulgaria, Iceland, and Luxembourg, annual growth in health spending outpaced GDP growth in all European countries over the past decade. This explains why the share of GDP allocated to health increased from 7.3% to 9.0% during that period.

In France and Germany, the health spending to GDP ratio increased from just over 10% in 2000 to 11.6% in both countries in 2010. Health spending *per capita* grew slightly faster in Germany than in France over the past decade, but so did GDP *per capita*. The share of GDP was relatively stable in both countries between 2003 and 2008, but it then increased by 1% in 2009 as health spending continued to grow while GDP fell in both countries. In the United Kingdom, the health spending share of GDP used to be below the EU average; but since 2006, it is now above the average. As in many other European countries, the share of health spending allocated to GDP in the United Kingdom increased by a full percentage point in 2009 following the financial and economic crisis, but came down slightly in 2010 (OECD 2012).

1.5 Private health insurance in the EU

Every EU country allows **private health insurance** (PHI) to be sold alongside statutory health insurance, but there is an enormous diversity in the role PHI plays within the healthcare system and in the size and functioning of different markets for PHI. PHI has been defined as insurance taken out voluntarily and paid for privately, either by individuals or by employers, on behalf of individuals (Mossialos and Thomson 2002). This definition recognises that PHI may be sold by a wide range of entities, both public and private in nature – including statutory 'sickness funds', nonprofit mutual, or provident associations and commercial for-profit insurance companies. In Europe, private health insurance plays only a limited, supplementary role. It enters the system for a number of reasons.

- Because of the exclusion of some social and professional groups (e.g., sole traders), a number of citizens remain outside the public healthcare system.
- The highest income groups may opt out of the public system.
- A number of medical services and products have been eliminated from the package guaranteed by the public system.
- In the public system, some services are partly funded by the system, partly paid for individually by patients.
- Access to services that are free of charge for patients or partly paid by them within the public system is limited.

Under the domination of the public health system, three main types of private health insurance may be distinguished:
- substitutive,
- complementary, and
- supplementary (parallel, alternative, ancillary).

Substitutive insurance provides coverage for the costs incurred to meet health needs resulting from staying outside of the public healthcare system. Complementary insurance offers coverage for the costs of services that are not offered within the public system or the payments required in the public system. Supplementary insurance is the insurance against the risk of limited access to services that are free or partially paid for in the public system.

Understanding these differences in the role of the market (summarized in table 1.2) is important for three reasons. First, the role a PHI market plays is closely correlated to its size, particularly in terms of its contribution to spending on healthcare, as we will discuss in the following section. Second, the market role largely determines the way in which it is regulated; this has implications in terms of EU competition and internal market rules. And third, as a result of its combined effect on the market size and on the public policy regarding PHI, the market role may tell us a great deal about the likely impact of PHI on health financing policy goals (Thomson and Mossialos 2009).

Tab. 1.2: Functional classification of PHI markets
Source: Adapted from Thomson, S., and E. Mossialos (2009). Private health insurance in the European Union, Article Retrieved June 21, 2011, p.16 (Final report prepared for the European Commission, Directorate General for Employment, Social Affairs and Equal Opportunities), p.15 and adopted from: Mossialos, E. and S. Thomson (2002). Voluntary health insurance in the European Union: a critical assessment. International Journal of Health Services 32(1): p.19–88 and Foubister, T., S. Thomson, E. Mossialos and A. McGuire (2006). Private medical insurance in the United Kingdom. Copenhagen, World Health Organization

Market role	Driver of market development	Nature of coverage	Examples
Substitutive	Public system inclusiveness (proportion of the population eligible for public coverage)	Covers people excluded from or allowed to opt out of the public system	Germany
Complementary (services)	Scope of benefits covered by the public system	Covers services excluded from the public system	Hungary, Denmark
Complementary (user charges)	Depth of public coverage (the proportion of the benefit cost met by the public system)	Covers statutory user charges imposed in the public system	Belgium, France, Latvia, Slovenia
Supplementary	Consumer satisfaction (perceptions about the quality of publicly financed care)	Covers faster access and enhanced consumer choice	Poland, Romania, UK

The role PHI plays in a given health system is largely determined by public policy. This in turn may reflect historical developments, a political ideology, the relative power and interests of different stakeholders (particularly providers and insurers, but also different groups in the population – for example, civil servants or higher earners), and government capacity to shape and develop the market. The size of the market will also be affected by these factors as well as by others, such as people's willingness and ability to pay for private coverage (Thomson and Mossialos 2009).

Tab. 1.3: Overview of markets for PHI: selected countries
Source: Adapted from Thomson, S., E. Mossialos (2009). Private health insurance in the European Union, Article Retrieved June 21, 2011, p.16 (Final report prepared for the European Commission, Directorate General for Employment, Social Affairs and Equal Opportunities)

Country	Market role(s)	Eligibility	Examples of benefits covered
Belgium	Complementary (user charges)	Whole population	Reimbursement of statutory user charges and extra billing for inpatient care
	Complementary (services)		CAM, dental and eye care, vaccines, prostheses and implants, treatment abroad, inpatient and outpatient care
Bulgaria	Supplementary	Whole population	Superior amenities in hospital, private room, faster access to care
	Complementary (services)		Dental care, medical devices, outpatient pharmaceuticals
Czech Republic	Supplementary	Whole population	Private room
	Substitutive	Nonresidents, self-employed migrants, children of migrant workers with residence permits, foreign students not entitled to statutory coverage	Similar to statutory cover, but excludes treatment of some chronic conditions, e,g,, HIV/AIDS, drug addiction, mental health, spa treatment, etc.
Estonia	Substitutive	Individuals not entitled to statutory coverage	Similar to statutory coverage, but commercial coverage offers different levels of benefit
Germany	Substitutive	Households with higher earnings, self-employed excluded from statutory coverage	Similar benefits to statutory coverage
	Complementary (user charges)	Civil servants	Reimburses healthcare costs not fully covered by the government
	Complementary (services)	Whole population	Dental care
	Complementary (user charges)		Reimburses statutory user charges for outpatient care
	Supplementary		Private hospitals, choice of specialist, per diem cash benefits for hospitalization
Poland	Supplementary	Whole population	Private care, faster access
Sweden	Supplementary	Whole population	Faster access, private elective care
	Complementary (user charges)		Reimburses statutory user charges for outpatient prescription drugs
UK	Supplementary	Whole population	Acute care (i.e., elective surgery), screening, 'employee health management' processes

Note: CAM: complementary and alternative medicine

1.6 EU healthcare systems: the patient perspective

One of the most comprehensive studies evaluating health systems in Europe from the perspective of the patient/client is the Euro Health Consumer Index (EHCI). It has established itself as the "industry standard" of modern healthcare monitoring since its start in 2005. The 2013 edition ranks thirty-five national European healthcare systems on forty-eight indicators, covering six areas that are essential to the health consumer: *patients' rights and information, accessibility of treatment* (waiting times), *medical outcomes, range and reach of services provided,* and *pharmaceuticals.* The 2013 Index has now introduced *prevention* as a new area, with eight indicators. The EHCI is compiled from a combination of public statistics, patient polls, and independent research conducted by the Sweden-based research company Health Consumer Powerhouse Ltd.

The results of the research presented in the latest report show that there is a group of European countries that all have good healthcare systems from the point of view of the customer/consumer. The total ranking of healthcare systems shows a much narrowed victory for The Netherlands, scoring 870 points out of 1000 and nineteen points ahead of runner-up Switzerland at 851 points. After the top two, there is more than a thirty-point gap down to three closely knit Scandinavian countries: Iceland third at 818 points, Denmark in fourth place with 815, and Norway fifth with 813 points (Euro Health Consumer Index Report 2013).

The report noted that Denmark gained a lot from the introduction of the e-Health sub-discipline. The Swedish score for technically excellent healthcare services is, as ever, dragged down by the seemingly never-ending story of access/waiting time problems, in spite of national efforts such as *Vårdgaranti* (National Guaranteed Access to Healthcare). In 2013, Sweden dropped to eleventh place with 756 points.

In southern Europe, Spain and Italy provide healthcare services where medical excellence can be found in many places. Real excellence in southern European healthcare seems to be a bit too dependent on the consumers' ability to afford private healthcare as a supplement to public healthcare. Also, both Spain and Italy show large regional variation. Some eastern European EU member systems are doing surprisingly well, particularly the Czech Republic and Slovakia, considering their much smaller healthcare spending in purchasing power adjusted dollars *per capita*. However, readjusting from politically planned to consumer-driven economies does take time. Consumer and patient rights are improving. In a growing number of European countries, there is healthcare legislation explicitly based on patient rights and a functional access to a patient's own medical record is becoming standard (*Euro Health Consumer Index Report* 2013).

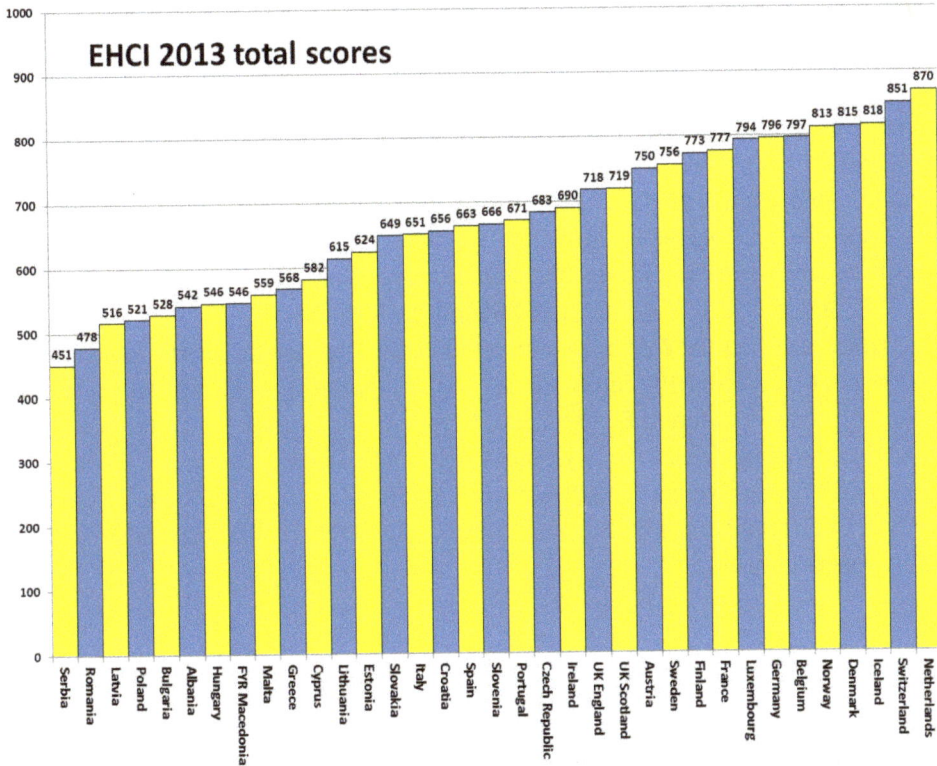

Fig. 1.3: EHCI 2013 total scores
Scource: Adapted from Euro Health Consumer Index Report 2013p. 23

Medical travel supported by the new patient mobility directive could accelerate the demand for performance transparency. After the cross-border directive, the criteria for this indicator have been tightened to reflect the implementation of the directive. Not unexpectedly, in 2013 the only countries among good-performance countries were The Netherlands and Luxembourg, who have been allowing cross-border care seeking for years. Generally, European healthcare continues to improve but medical outcome statistics are still appallingly poor in many countries. This is the case regarding the number one killer condition: cardiovascular diseases, where data for one very vital parameter; thirty-day fatality for hospitalized heart infarct patients had to be compiled from several disparate sources. If healthcare officials and politicians began looking across borders and "stealing" improvement ideas from their European colleagues, there would be a good chance that a national system would come much closer to the theoretical top score of 1000. As a prominent example, if Sweden could achieve a Belgian waiting time situation, that alone would suffice to lift Sweden to the level of The Netherlands at ~880 points (*Euro Health Consumer Index Report* 2013).

The report also indicates that the Bismarck model seems to be much more effective. The Beveridge model seemed to achieve good results only in small population countries, such as Iceland, Denmark, and Norway. For more than half a century, particularly since the formation of the British NHS, the largest Beveridge-type system in Europe, there has been intense debate over the relative merits of the two types of systems. Looking at the results of the EHCI from 2006 to 2009, it is very hard to avoid noticing that the top consists of dedicated Bismarck countries, with the small-population and therefore more easily managed Beveridge systems of the Nordic countries also squeezing in. Large Beveridge systems seem to have difficulties attaining really excellent levels of customer value. The largest Beveridge countries, the U.K. and Italy, rank together in the middle of the Index.

The rest of the book describes in detail issues concerning health systems and markets. The basis for the international analysis is the level of functioning of the health systems in different EU countries, in relation to: the adopted healthcare, the role of private health insurance, effectiveness, and patient opinion. For this discussion, five counties were selected: Germany, Sweden, Belgium, and the UK, as well as Poland as an example of a country with a completely revised healthcare system in the last twenty years.

References

Bukowska-Piestrzynska A. 2011: *Kierunki zmian w dostepnosci opieki zdrowotnej w województwie lodzkim u progu XXI w.*, Acta Universitatis Lodziensis, Folia Oeconomica Vol. 253, 117–127

Dietrich A.R.& Osak M., 2002: *Reforma reformy zdrowotnej w Polsce. Diagnoza wstępna*, Polityka Społeczna Vol. 29, 1–13

Encyklopedia PWN 1999: t. II, Wydawnictwo Naukowe PWN, Warszawa.

*Euro Health Consumer Index Report 20*13, Retrieved February 14, 2014 from: http://www.healthpowerhouse.com/index.php?Itemid=55, 1–102

Foubister, T., Thomson S., Mossialos E. & McGuire A., 2006: *Private medical insurance in the United Kingdom*. Copenhagen, World Health Organization, 1–125

Health at a Glance: Europe 2012, OECDiLibrary, Retrieved February 14, 2014 from: http://www.oecd-ilibrary.org/, 1–54

Healthcare Systems in EU. A Comparative Study. Working Paper, Public Health and Consumer Protection Series, European Parlament 1998, Retrieved February 14, 2014 from: http://www.europarl.europa.eu/workingpapers/saco/pdf/101_en.pdf, 1–130

Investing in Health. Commision Staff Working Document. Social Investment Package, European Commision 2013, 1–23

Jasiński G., 2001: *Wybrane aspekty organizacji i metod finansowania systemów ochrony zdrowia w państwach europejskich*, "Biuletyn Kas Chorych" kwiecień 2001, nr 3–4, 16–22.

Klos K., Pazdzioch S., Sidorowicz W. & Suski B., 2005: *Samorządowa opieka zdrowotna krajach Unii Europejskiej – kierunki i wytyczne dla polskich samorządów wojewódzkich*, Warszawa, 1–99

Poznański P., Konracka D., Skolimowska J., Gałczyński K. & Zbylut J., 2000:, *Analiza gospodarki finansowej Kas Chorych w aspekcie zapewnienia dostepnsci do wybranych świadczeń zdrowotnych*, Antidotum, Vol. 6, 6

Mossialos, E. & Thomson S., 2002: *Voluntary health insurance in the European Union: a critical assessment*. International Journal of Health Services 32(1), 19–88

Siwińska V., Brożyniak J. & Iłżecka J., 2008: *Modele systemów opieki zdrowotnej w Polsce i wybranych państwach europejskich*, Zdrowie Publiczne Vol. 118(3), 358–367

Suchocka J., 2008: *Regulacje publiczne i prawne, rownosci sektorów w ochronie zdrowia*, [in:] K. Ryc, Z. Skrzypczak Z. (Ed.) Ochrona zdrowia i gospodarka. Mechanizmy rynkowe a regulacje publiczne, Wyd. Nauk. WZ UW, Warszawa, 24

The World Health Report 2000 - Health systems: improving performance, WHO 2000, Retrieved February 14, 2014 from: http://www.who.int/whr/2000/en/, 1–215

Thomson S.& Mossialos E., 2009: *Private health insurance in the European Union*, Article Retrieved (June 21, 2011) Retrieved May 16 from: http://{ http://eprints.lse.ac.uk/25511/}, 1–333

Włodarczyk W.C., 1996: *Polityka zdrowotna w społeczeństwie demokratycznym*, Vesalius, Krakow, 95–96

Jagoda Gola

2 Investment Attractiveness of the Healthcare Markets in Europe

Abstract: The healthcare market is one of the most interesting areas of investment. Its attractiveness depends on many factors: the health model and a country's macro and micro characteristics, among others. Although the leading countries in healthcare are the USA and China, European countries have a huge potential to grow. It may be assumed that all the described markets – Belgian, German, Polish, Swedish and the United Kingdom – should be interesting for investors, though in different areas. Depending on the level of the market development, social changes, and accepted risk rate, different directions of investment are recommended in the areas of pharmacy, medical services, and medical devices.

Keywords: Healthcare system, Financing healthcare, European market

2.1 Introduction

Investment attractiveness can be perceived in many ways. It is important to indicate comparable units, which can be achieved by choosing only a few characteristics that are significant from the investor's perspective. In this chapter, the investment attractiveness of the medical sector is described. However, since there are many differences among some countries and similarities among others, four main health models were considered. As representative countries, Germany, for the insurance model; the United Kingdom and Sweden, for the tax model; Belgium, for the mixed model; and Poland, for the "post-communist" model, were chosen. All comparisons will be focused on these selected geographical areas and compared with Europe or the world. The aim of this chapter is to show the potential of these medical markets, with the stress on medical services, including treatment and wellness; pharmaceuticals; and medical devices, and indicate the future attractiveness of the markets, based on current data and forecasts.

2.2 Investment attractiveness – theoretical attitude

When deciding whether to undertake an investment or not, it is crucial to consider many circumstances in addition to financial efficiency. The investment process needs to consider various signals coming from the environment. This leads to the conclusion that every investment should be preceded by an analysis of the possible opportunities and threats coming from outside of the organization (Marcinek 2002: 19).

To make the best possible decision, an analysis of attractiveness, defined as something that gains interest or engages one's thought (Dictionary), should be considered. Market attractiveness can be defined as a measure of the profits that are possible to gain within the structure of a particular market (*Barron's Marketing Dictionary*). It is best represented by market potential and growth potential (Gleißner, Helm & Kreiter 2013: 60). However, more indicators can be useful – investment risk, progress of the marketing infrastructure, market intensity, market consumption capacity, economic freedom, market absorption capacity, commercial infrastructure, market diversity, and profit potential[1] (Gleißner, Helm & Kreiter, 2013: 6).

Factors that contribute to investment attractiveness may be divided into five main areas: market factors (e.g., size and growth rate), economic factors (industry saturation, investment potential, rate of inflation), technological factors (availability of raw materials, know-how), competitive factors (bargaining power, type of market, types of rival businesses), and environmental factors (degree of social acceptance for a product, existing regulatory climate) (*Barron's Marketing Dictionary*).

Investment attractiveness of a chosen sector can be examined from the perspective of home and foreign investors. The determinants influencing the level of foreign direct investments (**FDI**) can be divided into two main groups: macro-level factors and host country branch factors. Macroeconomic factors include political, economic, social, and legal factors. The second group includes **demand**, competition, and production conditions specific to a chosen sector (Turek 2003: 147–148).

Market **investment attractiveness** is strongly connected to market potential, which can be measured in many dimensions. As an example, an emerging economic market potential index can be mentioned. It covers areas such as market size (measured by urban population and electricity consumption), growth rate (measured by average annual growth rate of primary energy use and real gross domestic product growth rate), intensity (measured by GNI *per capita* and private consumption as a percent of GDP), market consumption capacity (measured by the percentage share of the middleclass in consumption/income), commercial infrastructure (measured by number of PCs, main telephone lines, paved road density, population per retail outlet, Internet users, cellular mobile subscribers, and percentage with TV sets), economic freedom (measured by the political freedom index and economic freedom index), country risk (measured by the country risk rating), and market receptivity (measured by trade as a percentage of GDP and *per capita* imports from the US) (*Market Potential Index*). Another example of measuring attractiveness is the EBA Investment Attractiveness Index, which is dedicated to Ukraine and its investment climate and is based on five aspects that indicate the investment climate: political, economic, legislative, regulatory and other factors, and risk levels and profit-

---

1 These indicators were analyzed in research conducted during the years 1992 to 2002 by different scientists analyzing market attractiveness.

ability of investment (European Business Association). These two examples show that it is difficult to create a comparable market attractiveness index that is accepted worldwide. Market attractiveness should instead be indicated from the point of view of a specific investor; and because of this, an analysis that considers selected aspects should be conducted.

Companies operating in an international environment need to evaluate the potential attractiveness of the market. This evaluation can be done on the basis of substantial amounts of information from many sources, statistical data suppliers or specialized sources. Such vast and diverse information is used very rarely in systematic ways in the decision process (Saaty & Vargas 2001: 135). Because of the limited range of this chapter, only selected aspects of the investment attractiveness of the medical market in Europe will be described.

The healthcare market is very different from others because of the nature of medical goods, which are not typical market goods. This is the reason that it sometimes is called a "quasi market" (Bukowska–Piestrzyńska 2011: 162). At the same time, this industry impacts everybody, every day.

2.3 Macro-level factors influencing medical market attractiveness

Macroeconomic factors are related to household life level, influences on income, working conditions, housing conditions, and life style. These factors directly influence health phenomena. It has been demonstrated that positive changes in one of them influences health effects even more than increasing expenditures on health. Moreover, the general condition of a country's economy influences the conditions of particular branch markets, which generate cash flow used in the healthcare sector (Rudawska 2007: 57).

Among economic factors, GDP, total health expenditures, share of total health expenditures in GDP, public and private health expenditures and their share in GDP, current expenditures on healthcare, and investment expenditures on healthcare should all be mentioned (CSIOZ 2009). Table 2.1 presents selected macro-level factors.

In 2013, according to OECD data (2014), GDP *per capita*, counted in USD current PPPs in constant prices, was on a similar level in Belgium, Germany, Sweden, and the United Kingdom. A much lower level of this indicator was observed in Poland – only a little more than half of the level of the remaining countries, although it is growing between 2% and 7%[2] per year. (In 2002, it was on average about 40% of the remaining countries GDP *per capita*.) At the same time, disposable income in Polish

---

2 Growth in 2007 to 2006 according do OECD data; moreover, from 2002 to 2012, only Poland didn't experience a decrease in GDP *per capita* level; and its growth was the highest of the selected countries.

and Swedish households was the fastest growing of the countries, while Belgium saw a decrease. Disposable income and the ability to pay for goods depend, among other things, on employment and unemployment – total and over the long term.

Since expenditures on health depend on two main sources, public and private, the governmental situation should also be considered. The lowest deficit was in the United Kingdom, minus 8.18% of GDP. The best situation was in Sweden and Germany, which had low deficits. The United Kingdom also had the highest general government debt, on a similar level as Belgium. The best situation was in Sweden and Poland.

Private expenditures on health are about 30% of public expenditures in Germany and Belgium, about 20% in Sweden and the UK, and almost 40% in Poland.[3] These figures indicate that in Poland, the situation of households – their income level and level of employment – will have a stronger impact on the healthcare market than in the other selected countries in comparison to public expenditures. Total expenditures on health are the highest in Germany – 11.6% of GDP. In Belgium, they exceed 10%; in Sweden and the UK, they are almost 10% of GDP. Only in Poland, expenditures do not exceed 7% of GDP. In absolute value, they are the highest in Germany, 371.7 million USD current PPPs; and in the United Kingdom, 210.6 million USD current PPPs. The lowest level was observed in Sweden, 37.3 million USD current PPPs. A health market segment in which POO is dominating is pharmacy; about 65% of drugs were financed from patients' private sources (Jakubiak).

Tab. 2.1: Selected macroeconomic indicators describing Belgium, Germany, Poland, Sweden, and the United Kingdom in 2011
Source: Adapted from OECD (2014) (date: March 25, 2014)

Indicator	Unit	Belgium	Germany	Poland	Sweden	United Kingdom
GDP *per capita*	USD current PPPs	32 899.44 ***	34 807.63 ***	18 298.76 ***	35 130.44 ***	32 662.73 ***
Household disposable income	Annual growth %	– 1.07 **	0.86 *	2.65 *	3.01 **	0.46 *
Government deficit	% of GDP	– 4.0 ***	0.1 ***	– 3.9 ***	– 0.2 ***	– 6.1 ***
General government debt	% of GDP	99.8 ***	81 ***	99.8 ***	38.2 ***	88.7 ***
Public expenditure on health	% of GDP	7.99 **	8.38 **	4.53 **	7.33 **	8.01 *
Private expenditure on health	% of GDP	2.54 **	2.51 **	1.86 **	1.65 **	1.61 *

* 2010, ** 2011, *** 2012

---

3 The ratio of private to public expenditures on health also depends on the model of financing in specific countries.

The tax system also remains important from the investor's point of view.

Table 2.2 presents selected elements of the tax system, focusing attention on the rates of the most commonly paid taxes.

Entities operating in local markets are interested in the profits they can gain; however, in every country, profits are reduced by taxes. Depending on the legal form of the entity and considering the sources of profits, a wide spectrum of tax rates apply.

Tab. 2.2: Selected elements of the tax system in Belgium, Germany, Poland, Sweden, and the United Kingdom
Source: Adapted from Ernst & Young (140, 1031, 1244, 1347), Stawki i regulacje dotyczące podatku VAT

Factor		Belgium	Germany	Poland	Sweden	UK
Corporate Income Tax Rate	%	33	15	19	22	24
Corporate Gains Tax Rate	%	0.4/25/33	14	19	22	24
Branch Tax Rate	%	33	15	19	22	24
Withholding Tax						
Dividends	%	10/15/25	25	19	30	0
Interest	%	15/25	0	20	0	20
Royalities	%	25	15	20	0	20
Net Operating Losses	Years					
Carryback		0	1	0	0	1
Carry forward		unlimited	unlimited	5	unlimited	unlimited
VAT	%	21	19	23	25	20

Table 2.2 presents information on the tax systems. As can be observed, the CIT rate is different among the countries – the lowest is in Germany; the highest is in Belgium. Since the tax system in all these countries is subject to many changes, it needs to be evaluated taking into account predicted improvement. A good example is the UK, where since January 1, 2014, the CIT rate has been reduced to 22%.

In addition, the VAT rate varies from 19% up to 25%. In some countries, medical services are exempt from the VAT (e.g., Poland). Thus all costs are treated as gross – the VAT is not deductible at all or is only partly deductible if the business area of an entity is more diversified and covers other services.

Among the social factors important for running a business are employment rules, personal attitude, trade union power, and strikes.

The unemployment rate is the highest in Poland – more than 10% – and the lowest in Germany – less than 6%. There is not a big difference among the remaining countries – the average is 8.2%. Long-term unemployment is important when considering the work flexibility of the population – the larger the share of long-term unemployment in total unemployment, the lower the possibility that the situation in the labor market will change in the near future (Table 2.3).

Tab. 2.3: Selected social indicators describing Belgium, Germany, Poland, Sweden, and the United Kingdom
Source: Adapted from OECD (2014)

Indicator	Unit	Belgium	Germany	Poland	Sweden	United Kingdom
Unemployment rate: total labor force – year 2013	%	8.4	5.3	10.3	8.0	7.9*
Long-term unemployment: total unemployed – year 2012	%	48.31	47.96	31.59	17.17	33.45

*2012

In Germany, employment relations are regulated by statutory legislation, collective bargaining agreements, case law, and individual employment agreements. Trade unions play a significant role in labor relations. In medicine, the dominance of and membership in trade unions is overwhelming (IndexMundi). In the United Kingdom, organized interest groups such as trade unions are not formally involved in health policy making; however, groups such as the British Medical Association or the Royal Colleges may exert influence informally (Boyle 2011: 8).

Also of interest to a potential investor is the level of contract transparency and corruption. According to transparency.com data (2013), the lowest level of corruption among analyzed countries is in Sweden; and the highest is in Poland (Table 2.4).

Tab. 2.4: Level of corruption and its control in Belgium, Germany, Poland, Sweden, and the United Kingdom in 2011
Source: Adapted from transparency.org data

Country	Belgium	Germany	Poland	Sweden	UK
Points	75	79	58	88	74
Ranking position (of 176 countries)	16	13	41	4	17
Control of corruption level (2010)	90%	93%	70%	99%	90%

The political structure is important for running a business – its stability and development perspective. In this chapter, the political structure is described along with legal factors. The legal framework is important because it creates the environment in which a company exists. It creates the list of possible legal forms of entities and delivers a variety of rules governing their existence. In addition, taxation, which is both an economic and a legal factor, plays an important role in the amount of profits and the possible ways of optimizing profits.

Also interesting for a potential investor is the condition of the healthcare market itself and the areas on which local medical entities focus their attention.

The development of companies operating in the healthcare market should be focused on solving the problems of an aging population (taking care of elderly people, delivering health services at patients' homes), treating chronic diseases (the increasing incidence of chronic diseases has been observed worldwide, so competition will increase around the world in this market segment; however, this is also an area that allows going global more easily than in the case of other products), emerging market exploration (developing markets create new needs for patients and also develop segments that are saturated in mature countries; this creates new perspectives for new companies that try to find a **market gap** and increase their market share as well as for experienced players that already implement solutions and are trying to modify their products and gain new markets). Technological changes and putting more stress on product innovation has been observed worldwide. For this reason, cooperation between medical entities and IT companies should be considered. On the one hand, this allows for better needs fulfillment; on the other hand, it results in new solutions and new needs (Sławatyniec 2010).

In The Federal Republic of Germany, the Basic Law divides power between the states and the federal level. The power is divided at both levels into three branches – legislative, executive, and judicial. The head of the federal government is the chancellor. Important for running a business is that the states themselves are parliamentary republics (IndexMundi). In 2013, Angela Merkel was chosen for the third time to be the chancellor of Germany (Scholz, Matzke 2013). This can be viewed as a sign that the political situation in the country is stable. The German legal system is based on civil law. According to the Basic Law, all legislative power remains at the state level unless otherwise designated by the act itself. Therefore, many fundamental matters remain within the jurisdiction of the states (IndexMundi). This arrangement allows for achieving faster solutions. In the area of healthcare, the sharing of decision-making powers among the states, legitimate civil society organizations, and the federal government is common. In practice, responsibilities are delegated by the government to membership-based, self-regulated organizations of providers and payers. The sickness fund has the status of a quasi-public corporation, with a self-regulated structure. The most important organizations for medical service providers are SHI-affiliated physicians' and dentists' associations and the German Hospital Organization (Busse & Reisberg 2004: 29–30, 34). The German health system is decentralized – competence and responsibility is shared by federal authorities and the states. The copayment is accepted by the public. The most important payers are health-insurance funds (sickness funds) (Domagała 2012 b: 42), while the main collection of the pooled health insurance contributions is managed by the national social health insurance fund (Jakubowska & Saltman 2013: 32). Every individual can freely choose a sickness fund (Kaiser Permanente International 2010). Public sources cover three-fourths of expenses for healthcare. The benefits list is regulated by law (Domagała 2012 b 2012: 42–45 b). The benefits package excludes, among other things, funeral benefits, OTC medicines, patient transport, glasses, and lifestyle medications (Kaiser Permanente International

2010). Germany spends more on health than most of the other European countries (counted as a proportion of GDP); and costs are increasing, mainly as a result of increasing levels of OOP spending (Thomson, Foubister & Mossialos 2009: 141). Almost 10% of the population buys full-coverage private insurance to cover items that are not part of the common benefit package (Kaiser Permanente International 2010). Germany ranked in seventh place in the Euro Health Consumer Index 2013 Report, prepared by the Health Consumer Powerhouse (2013). The people of the country are learning to pay for health services; and since their disposable income *per capita* is at a high level and health expenditures, compared to the total expenditures of a household, are relatively high compared to less developed countries, it can be predicted that investing should bring profits, especially for entities that stress quality. Germans are used to seeking almost any type of care they wish at any time, so efforts should be focused on delivering complex solutions or specialized services, provided in cooperation with other entities. In recent times, the waiting time for primary care service has been counted in minutes. This shows that the market is highly saturated in the area of primary care.

The United Kingdom is a constitutional monarchy. It is governed by a parliament made up of two houses. The head of the government is the prime minister (Boyle 2011: 7). The healthcare market in the UK is rather a public sector; however, nowadays many changes are in progress. Medical services are available for everybody; there is no list of guaranteed benefits. Most of the benefits are free-of-charge; but for some, the patient has to pay an extra fee or the fee is paid by private medical insurance, which is voluntary.[4] The general practitioner (GP) plays the role of gatekeeper (Kaiser Permanente International 2010). Services are financed from taxes and national insurance contributions (NIC). Expenditures on health have increased from £231 *per capita* in 1980 to £1872 in 2008. The global financial crisis has demonstrated that further increases of expenditures are impossible. The government undertook a new plan of reform, stressing cost reduction, increased competition, improvement of effectiveness, bureaucracy reduction, and changes in contracting services. In addition, the structure has changed; new bodies have appeared – the NHS Commissioning Board and Clinical Commissioning Groups, working on the local level. They are responsible for buying services. The responsibilities of entities have changed as well. Suppliers of benefits may be anybody with proper qualifications. The reform has abolished preference. The new rule allows any qualified provider instead of preferred providers. It is estimated that in the near future, 49% of medical services will be delivered by private suppliers. The reform will be completely implemented by the end of 2014 (Domagała 2013 b: 46–47). In the UK, trusts concentrate hospitals.[5] However, since 1997, Private Finance

---

4 Includes, among others, medical treatment in NHS posts, part of drug costs, and ophthalmological treatment.

5 Statistics show numbers of trusts, not of hospitals.

Initiatives (PFI) are becoming more popular. Earlier, cost-effectiveness and legal barriers made their existence in the health sector difficult. Nowadays, they have become a way to raise capital for health entities, rebuild, and replace of hospital trusts. The range of PFI coverage is very wide and includes, among others, hospitals, homes for the elderly, primary healthcare schemes, services, ICT (information and communications technology), and equipment. These are contracts typically set up for periods of thirty years (Rechel, Erskine, Dowdeswell, Wright & McKee 2009: 124–125). When considering the United Kingdom as a place for investment, attention should focus on choosing the area – for example, Scotland has its own National Health Service; and Scots spend on average 10% more on health services than the English do. Lack of comparable data may be a problem when comparing Scotland to European countries because England and Scotland prepare adjusted statistics. One of the problems for Scots that remains unsolved is heart disease; others are depression and alcohol consumption. On the other hand, Ireland, which has a high ranking, has a very high level of duplicate health insurance bought by households. This may be connected to tax optimization strategies or high levels of dissatisfaction with the healthcare products and services currently offered (Health Consumer Powerhouse 2013).

The principle of equal access to healthcare benefits is in force in Sweden. The system has been regulated by the Health and Medical Services Act since 1982 and the Social Services Act since 1980. Benefits are financed mainly from taxes (80%) and patients' fees – OOP (17%). The rest are financed from voluntary insurance and subsidies. OOPs are established locally. There is a maximum level of fees paid by the patient, regulated by the government. In Sweden, an important role is played by telephone information services and local websites, which deliver information about medical services, consulting, and renewing prescriptions (Domagała 2013 a: 44–46). No basic health package is defined – the basis of delivery is based on three principles: need and solidarity, human dignity, and cost-effectiveness. There are geographical restrictions in choosing primary care physicians, who do not play the role of gatekeeper. The fee for seeing a GP is lower than for a specialist. Most healthcare personnel are publicly employed (Kaiser Permanente International 2010). The healthcare system in Sweden is working well. Much attention is paid to cardiovascular diseases and diabetes, tobacco use, asthma, anxiety, dental problems, and home violence. However, new areas of importance are, among others, mental illness, alcoholism, and obesity (Domagała 2013 a: 44–46). Sweden is also one of the top countries in the EHCI 2013 (eleventh position). Swedish patients are used to little contact with a doctor unless they are "really" unhealthy. Their accessibility to health services is poor. The government stimulated the creation of a decentralized healthcare system and this may be one of the areas of possible investment (Health Consumer Powerhouse 2013). Because of the geographical characteristics of the country and the problem of poor accessibility, e-health solutions may be a good area for investing.

In Belgium, both the country and the regions are responsible for health policy. The government is responsible for, among others, financial aspects, accreditation criteria, legislation connected with occupations, and drug policy. Regions are responsible for prevention, mother and child treatment, coordination of benefits on the basic treatment level, and others. Decisions connected to insurance and finance are made by government representatives, health insurance funds, employees, and employers. Expenditures are financed mainly from common insurance and taxes (together 66%), subsidies (10%), and value added taxes (14%). A list of refunded benefits includes about 8000 items and is called nomenclature. The level of the refund depends on many factors – among others, the income and social status of the patient and the purpose of the medical treatment. There is a maximum level of fees paid by the patient; the government regulates these payments. GPs are not gate-keepers. This results in little or lack of a wait time. Sixty-five percent of the society is satisfied with the level of medical services (Domagała 2012 a: 44–45). Almost 100% of the population of Belgium is covered by the publicly financed health insurance scheme. Before 2008, that figure was 99% because self-employed people were excluded (Mossialos 2008: 115–117). Belgium ranked sixth in the Health Power House Index in 2013. It is described as the country with the most generous healthcare system in Europe and of a high quality. This leads to the supposition that in the near future the situation will not change and investing in this market will be profitable. Disadvantages are the market size and its possible rapid saturation connected with a vision of high profits (Health Consumer Powerhouse 2013).

The Republic of Poland is a democratic state with Parliament divided into a lower and upper house (Health System in Transition Poland, 2011, p. 6). Since 2003, the Polish healthcare system is based on a third party, called the National Health Fund (NFZ). The payer, NFZ, is a monopoly. Access to specialists is limited by contracts. This results in long wait times and increasing interest in private services (Rudawska 2007: 57–60). It is predicted that in 2014 to 2015, the National Health Fund will be replaced by the Health Insurance Office, which would be responsible for, among other things, ordering services and determining their valuation. A project of reform was announced in March 2013 and is currently being consulted. It is predicted that local departments will be more independent. One of the most important issues of reform is creating a map of health in Poland. This would support effective resource distribution. At the same time, investors would know in what regions their services are needed and contracted by the public payer (Rynekzdrowia.pl 2013). From 1989 to 1998, a slow process of medical unit privatization was in force. In 1999, as a result of reform, the functions of employer, payer, and service provider were divided. At that time, seventeen healthcare management offices were implemented (Dom Maklerski DFP 2013: 39). The main weaknesses of the Polish healthcare system are local conditions in hospitals; patient safety and gaps in discussions of medical errors; an ineffective information system that does not allow collection of appropriate data on a detailed enough level, which would be useful for finding out where potential problems are hidden; and an ineffective chip-card system. There is also the problem of not enough human capital, especially doctors and nurses (rynekzdrowia.pl). More than 1% of economic entities with foreign capital in Poland operate in the manufacture of pharmaceutical products (Tobolewska 2013: 115). Particularly attractive regions are mazowieckie, śląskie, dolnośląskie, and wielkopolskie voivodaship (Tobolewska 2013: 121). The pharmaceutical market is growing rapidly in Poland. It was predicted to grow between USD 1 to 5 billion per year (www.imshealth.com).

2.4 Micro-level factors influencing medical market attractiveness

Market factors include, among others, market size and growth potential. However, it is currently being discussed whether or not market size is still one of the most important factors in the era of globalization (CUTS 2002: 22–23). New market entry was more important for investors at the end of the twentieth century than cost reduction, when considering CEEs as host countries. However, these two factors were leading ones, according to much research.[6] In the early '90s, the reasons companies were entering CEE countries were mainly access to large local markets, high market potential, lower production costs, and access to raw materials (Karaszewski 2003: 16–23). At that time, the **supply** side of the market had not been developed yet. A similar situation in the healthcare market may be observed nowadays. For example, the process of privatization started in the '90s in Poland[7] (Dubik 2003: 193) in the medical sector was strengthened at the beginning of twenty-first century in basic healthcare entities (ZOZy). Nowadays, we can observe a new trend – privatization of the hospital sector. All this results in low saturation of the market.

Among the factors influencing the healthcare sector evaluation in the selected countries should be, among others, the following:
- demographic: population structure (sex and age, with indications of working age and non-working age numbers), population growth rate, real growth rate, fertility rate, urbanization ratio, level of education, level of unemployment, and income level of inhabitants;
- epidemic: mortality rate, average life expectancy, health adjusted life expectancy, potential years of life lost, infant mortality, mortality from main causes, reasons for hospitalization, absenteeism due to illness;
- service level usage: hospitalization ratio, ratio of medical advice, ratio of dental advice, average hospitalization duration, usage of hospital beds, vaccinations;
- medical resources: number of doctors with an indication of specialists and GPs, number of nurses and other medical personnel, number of beds for short- and long-term treatment, number of private beds (this is the ratio of beds owned by

---

6 Among others, research conducted by the OECD in 1993, Bundesverband der Deutschen Industrie and Ost-Ausschuß der Deutschen Wirtschaft in 1996, and by K. Meyer in 1998.

7 The most important low act was the privatization law in 1990.

private entities to the total number of beds in the health sector), selected medical device numbers – such as MRI, CT, and others;
– lifestyle: alcohol consumption, smoking, fat consumption; and
– opinions regarding the healthcare sector – social evaluation of the medical sector, expectations for changes in the sector (CSIOZ 2009).

The size of the medical market can be described by the number of potential patients (e.g., population, life expectancy at birth), the structure of demand (e.g., consumption of pharmaceutics), availability of medical personnel and their engagement (e.g., doctors' consultations), and infrastructure (e.g., hospital beds per person).

Table 2.5 presents a selection of micro factors.

Tab. 2.5: Selected micro indicators describing Germany, the United Kingdom, Sweden, Belgium, and Poland
Source: Adapted from OECD (2014)

Indicator	Unit	Germany	United Kingdom	Sweden	Belgium	Poland
Total population (2013)	'000 inhabitants	82,021	63,896	9,556	11,162	38,533
Life expectancy at birth (2012)	Years	78.6	79.1	79.9	77.8	72.7
Hospital beds density (2011)	Per 1 000 population	8.3	3.0	2.7	6.4	6.6
Doctor's consultations	*Per capita*	9.7	5.0*	3.0	7.4	6.8
Antibiotics consumption (2010)	Defined daily dose, per 1 000 people per day	14	18	16	28	24
Antidiabetics consumption (2010)	Defined daily dose, per 1 000 people per day	81	75	51	57	n/a
Antidepressants consumption (2010)	Defined daily dose, per 1 000 people per day	47	66	76	69	n/a

* (2009)

The largest potential markets, considering the number of possible patients, are in Germany and the United Kingdom, while the smallest is in Sweden.

When considering life duration, the longest living patients reside in Sweden. Over thirty years, the greatest change took place in Germany, where the life expectancy increased from 73 to 78.6. The smallest change was in Sweden – from 76 to 79.9 (World Bank 2014). Prolonging life leads to a situation in which the number of payers will be smaller than the number of patients. Moreover, the costs of medical treatment will increase as a result of changes in the average patient profile. For example, nowadays people burdened with more than three diseases require consultations with eighteen specialists within one year. Elderly people very often suffer from multiple diseases (Jakubiak, 2013).

The highest number of beds per inhabitant is in Germany, and the lowest number is in Sweden and the UK. Doctors' consultations are most popular in Germany and Belgium. The highest consumption of antidepressants is in Sweden; however, in recent years, the increase in this country was the slowest (about 60%), while the highest increase was in Germany (more than 130%). The highest consumption of antibiotics is in Belgium, while the fastest growing market from 2000 to 2010 was the United Kingdom (about 30% in ten years, while the remaining markets increased by an average of 6%).

Also important when discussing market factors is the technical and technological potential. Patients' behavior in recent years has changed, among others, in their relations with medical entities, which can be active or passive; the channels of medical services usage, which can be a PC, mobile electronic device, or a phone; their contact with medical entities, which is direct, personal contact, mixed, or virtual; and the reduction of uncertainty in the virtual environment, which means avoiding uncertainty and seeking information, marketing communication, and recommendations (Matysiewicz & Smyczek 2012: 122). Because of its important role in market potential, the evaluating process should include information about access to the Internet and the number of PCs or other devices allowing for virtual contact with medical entities. Also the destination of Internet users is important information for companies. It allows the addressees to have needed information about e-consumers. The Internet is a tool that allows people to find information, work, and do many other things. It is a kind of "window" to the world. Since the economy is becoming more and more digitalized and e-services are becoming more and more popular, it is important to focus appropriate attention on the supply of e-services. Table 2.6 presents selected indicators of Internet availability and its usage.

The highest rate of Internet access, frequency of its usage, and use for finding information about goods and services is in Sweden; and the lowest is in Poland.

Demand for medical goods is not based on fulfilling a desire, but instead is a necessity that people may wish to avoid. There is an asymmetry of information between patient and doctor, which drives patients to buy trust. As an additional feature of a medical good, the demand curve is deformed because of overconsumption; and, moreover, the factor creating demand is not price, just supply (Wiercińska 2010: 167). Determinants of demand for healthcare services may be divided into four main groups: economic (income, prices of alternative goods, time), demographic (age, education level), health (health of consumer), psychological (individual values hierarchy;

desire to be healthy; barriers connected to, among others, mastering the bureaucracy) (Rudawska 2007: 18). It is often emphasized that demand for medical goods depends highly on doctors, and this is harmed by overconsumption (Wiercińska 2010: 167). Changes in demand – its direction and intensity – are important information for suppliers.

Tab. 2.6: Selected micro indicators describing Germany, the United Kingdom, Sweden, Belgium, and Poland – access to and usage of the Internet
Source: Adapted from Eurostat (2013)

Indicator	Unit	G	UK	S	B	Pl
Households having access to the Internet via broadband connection	%	82	86	87	75	67
Individuals frequently using the Internet in 2012	% of individuals aged 16 to 74	65	73	80	65	46
Individuals never having used the Internet in year 2012	% of individuals aged 16 to 74	15	10	5	15	32
Individuals using the Internet for finding information about goods and services in 2012	% of individuals aged 16 to 74	75	72	83	65	51

* 2010

Nowadays, patients are becoming more and more demanding. Aging and overweight populations will result in a re-examination of resources and priorities in the medical sector. Overweight will result in worse health in the population and higher expenses for treatment. The changing nature of disease directly influences fulfilling the needs of ill people – about 75% of the health resources of developed countries are consumed by patients with chronic illnesses. Chronic diseases are also responsible for most deaths in developed countries. Chronic conditions require ongoing care and management, and most health systems nowadays are focused on providing episodic care. New medical technologies and treatments drive change in healthcare by increasing the quality of care, among other things. This also results in higher unit costs and greater demand. The most important and rapidly emerging technologies are genomics, regenerative medicine, and information-based medicine. They will be major drivers of changes in the medical sector (IBM: 4–11).

Based on Maslow's hierarchy of human needs, a hierarchy of healthcare needs model was created (IBM: 21). The first stage includes environmental health needs that are rudimentary healthcare needs (clean water, adequate food, clean air, etc.). The second level is basic healthcare needs that include basic medical care (immunizations, preventive screenings). The third level – medically necessary needs – includes medical treatment of acute injury, episodic illness, and chronic disease. This level includes treatments that are affordable for the society and enable patients to perform the activities of daily living. Health enhancement is the next level and covers treatments that are not strictly medically necessary; however, they improve overall health and quality of life (cosmetic surgery, lifestyle drugs, etc.). The top level is optimal health, and it encompasses an understanding of health through which the individual attains optimal physical and mental health. This could also be understood as an absence of symptoms or disease. Treatments attributed to this level include personalized wellness plans and genetic testing. These levels are different in different countries, according to the level of their development. Figure 2.1 presents a graphic illustration of potential areas of growth and the relative importance of different needs.

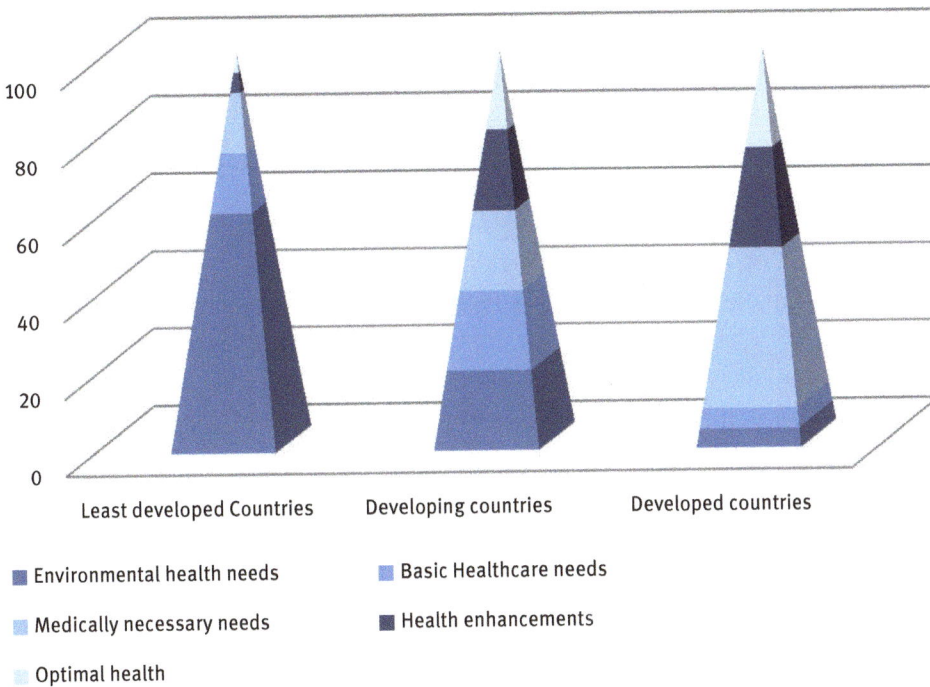

Fig. 2.1: Relative needs in developed, developing, and least developed countries
Source: Adapted from IBM (23)

All of the countries being analyzed can be treated as developed or developing. The health **needs** of people remain the same; only their share of the needs structure changes. This results also in focusing attention on more diversified means and high technology solutions.

   Expenditures on healthcare are increasing yearly around the world. Rapid increases were observed in the USA for the first time in the mid-1960s. Later the phenomenon also began in Europe, first in developed countries (Hady & Leśniowska 2011: 250). Nowadays, increasing expenditure on healthcare is a phenomenon observed globally (Hady & Leśniowska 2011: 25). Countries experiencing changes later were depending on economic transformation changes to deal with increasing expenditures, as in the example of Poland (Hady & Leśniowska 2011: 250). The most important cost drivers are innovation in health technology and aging of the population. New technologies allow for interventions that were unavailable before and are better now or available at a lower cost. As result of their implementation and frequent usage, total treatment costs increase. The population structure is also important. As the share of older people in the population grows, their health services take a larger amount of healthcare spending. This results in higher demand for health and an increase in expenses (Thomson & Foubister & Mossialos 2009: 2).

Healthcare is financed from two main sources: public, including tax and social insurance contributions; and private, paid by out-of-pocket payments (OOP), private health insurance, medical savings accounts, cost sharing for services that are covered by the benefits package, and informal payments (Thomson, Foubister & Mossialos 2009: XVII, 68–69). Private payments are classified in cross-country statistics into two main categories: HF 3.1., out of pocket excluding cost sharing; and HF 3.2, cost-sharing with third-party payers. Informal payments are not taken into consideration in the official statistics (Bem 2012: 19). This indicates that the financial liquidity of the sector and of a single medical unit depends on the condition of the government and the whole economy as well as on the condition of households. Increases in GDP, government support, and income *per capita* are expected to drive the demand for the medical services and equipment industry (Market Research Reports). Map 2.1 presents the level of expenditures on health, without distinguishing the source – private or public – as a percent of GDP worldwide.

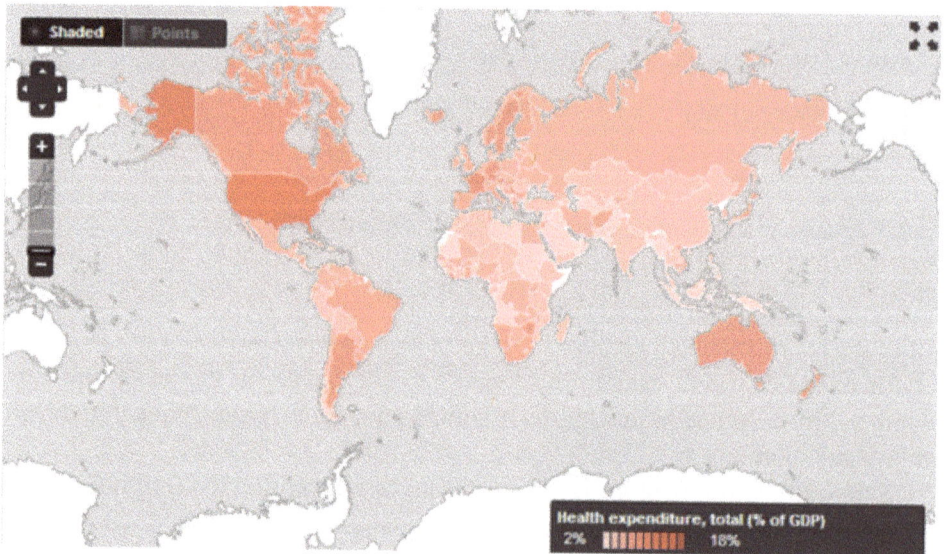

Map 2.1: Health expenditures, total (% of GDP) from 2009 to 2013
Source: Adapted from World Bank (2014)

It can be observed that the highest expenditure on health as a percent of GDP in 2012 was in the USA – almost 18%, and the lowest was in Myanmar– 1,8% of GDP. The share over 10% included Germany (11,3%) and Belgium (10,8%). The world mean of expenditures on health was 6,8% of GDP in 2012. In Sweden the ratio was 9,6%, in the United Kingdom, 9,4%; and in Poland, it was 6,7% in 2011. An illustration of trends in expenditures on health in Belgium, Germany, Poland, Sweden, and the United Kingdom compared to world changes is presented in Figure 2.2.

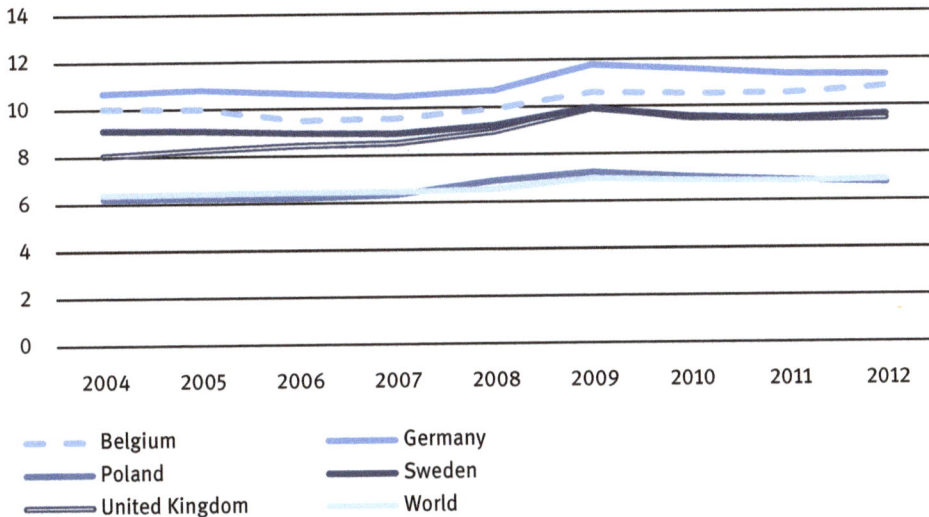

Fig. 2.2: Health expenditures in selected European countries during 2004 to 2012, total (% of GDP)
Source: World Bank (2014)

The general trend is an increase in expenditures. In the world, expenditures have increased from 6,4% in 2004 to 6,9% in 2012. In 2009, expenditures were at the highest level. This was the year of a change in the trend, a result of the overall economic situation. Medium increases were observed in Belgium – 0,5% (5% increase) and Germany – 0,5% (5% increase). A high increase was observed in the UK – 1,4% (17% increase) and Poland – a 0,6% (10% increase) in 2012 compared to 2004. In Sweden, the situation is changing only slightly. This is connected with high health spending in the entire period of analysis.

The supply is in many areas controlled by external entities, which is typical for a regulated market. For example, external entities control access to professional titles, specializations, the tools of communication with the market, and other things (Bukowska–Piestrzyńska 2011: 162). Sources of uncertainty in healthcare markets are mainly government regulations, new information technology, tighter margins, and new consumer behavior (Keckley). All of this influences the market's investment attractiveness compared to other sectors of the economy. The supply in this market depends on, among other things, the value of money streams coming into the health system of a selected country; medical human capital, its amount, qualifications, spatial placement and functional effectiveness; the availability of medical technology, its distribution, degree of utilization and efficiency; and access to medical know-how (Rudawska 2007: 20). This can be assumed: that the structure of the healthcare market financing directly influences the market's attractiveness (Rudawska & Urbańczyk 2012: 18).

Competition in the market is another important factor influencing both supply and demand. In the healthcare market, improvement was attempted by implementing the third-party payer. This is in accordance with the internal market concept, created by A. Enthoven. In his theory, the buyer is not the patient himself, but a third-party payer, while suppliers are public and private entities, delivering services on the basis of contracts. As a result, competition in this market may be present on four main levels: public and private service suppliers in relation to patient, public and private service suppliers in relation to a third-party payer, a third-party payer in relation to a patient, and relations between service suppliers and the central organ, for example, the Health Ministry. The subject of the competition may receive access to a certain number of patients; to public financial sources, connected directly with contracts' conditions; to patients' financial sources, insurance fee or tax[8]; and to financial sources that finance highly specialized medical services. These competitive interactions are present in all European countries, but with a different intensity and configuration (Rudawska 2007: 75–76). Because of the full reach of the EU's Internal Market rule, this competition is not only on the country level, but also is among entities from different countries, since the EU patient has the right to receive treatment in other Member States (Thomson, Foubister & Mossialos 2009: 1). In October 2013, an EU directive (Directive 2001/24/EU) came into force; and based on the directive, patients can receive treatment in medical entities of other Member States. The competition in the market is not only based on price character, in the case of medical goods, the catalogue of important factors influencing the choices is wide. As an example, it includes quality, price, technical value, aesthetic and functional value, influence on ecology and environment, cost of exploitation and LCC[9], profitability, service conditions, time of delivery, spare parts availability, and others (Szefke 2013: 6).

Companies operating in the free market treat owners' profit maximization as the most important aim of their existence (Pierścionek 2006: 79). In the healthcare market, profit is not the most important target influencing the decision process

---

8 Depending on the model of financing; for example, France and Germany, which represent the insurance model, have the highest level of health expenditures; and the quality of medical services in these two countries is evaluated as the best in the European Union.
9 Life Cycle Cost.

(Wiercińska 2010: 167). Because of the great importance of the health sector to the overall economy in many countries, subsidies are available for investors. As an example, European Union funds may be mentioned. In the perspective for 2007 to 2013, healthcare entities were indicated directly for the first time; and part of the fund was reserved for developing health infrastructure, among other things. In the new funding perspective for the years 2014 to 2020, further support of this segment is predicted. One of the aims of EU policy is to even out the health condition of the inhabitants of Member States (Hnatyszyn–Dzikowska 2007: 57).

Even though the healthcare sector is strongly public in Europe, many are of the opinion that the medical market should be privatized. It is believed that this will result in an increase of supplier offers, better fulfill demand, improve the quality of medical services, improve the investment possibilities of medical entities, and strengthen the sector itself (Wiercińska 2010: 167). Because of this, the trend of healthcare privatization is becoming more and more popular (i.e., Poland, Great Britain). In the CEE countries alone, the value of the private healthcare market was € 24.1 billion in 2011, according to Raiffeisen Investment data (Gerber).

2.5 Available market attractiveness measures

FDI is one of the factors illustrating a country's investment attractiveness and can be treated as its measure. According to OECD, Belgium realized the highest interest of foreign investors in 2008 and the greatest decrease from 2008 to 2012, decreasing from USD 193.6 billion to USD 1.6 billion. The most stable situation was in Poland. The most favorable country was the United Kingdom in 2012, the least favorable was Belgium. Figure 2.3 presents the graphic illustration of FDI inflows to these countries. It can be assumed that Belgium, Germany, Sweden, and the UK are parent countries, while Poland is a host country – inflows are higher than outflows. When considering the ratio of FDI as a percent of GDP, the highest share of inflows in 2012 was observed in Sweden and the UK, 2.6%; in Poland, it was 0.7%; in Germany, 0.2%; and in Belgium, 0.0%.

Another measure of attractiveness for investors may be different rankings. According to the report "European Cities and Regions of the Future 2012/2013," published by fDi Magazine (2012), London as a city and the United Kingdom as a country were on the top of the list. The list of top twenty-five European cities overall included places from the UK, Germany, Sweden, Belgium, and Poland. Cities from the UK also dominated the rankings of top ten small European cities, micro, and Northern European cities in general. Major cities from the UK, Germany, Sweden, and Belgium were mentioned on lists of top ten major cities when considering economic potential, human resources, quality of life, and infrastructure. Additionally, a major Polish city was mentioned as one of the top ten when considering business friendliness. In the rankings of major cities' FDI strategy, places from Germany, the UK, and Poland were mentioned. When evaluating regions, the list of the top twenty-five regions overall includ-ed places from Sweden, the UK, Germany, and Belgium. On the list of the top twenty-five regions in terms of FDI strategy, an additional region from Poland was included. It may be assumed that Germany, the United Kingdom, Sweden, and Belgium are seen as interesting places for running a business. Poland, although included in many rank-ings, still needs to improve many indicators.

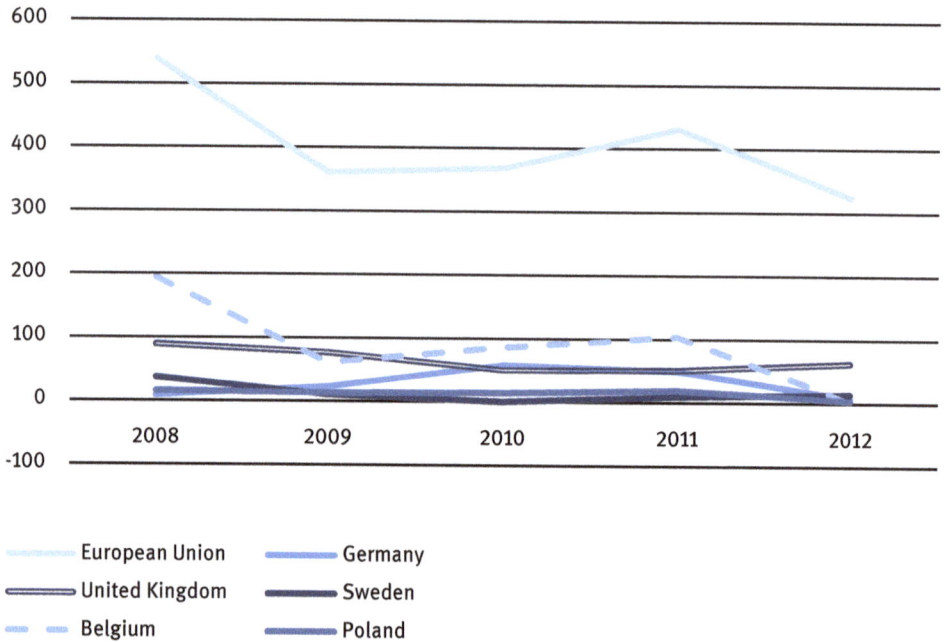

Fig. 2.3: Foreign direct investment inflows in selected European countries in 2008 to 2012 [USD billions] *Source: Adapted from OECD (2013)*

According to The Euro Health Consumer Index 2012, the situation in the health sec-tor in Europe is quite diversified. The Netherlands received the best score result, and the worst was Serbia – out of 1000 points, Serbia received only 451. Belgium re-ceived 783 points; Sweden, 775; the UK, 721; Germany, 704; and Poland, only 577 (Health Power House 2013: 3). The spread between these countries is the result of many factors, including macroeconomic factors that influence the economy of a country as a whole, not only the health sector. The results of the EHCI confirm that Poland needs to catch up with the other countries being discussed.

2.6 Forecasts – potential areas of investment

It is predicted that the healthcare industry will change through 2020 because of the increasing importance of large data networks, cloud computing, and mobile devices, among other reasons. This will improve the integration of all involved parties, including patients, care providers, health insurers, pharmaceutical companies, and others. The result will be increased importance of the patient-centric model, decreased costs of providing goods, and increased innovation (Meissner).

Demographic changes will also influence the future of the healthcare industry. In emerging markets new growth opportunities will occur, while the aging population in most developed countries will lead to the increased importance of chronic diseases (Meissner).

It is predicted that in the near future, European countries will face a shortage of doctors – generally or in specific locations or for certain categories of doctors (OECD 2012: 68). Already some regions are dealing with this problem. In 2010, the highest doctor *per capita* ratio was in Greece, with 6.1 doctors per 1000 population. Sweden was also very high. The lowest was in Montenegro and Turkey, followed by Poland. In 2010, the UK ranked sixth from the bottom; in 2011, the ratio exceeded 2.8 doctors per 1000 population. This was highly associated with increased registration of foreign-trained doctors since 2003; also the number of medical school graduates increased from 2003 to 2011. The balance between GP and specialist doctors is changing in nearly all countries; the number of GPs is increasing, but more slowly than the number of specialists. This has resulted in a larger population of specialists than family doctors, except for in Ireland, Portugal, Malta, and Norway. This change affects the healthcare system. Some countries are considering new roles for other healthcare providers in order to respond to the growing demand for primary care. In Germany, GPs are 42% of the physician population; in Belgium, 38%; in the EU, 30%; in the UK, 30%; in Poland, 21%; and in Sweden, 17% (OECD 2012: 68–69).

In the future, more attention will be paid to healthcare delivered at home, since most people would choose to stay in their home instead of receiving care in an institution. In addition, home care is more cost-effective. One of the reasons for this likely change is the implementation of new technologies that allow care coordination and growing possibilities for distant monitoring and more complex treatment in the home situation. Also the demographic changes and social developments resulting in higher demand for healthcare supports this solution – it is predicted that by 2050, for every person over the age of sixty-five, there will be only two people of working age; nowadays it is four. This will result in increasing demand for long-term care and more private initiatives. Simultaneously, informal care is becoming scarcer in many countries as a result of growing mobility, women's increasing participation in the labor market, and urbanization. When considering the problem of taking care of an aging society requiring long-term care, people believe that the public or private service provider should see them and provide appropriate help; 60% of Swedish, 38% of

Belgians, 35% of the UK, 29% of Germans, but only 8% Polish hold this opinion (Genet, Boerma, Kroneman, Hutchinson & Satlman 2012: 2–5).[10]

The medical device (MD) industry has experienced significant growth worldwide over the last five years. In the forthcoming years, it is expected to continue its growth, reaching approximately USD 302 billion in 2017 (Global Medical Devices Industry 2012–2017: 2012). The high-tech medical device sector, which covers a range of diversified items, is a key component of the healthcare system. It is estimated that the European market has about a 30 to 34% share of the total world value of this sector. The provision of health insurance has been key to innovation in MD. The expansion of insurance in all national systems has nourished innovation in medical technology; at the same time, new technologies and new medical capabilities resulted in increased demand for insurance (Pammolli, Riccaboni, Oglialoro, Magazzini, Baio & Salerno 2005: 7–12).

The annual revenue from the vaccine industry is forecast to reach USD 41.85 billion by 2018. The next five years are forecast to be a time of high growth (Global Human Vaccine Industry 2013–2018). It is predicted that in Germany and the UK, annual *per capita* drug spending will be about USD 375; in Belgium and Sweden, about USD 321; and in Poland, USD 96 (IMS 2012).

The European pharmaceutical market is worth about USD 121 billion counted as a share in global pharmaceutics. The most important European markets – France, Germany, Italy, Spain, and the UK (top five) – are forecast to slow down in the following years. Their growth is predicted to be 1 to 3% (IMAP 2011: 3). Pharmerging countries will double their pharmaceutical markets during 2006 to 2016 (IMS 2012). Poland is seen as an important market player, belonging to the third tier of the pharmaceutical market (the group is also called fast followers) because, in the near future, Poland's market value is predicted to grow rapidly and create investment possibilities for new players (IMAP 2013: 5). This means that the top five European pharmaceutical markets are very strong and highly saturated; while the Polish market is growing, and there are still market gaps to be filled.

Rehabilitation will also be one of the very important areas of potential investment. For example, in Poland, the average waiting time for rehabilitation services is three months. The number of people who need rehabilitation is increasing yearly, but public medical entities do not support their treatment. The most important barriers are lack of financial support and a deficit in the supply of specialized entities (Dom Maklerski DFP 2011: 41).

Trends for the whole healthcare market include continuing increased spending; a degree of rationing and consolidation of facilities; increased importance of GPs as gatekeepers and coordinators of treatment for patients with multiple health issues; promotion of healthy behavior through preventive measures; increased responsibil-

---

10 Results of the survey show that home care is a relatively new phenomenon in CEE countries.

ity of patients for individual health, treatment, and care (Economist Intelligence Unit 2011: 14–21); development of the idea of healthcare as a societal right and an area of market service; and collaboration with governments for change and reform implementation (IBM,:2 -4).

Conclusions

The European healthcare market is strongly diversified. When answering the question as to whether it is attractive for investors, an analysis of selected countries should be considered instead of the whole continent. It may be assumed that all described markets – Belgian, German, Polish, Swedish, and the UK – should be interesting for investors, however in different areas.

First of all, these markets will grow in the future. The Polish pharmaceutical market will grow rapidly in the near future. In addition, areas of medical services such as wellness will develop in the near future as a consequence of the growing purchasing power of society and changing medical service consumption patterns. In Germany and the United Kingdom, the primary healthcare and home delivery services area will grow and create chances for new investments. Belgium is growing steadily and will attract capital for caring for the elderly as well as for solving internal health problems. Disadvantages of Belgium are the market size and its possible rapid saturation. In Sweden, the main problem continues to be waiting time. This creates opportunities for two areas of innovation: one connected with e-health services and a second with filling the need for more and easier access to specialists and physicians (e.g., by opening a network of health service suppliers).

Second, because the healthcare markets in these countries were subject to huge reforms that influenced the existing models, new market niches were created. Also important is the development level of a country. According to the hierarchy of health needs, it is possible to predict which areas of the market will develop more rapidly in the different countries. Moreover, the general economic situation indicates which areas are likely to be developed in the near future by governments, the healthcare sector included. In comparison to the size and potential of the most highly developed healthcare market, the USA, as well as compared to fast growing markets, such as China and India, European countries are not in the most favorable position. Nevertheless, there is still a huge potential for investment. According to macro factors and its stable position, Germany is the safest country to invest in. Considering the predicted pace of change and new possibilities, Poland may provide the best investment opportunities. The form of investment depends on the area of interest. In the case of the pharmaceutical market, investment can be connected to implementing new products or green field investments. In developed countries, the labor cost is too high to make green field investments. It is easier and cheaper to build a factory in developing countries such as India or China and hire specialists from all over the world. Taking into consideration growing labor costs in Asian countries, it can be predicted that they will lose their competitive strength; and in a few years, Poland may be more attractive for green field investment because of a favorable location, good logistic conditions, high technology, and a comparatively low cost of labor.

Moreover, high technology will play a more important role in the healthcare market in the future than it does today. This will increase competition among medical entities and will result in higher expenses for R&D in ICT. Information technology development will be particularly noticeable in the medical device and treatment (e-health) sectors.

It may be concluded that Germany and Sweden are the most developed countries among these selected ones. They have high potential and resources. From a general economic investment perspective, they are advantageous for investments dedicated to a mature market. Investments in these markets should be focused on high quality and innovative solution development or on home delivery services. Among less developed countries, Poland seems to have the greatest potential for development. Trends connected to catching up with the developed countries indicate potential gaps and areas of investment, including access to the Internet and, from the health perspective, efforts to increase life expectancy. Investments should be directed toward medically necessary needs fulfillment, health enhancements, and optimal health. Finally, investments in pharmacy will likely result in profits.

References

Badania kliniczne w Polsce – główne wyzwania, PWC. Retrieved June 11, 2013 from: http://www.medicamo.pl/pliki-do-pobrania

Barron's Marketing Dictionary. Dictionary of Marketing Terms. Retrieved April 25, 2013 from: http://www.answers.com

Bem, A., 2012. Katastrofalne wydatki w ochronie zdrowi. In: Rudawska, I., Urbańczyk, E. (Ed.) Opieka zdrowotna. Zagadnienia ekonomiczne, Warszawa: Difin, 19

Boyle, S., 2011. Health Systems in Transition. United Kingdom (England) Health system review: 8, vol 13 no. 1

Bukowska – Piestrzyńska, A., 2011. Reputacja jednostek opieki zdrowotnej, Prace Naukowe Uniwersytetu Ekonomicznego we Wrocławiu, Wrocław, Wydawnictwo Uniwersytetu Wrocławsiego, no 226, 162

Busse, R., Reisberg, A., 2004. Healthcare Systems in Transition. Germany. Retrieved June 21, 2013 from: http://www.euro.who.int/__data/assets/pdf_file/0018/80703/E85472.pdf

Campbel, D. 11., Pharmerging shake-up. New imperatives in a redefined world, IMS. Retrieved June 15, 2013 from: http://www.bvgh.org/LinkClick.aspx?fileticket=kMaOKGUbqgl%3D&tabid=168

Dictionary. Retrieved 10 June, 2013 from: http://dictionary.reference.com

Domagała M., 2012 a. Belgia – kraj skomplikowany, dobrze poukładany. Gazeta Lekarska, 11/ 2012, 44–45

Domagała M., 2012 b. Niemcy: trwałość, decentralizacja i autonomia. Gazeta Lekarska, 05/2012, 42–45

Domagała M., 2013 a. Wielka Brytania – czas wielkich reform, Gazeta Lekarska, 6/2013 46–47

Domagała M., 2013 b. Szwecja – wszystkim według potrzeb. Gazeta Lekarska, 3/2013, 44–47

Dubik B. M., 2003. Podstawowe motywy podejmowania inwestycji zagranicznych w Polsce. In: Diagnoza i perspektywy procesów inwestycyjnych w krajach Europy Środkowej, Henzel H. (Ed.), Katowice, AE w Katowicach, 193

Emerging Markets. As growth opportunities continue to dwindle in more developed economies, large healthcare companies have made the emerging markets a strategic priority. Retrieved December 31, 2013 from: http://www.imshealth.com/portal/site/ims/menuitem.edb2b81823f67dab41d84b903208c22a/?vgnextoid=2f78cb79461bf210VgnVCM100 00071812ca2RCRD

European Business Association. Homepage. Retrieved June 05, 2013 from: http://www.eba.com.ua/en/about-eba/indices/investment-attractiveness-index

European Cities and regions of the future 2012/2013, fDi Magazine Ranking 2012. Retrieved June 13, 2013 from: http://en.invest.katowice.eu/events/32/fdi_magazine_ranking.html

Eurostat. Retrieved March 25, 2014 from: http://epp.eurostat.ec.europa.eu/portal

European Parliament, 2011. Directive 2011/24/EU of the European Parliament and of the Council of 9 March 2011 on the application of patients' rights in cross-border healthcare. Retrived June 14, 2013 from: http://eur-lex.europa.eu/LexUriServ/LexUriServ.do?uri= OJ:L:2011:088:0045:0065:EN:PDF

Financial healthcare in the European Union. Challenges and policy responses, Thomson, S., Foubister, T., Mossialos, E., (Ed.) Observatory Studies Series no 17, WHO, Copenhagen 2009. Retrieved June 9, 2013 from: http://www.euro.who.int/__data/assets/pdf_file/0009/98307/E92469.pdf

Foreign Direct Investment in Developing Countries: What Economists (Don't) Know and What Policymakers Should (Not) Do!, Monographson on Investment and Competition Policy, #11CUTS Centre for International Trade, Economics and Environment, Jaipur 2002. Retrieved June 13, 2013 from: http://www.cuts-international.org/FDI%20in%20Developing%20Countries-NP.pdf

Gerber, P., Szpitale prywatne w Europie Środkowo – Wschodniej, Polish assotiation of Private Hospitals. Retrieved June 11, 2013 from: http://www.szpitale.org/konferencja/file/pdf/Gerber-Europejski_Kongres_Gospodarczy.pdf

Germany Pharmaceutical Market Overwiev, Datamonitor 2010. Retrieved April 17, 2013 from: http://www.google.pl/url?sa=t&rct=j&q=&esrc=s&source=web&cd=10&cad=rja&sqi=2&ved =0CHQQFjAJ&url=http%3A%2F%2Fwww.datamonitor.com%2Fstore%2FDownload%2FBrochur e%2F%3FproductId%3DHC00002-001&ei=NQm-UeP3EYiv4QSOo4HYDg&usg=AFQjCNFt0qMgHn-xMhYGWPGFPfFsyoeFsw

Gleißner, W., Helm, R., Kreiter, S., 2013. Measurmement of competitive advantages and market attractiveness for strategic controlling, Manag Control 24, 60–62

Global Human Vaccine Industry 2013–2018: Trend, Profit, and Forecast Analysis. Retrieved June 1, 2013 from: http://www.lucintel.com/reports/medical/global_human_vaccine_industry_2013-2018_trend_profit_and_forecast_analysis.aspx

Global Medical Device Industry 2012–2017: Trend, Profit, and Forecast Analysis. Retrieved June 1, 2013 from: http://www.lucintel.com/reports/medical/global_medical_device_industry_2012_2017_trends_foreacast_february_2012.aspx

Hady, J., Leśniowska, M., 2011. Healthcare expenditure and the state of healthcare sector in selected European union countries, eFinanse, vol. 7, no 4. Retrieved November 30, 2013 from: https://www.econstor.eu/dspace/bitstream/10419/66751/1/688849415.pdf , 25

Health at a glance 2012. Retrieved June 13, 2013 from: http://www.oecd-ilibrary.org/social-issues-migration-health/health-at-a-glance-europe-2012_9789264183896-en;jsessionid= 37phau4ikmkaa.x-oecd-live-02

Health Consumer Powerhouse, 2013. Euro Health Consumer Index 2013. Taby. Retrieved May 30, 2013 from: http://www.healthpowerhouse.com/index.php?Itemid=55

Health Systems in Transition. Poland. Health system review, vol. 13 no. 8 2011. Retrieved 1 April, 2013 from: www.euro.who.int/__data/assets/pdf_file/0018/163053/e96443.pdf

Healthcare 2015: win-win or lose-lose? A portrait and a path to successful transformation, IBM Global Business Services. Retrieved June 15, 2013 from: http://www-935.ibm.com/services/us/gbs/bus/pdf/healthcare2015-win-win_or_lose-lose.pdf

Hnatyszyn – Dzikowska, A., 2007. Fundusze strukturalne UE dla systemu opieki zdrowotnej w perspektywie budżetowej 2014 – 2020. In: Opieka zdrowotna, aspekty rynkowe i marketingowe, Rudawska I. (Ed.). Warszawa, Wydawnictwo Naukowe PWN, 57

Home Care across Europe. Current structure and future challenges, Genet, N., Boerma W., Kroneman, M., Hutchinson, A., Satlman, R. B., 2012. Copenhagen, European Observatory on Health Systems and Policies, WHO. Observatory Studies Series 27. Retrieved June 8, 2013 from: http://www.euro.who.int/__data/assets/pdf_file/0008/181799/e96757.pdf, 2–5

IMAP's Pharma & Biotech Industry Gobal Report 2011, IMAP. Retrieved December 31, 2013 from: http://www.imap.com/imap/media/resources/IMAP_PharmaReport_8_272B8752E0FB3.pdf

Jakie mogą być efekty? Retrieved June 11, 2013 from: http://www.rynekzdrowia.pl/Rynek-Zdrowia/Jakie-moga-byc-efekty,129897,3.html

Jakubiak, L., Czeka nas bardzo trudne nadążanie za demografią. Retrieved June 11, 2013 from: http://www.rynekzdrowia.pl/Rynek-Zdrowia/Czeka-nas-bardzo-trudne-nadazanie-za-demografia,126986.html

Jesień na rynku aptecznym. Retrieved June 11, 2013 from: http://www.rynekzdrowia.pl/Rynek-Zdrowia/Jesien-na-rynku-aptecznym,126714.html

Karaszewski, W., 2003. Motywy podejmowania przez inwestorów zagranicznych inwestycji bezpośrednich w krajach Europy Środkowowschodniej. In: Diagnoza i perspektywy procesów inwestycyjnych w krajach Europy Środkowej, Henzel, H., (Ed.). Katowice, AE w Katowicach, 16–23

Keckley P., Healthcare Industry Megatrends. A Deloitte Center for Health Solutions discussion, a video presentation. Retrieved June 6, 2013 from: http://www.deloitte.com/view/en_US/us/Industries/health-care-providers/aae30d2ff6b2a310VgnVCM1000003156f70aRCRD.htm

Marcinek, K., 2002. Finansowa ocena przedsięwzięć inwestycyjnych przedsiębiorstw. Wydanie V. Katowice, Wydawnictwo Akademii Ekonomicznej w Katowicach, 19

Market Potential Index (MPI) for Emerging Markets – 2013. Retrieved June 1, 2013 from: http://globaledge.msu.edu/mpi

Market Research Reports. Retrieved June 5, 2013 from: http://www.lucintel.com/reports/medical/global_medical_equipment_industry_2012_2017_trends_foreacastjuly_2012.aspx

Matysiewicz, J., Smyczek, S., 2012. Modele relacji jednostek medycznych z pacjentami w otoczeniu wirtualnym. Warszawa, Placet, 122

Meissner A., The Global healthcare Industry in the year 2020. Retrieved June 6, 2013 from: http://www.mddionline.com/article/global-healthcare-industry-year-2020

Menedżerowie z unijnych szpitali – jak widzą nasz system? Retrieved June 11, 2013 from: http://www.rynekzdrowia.pl/Finanse-i-zarzadzanie/Menedzerowie-z-unijnych-szpitali-jak-widza-nasz-system,131181,1,2.html

Pammolli, F., Riccaboni, M., Oglialoro, C., Magazzini, L., Baio, G., Salerno, N., 2005. Medical devices competitiveness and impact on public health expenditure. Retrieved June 15, 2013 from: http://www.imtlucca.it/whos_at_imt/faculty/_publications/Medical_Devices_Competitiveness_and_Impact_on_Public_Health_Expenditure.pdf

Pharmaceuticals & Biotechnology Industry Global Report 2011. IMAP healthcare report. Retrieved
June 16, 2013 from:
http://www.imap.com/imap/media/resources/IMAP_PharmaReport_8_272B8752E0FB3.pdf

Pierścionek Z., 2006. Strategie konkurencji i rozwoju przedsiębiorstwa, Warszawa, Wydawnictwo
PWN, 79

Prospekt emisyjny Polmed Spółka Akcyjna, Dom Maklerski DFP sp. z o.o., 2011. Retrieved June 15,
2013 from: http://www.polmed.pl/pub/pl/uploaddocs/POLMED_Prospekt_Emisyjny
_13122011.pdf

Rechel B., Erskine J., Dowdeswell B, Wright S., McKee M., 2009. Capital investment for health. Case
studies from Europe, WHO. In: Observatory Studies Series No 18, Copenhagen 2009. Retrieved
June 8, 2013 from: http://www.euro.who.int/__data/assets/pdf_file/0014/43322/E92798.pdf

Rudawska I., 2007. Opieka zdrowotna, aspekty rynkowe i marketingowe. Warszawa, Wydawnictwo
Naukowe PWN, 18–20, 75–60, 75–76

Rudawska, I., Urbańczyk, E., (ed.), 2012. Opieka zdrowotna. Zagadnienia ekonomiczne, Warszawa
Difin, 18

Rynek prywatnej opieki zdrowotnej w Polsce: wzrost o 5% w latach 2012–2014. Informacja prasowa,
2012. Retrieved June 11, 2013 from: http://www.medicamo.pl/pliki-do-pobrania

Saaty, T.L., Varga, L. G., 2001. Models, Methods, Concepts & Application of the Analytic Hierarchy
Process. In: International Series in Operations Research & Management Science 34. Retrieved
June 5, 2013 from: http://www.springer.com/business+%26+management/operations+
research/book/978-1-4614-3596-9, 135

Scholz, K., Matzke, M., 2013. Angela Merkel zwycięża w wyborach. Retrieved June 15, 2013 from:
http://www.dw.de/angela-merkel-zwyci%C4%99%C5%BCa-w-wyborach/a-17104174

Selected European Countries' healthcare Systems, Kaiser Permanente International, 2010. Retrieved June 14, 2013 from: xnet.kp.org/kpinternational/docs/European Healthcare Systems
Comarison.pdf

Sławatyniec, Ł., 2013. Investing in Life Sciences in Poland. Opportunities and risks. Warsaw,
Deloitte, Warsaw. Retrieved December 30, 2013 from:
http://www.wdmcapital.com/uploads/lsc_slajdy/Deloitte_Investing_in_LS_in_Poland.pdf

Stawki i regulacje dotyczące podatku VAT, VAT i cennik. Retrieved June 8, 2013 from:
http://www.vistaprint.pl/customer-care/vat-
podatek.aspx?&GP=10%2f1%2f2013+9%3a34%3a13+AM&GPS=2968569564&GNF=0

Sygut, M., Kto zyska, kto straci? Retrieved June 11, 2013 from: http://www.rynekzdrowia.pl/
Rynek-Zdrowia/Kto-zyska-kto-straci,126977.html

Szefke, W., 2013. Praktyczne wykorzystanie innego niż cena kryterium w postępowaniu o udzieleni
zamówienia publicznego na rynku ochrony zdrowia, Liderzy rynku medycznego 2013. In:
Medinfo,. Retrieved June 7, 2013 from: http://data.axmag.com/data/201301/
U44018_F186320/FLASH/index.html

The changing National Role in Health System Governance. A case – based study of 11 European countries and Australia, Jakubowski, E., Saltman, R.B. (ed.), 2013. European Observatory on Health
Systems and Policies. In: Observatory Studies Series 29. WHO. Retrieved June 8, 2013 from:
http://www.euro.who.int/__data/assets/pdf_file/0006/187206/e96845.pdf [8th June 2013]

The future of healthcare in Europe, Economist intelligence Unit, The Economist 2011. Retrieved June
16, 2013 from: http://www.janssen-emea.com/sites/default/files/The-Future-Of-Healthcare-
In-Europe.pdf [16th June 2013]

The Global Use of Medicines: Outlook Through 2016, IMS Institute for Health Informatics, 2012.
Retrieved June 10, 2013 from: http://www.imshealth.com/deployedfiles/ims/Global/Content/
Insights/IMS%20Institute%20for%20Healthcare%20Informatics/Global%20Use%20of%20
Meds%202011/Medicines_Outlook_Through_2016_Report.pdf

Time to learn from the Dutch champions how to build value for- money healthcare! Retrieved June 4, 2013 from: http://www.healthpowerhouse.com/files/ehci-general-press-release.pdf

Tobolewska, A., 2013. Structure of foreign investment in the industry of Poland at the beginning of the second decade of the 21st century. In: Bulletin of Geography. Socio-economic series 22. Retrieved December 31, 2013 from: http://www.bulletinofgeography.umk.pl/22_2013/09_Tobolska.pdf

Transparency.com. Homepage. Retrieved June 3, 2013 from: http://www.transparency.org/country#SWE

Turek, I., 2002. Uwarunkowania i rozwój bezpośrednich inwestycji zagranicznych w Polsce w latach 1991 - 2002, in: Diagnoza i perspektywy procesów inwestycyjnych w krajach Europy Środkowej, Henzel, H. (ed.). Katowice, Wydawnictwo AE w Katowicach, 147–148

W 70 wskaźników dookoła zdrowia, CSIOZ, 2009. Retrieved June 16, 2013 from: http://www.csioz.gov.pl/publikacja.php?id=5

Wiercińsk,a A., 2010. Specyfika rynku usług rynkowych. In: Zarządzanie i finanse no 287 (63)

World Bank, Homepage. Retrieved June 5, 2013 from: http://data.worldbank.org/indicator/

Worldwide corporate tax guide 2013, Ernst & Young. Retrieved June 5, 2013 from: http://www.ey.com/Publication/vwLUAssets/Worldwide_corporate_tax_guide_2013/$FILE/Worldwide_corporate_tax_guide_2013.pdf;

Artur Turek and Aleksander Owczarek

3 Consumption and Consumer Behavior in the European Healthcare Market

Abstract: Many variables influence consumption of medication and the behavior of consumers who use medication. The aim of this study was to compare these parameters in various insurance models. The results have been estimated on the basis of medication sales from pharmaceutical wholesalers to community pharmacies and hospitals. The data were obtained from IMS Healthcare, and the database of IMS MIDAS Market Segmentation was used. It was revealed that consumption and consumer behavior depend rather on the type of medications (OTC and Rx) and the setting of consumption. When analyzing the results, the influence of macroeconomics and epidemiology was also taken into consideration.

Keywords: Consumption, Consumer behavior, Cardiovascular medications, Hospital, Community pharmacy

3.1 Introduction

Consumption and consumer behavior in the pharmaceutical market is an interesting topic in health, social, and economic sciences. To generalize, it can be said that everyone takes a medication, anytime and anywhere.

It should also be explained that from the pharmaceutical and medical point of view, using the term 'consumption' is highly controversial. This is so because the term is clearly associated with the abuse of drugs. It is better to say that medications are rather used or taken. However, the study on medication sales concerns patients as consumers; therefore, use of the term 'consumption' is reasonable. Holdford (2007: 109) coined the term 'healthcare consumers', which seems to be the most appropriate.

Medication consumption and the behavior of healthcare consumers belong to very complex phenomena. Many variables *de facto* influence the consumption rate of medications and the behavior of healthcare consumers. Data in the literature on medication consumption may be analyzed in terms of sector, i.e., hospital or community pharmacy; kind of medication, i.e., brand medications and generic medications, over-the-counter (OTC) medications and prescription (Rx) medications; country income; illness, i.e., the presence of acute or chronic disease; medication reimbursement; and access to medical care (Cameron et al., 2009: 240; Cameron et al., 2012: 664; Millier et al., 2013: e84088; Turek and Owczarek, 2014: 25).

Overall, various determinants influence the behavior of healthcare consumers. The factors found in the literature include, but are not limited to, gender, age, number of persons and children in the household, place of residence, salary, pension, employment status, level of education, and health condition assessment (Holdford, 2007: 109; Smith et al., 2009: 17; Turek and Owczarek, 2014: 25).

According to IMS Health data, the medicinal products used in the treatment of the alimentary track and metabolism, cardiovascular system, central nervous system, respiratory system, and sensory organs belong to the major categories of currently used medications.

It should be pointed out that cardiovascular diseases are a significant problem in the European Union (WHO, 2013; Eurostat, 2013). Namely, cardiovascular diseases are a significant cause of death. According to the World Health Organization, cardiovascular diseases caused the death of nearly 17 million people in 2011 all over the world. They were the cause of three out of every ten deaths (WHO, 2013). Ischemic heart disease caused death in the case of nearly 7 million people in the world (WHO, 2013). In the European Union, ischemic heart diseases accounted for 76.2 deaths per 100,000 inhabitants in 2010 (Eurostat, 2013). Diseases of the circulatory system include those related to high blood pressure, cholesterol, diabetes, and smoking. However, the most common causes of death are ischemic heart diseases and cerebrovascular diseases (Eurostat, 2013).

In 2010, the standardized death rate (1 per 100,000 inhabitants) for circulatory disease and heart disease varied. The average value for the twenty-seven European Member States was 209.90 and 76.50 for circulatory diseases and heart diseases, respectively. Differences could be observed between the European Union average and the particular states that were analyzed: in the case of Germany, values were 208.70 and 80.90; Great Britain, 164.40 and 77.30; Sweden, 186.90 and 83.70; Belgium, 182.70 and 59.50; and Poland, 336.90 and 90.60 for circulatory diseases and heart diseases, respectively (Eurostat, 2010).

The consumption of cardiovascular medications and the behavior of healthcare consumers who take these medicinal products depend on the kind of medication and the sector of distribution. Overall, healthcare consumers use two categories of cardiovascular medications: OTC medications and Rx medications. OTC medications are products that are sold directly to a consumer without a prescription from a healthcare professional. In most cases, it is up to healthcare consumers to make the decision to purchase, and they use their liberty. These medications may also be professionally prescribed. OTC medications give the consumer the possibility of conducting a therapy for a general medical problem or addressing health issues in the period before consultation with a doctor. OTC medicinal products must be safe during the administration period (usually three to five days). They are also used in the case of easy symptom self-diagnosis by the patient. However, the decision to prescribe Rx medications lies with the doctor. In this case, consumers are not fully and directly responsible for the choices made. Moreover, consumers often do not cover the full cost of the medications themselves. They benefit from refunds. The consumption of these medications is not typically decided upon by the consumer himself.

In the case of OTC medications, consumption is thus mainly in the hands of the patient and, to a lesser degree, in the hands of a pharmacist or doctor. However, the consumption level of Rx medications is regulated by medical prescription. It can be stated that, in the first case, the patient can be called more a consumer and, in the second, more a patient.

OTC and Rx cardiovascular medications are available in the non-hospital sector, i.e., in community pharmacies (retail market) and in the hospital sector, i.e., in hospital pharmacies. However, there are some medicinal products that are used only in community pharmacies and some medicinal products used only in hospitals.

It should be noted that in community pharmacies, healthcare consumers make independent decisions about purchases; whereas, in hospitals, they do not have a choice.

The aim of this study was to compare the consumption of cardiovascular medications and the behavior of healthcare consumers during the period 2008 to 2012 in various models with various kinds of insurance: (i) in the typical insurance model applicable in Germany, (ii) in the tax model in place in Great Britain and Sweden, (iii) in the mixed model operational in Belgium, and (iv) in the post-communist model functioning in Poland.

In the current study on the consumption of cardiovascular medications and the behavior of healthcare consumers, the following aspects have been estimated: the rate of Rx and OTC medication sales, the value of the total sales of medications, the average price of the medication package, and the number of medication packages sold per inhabitant.

The justification for the topic under discussion is the fact that the insurance model may exert significant influence on the consumption of cardiovascular medications and on the behavior of the healthcare consumers who use these medications. In the available literature, it has been emphasized that what plays the deciding role in medication consumption is the efficiency of medical care and also reimbursement levels (Ward and Ozdemir, 2012). It should also be noted that in the European Union Member States, standardization of certain rules has been in place for a long time in the field of medication reimbursement. It seems that the type of insurance model in place over the last years may play a secondary role. However, taking into account the fact that the behavior of healthcare consumers is deeply rooted in the insurance model, the topic is worthy of analysis. In addition, age, income of consumers, and the government may also be of significance.

3.2 Medication reimbursement systems

EU law regulates the reimbursement system for medications only for the basic procedures. The choice of a particular model of reimbursement rests with particular Member States. In European Union countries, there are different reimbursement systems, e.g., based on percentage or quota. This determines the price of Rx medications. However, the standardization of certain rules has been in place for a long time in this area. Nowadays, there are many common elements in the reimbursement systems of Germany, Great Britain, Sweden, Belgium, and Poland that are important for this study: inter alia (i) a fixed charge for Germany, England, Sweden, and Belgium; (ii) a reference pricing system for Germany, Belgium, and Poland; and (iii) no reference pricing system for Great Britain and Sweden (Vogler et al., 2011a: 183; Vogler et al., 2011b: 69; Zimmermann, 2013: 339).

In the case of reimbursable medications, most consumers are compensated from insurance. Thus they do not experience the full financial consequence of purchase. Moreover, the government intervenes heavily in the market at all levels of the supply chain. Undoubtedly, the total consumption of cardiovascular medications is largely dependent on reimbursement and access to medical care.

It should be emphasized that each model has undergone changes; but in the last decade, the Polish 'post-communist' model has been subject to the greatest transformation (Vogler et al., 2011a: 183; Vogler et al., 2011b: 69; Zimmermann, 2013: 339).

In Germany, reimbursement covers all medications for which a market authorization has been granted within the framework of the Statutory Health Insurance. However, the Quality Assessment Institute may exclude medications that are deemed non-cost-effective or that do not provide additional benefit. Generally, healthcare consumers pay 10 percent of the price of medications. However, there is a minimum of € 5 and a maximum of € 10 per prescription up to an annual upper limit based on the consumer's income. Exception is made for medications whose price is 30 percent below the reference price. It is interesting, from the consumer's point of view, that OTC medications may be reimbursed. In Germany, Rx medications and a few OTC medications with specific indications are fully reimbursed (100 percent), notwithstanding that in general there is a co-payment. For children under twelve years of age, Rx medications and OTC medications are fully reimbursed. Both groups of medications, for a few specific indications, are also fully reimbursed for children less than eighteen years of age (IMI_EFPIA, 2012).

In contrast to the German market, only Rx medications are fully reimbursed in Great Britain. Healthcare consumers pay a flat fee per prescription. They may also get a discount on the fee per prescription by buying a prescription prepayment certificate for three or twelve months.

In Sweden, there is a list of reimbursable medications. From a consumption and consumer point of view, the solution in place in Sweden is interesting. The consumer pays a maximum of € 244 for prescribed medications per year. Healthcare consumers cover the full cost up to a ceiling. Depending on the consumer expenditure, the co-payment is progressively reduced, i.e., from 50 percent, to 25 percent, to 10 percent. Five levels of reimbursement are distinguished in Sweden, i.e., 0 percent up to a ceiling; and 50 percent, 75 percent, and 90 percent above the ceiling. However, several OTC medications may also be reimbursed (IMI_EFPIA, 2012).

In Belgium, there is a list of medications that are reimbursed, subdivided into different chapters according to the indication for use. The co-payment includes a flat fee for the medicine and a percentage of the real cost, limited by a specific ceiling. The flat fee varies by the reimbursement category. There are five categories of medication reimbursement rates, i.e., A (100 percent), B (75 or 85 percent), C (50 percent), Cs (40 percent), and Cx (20 percent) (IMI_EFPIA, 2012).

In Poland, there is also a list of reimbursable medications. There are four reimbursement categories with different reimbursement rates: 100 percent, 50 percent, 30 percent, and between 30 percent and 50 percent (IMI_EFPIA, 2012).

It should be noted that a review and critique of reimbursement systems in the states being analyzed is not the aim of this work. The above description has only been provided to allow an understanding of the environments in which healthcare consumers make decisions about the purchase of cardiovascular medications.

3.3 Changes to the pharmaceutical market in the period 2008 to 2012

The period from 2008 to 2012 resulted in significant changes in the European pharmaceutical market. Greater or lesser changes took place in the states being analyzed. The changes had various characters, which could influence medication consumption levels and the behavior of healthcare consumers.

In Germany, the following changes occurred that proved to be relevant for consumers. Pursuant to the amendments of the legislative act that came into force on January 1, 2011, two major changes in the pricing system in Germany were introduced, i.e., a 0.30 Euro reduction of the fixed fee for pharmacies and a reduction from 6 percent to 5.15 percent of the wholesale margin (Vogler et al., 2011a: 183; Vogler et al., 2011b: 69). The changes in medication pricing yielded varied reactions (Paris et al., 2008; Ognyanova et al., 2011: 11; Vogler et al., 2011a: 183; Vogler et al., 2011b: 69). Undoubtedly, the change in pricing is perceived positively by consumers while negatively by those participating in the distribution channels.

In Great Britain, no significant changes took place in the period from 2008 to 2012.

In Sweden, the state-owned company Apoteket AB had possessed a monopoly in retail sales of medications since 1971. This monopoly was the reason for the lack of competitiveness and limited access to pharmaceutical services. In 2009, privatization of the community pharmacies sector took place. The re-regulation also allowed new units to open. This change was intended to lead to longer hours of operation and lower prices. Moreover, OTC medications were to be available in grocery stores and gas stations (Anell et al., 2012: 1; Läkemedelsverket, 2014).

In Belgium, on April 1, 2012, the system based on digressive margins in community pharmacies was replaced by a system of fixed fees for each medication. A small linear margin was added to the fixed fee.

In Poland, on January 1, 2012, new legislation on the reimbursement of medications, food products for special nutritional purposes, and medicinal products came into force. This legislation resulted from the tightening of the medication reimbursement system. The act significantly changed the previous principles in the area of retail marketing of medicinal products funded from public reimbursement. Fixed margins and prices were introduced for the retail market (Vogler et al., 2011a: 183; Vogler et al., 2011b: 69). For hospitals, the prices announced by the Ministry of Heath are the maximum prices. As Zimmermann (2013) highlights, new regulations should be introduced with the intention of abolishing price competition. Moreover, these regulations should replace competition in pricing with competition in the quality of services provided by pharmacies (Vogler et al., 2011a: 183; Vogler et al., 2011b: 69; Zimmermann, 2013: 339). Prior to the introduction of the new pharmaceutical law, 'wild' competition was observed in the area of reimbursed products. Medication sales were not directly dependent on actual consumption. In this period, consumers often took advantage of bargain sales of reimbursed products called 'medicine for one penny'. Medications were bought regardless of whether they were actually needed. Nowadays, the community pharmacies compete with each other on non-reimbursed products. It is difficult to claim that this is competition in terms of service quality.

3.4 Materials and methods

The sales data concerning cardiovascular medications for each state were retrieved from the database of IMS MIDAS Market Segmentation. This is a program of next-generation market measurement services developed by IMS Health. This company belongs to the sector of global providers of information services within the healthcare industry. IMS Health collects data on hospitals and community pharmacies in various ways. Sampling at the hospital level is a combination of indirect sales and direct sales. Indirect sales involves measuring sales from wholesalers to hospital pharmacies, and direct sales involves measuring sales from manufacturers to hospital pharmacies. In the case of community pharmacies, a number of pharmacies and wholesalers are chosen for sampling; and sales data are collected on a regular basis. The data are projected to estimate sales for the total number of community pharmacies in a given state. IMS MIDAS Market Segmentation collects data for the database according to the Anatomical Therapeutic Chemical (ATC) Classification System. The first classification of this type was published in 1976 and thereafter has been controlled by the Collaborating Centre for Drug Statistics Methodology of the World Health Organization (WHOCC, 2014). IMS Health uses an analogous classification, which was published by the European Pharmaceutical Market Research Association (EphMRA, 2013) and applied in this work. This classification system subdivides products into groups and levels.

In this study, the sales within C group (i.e., the group used in the treatment of illnesses of the cardiovascular system, called cardiovascular medications in this work) have been analyzed. C group consists of C1, cardiac therapy; C2, antihypertensive medications; C3, diuretics; C4, cerebral and peripheral vasotherapeutics; C5, antivaricose/anti-hemorrhoid preparations; C6, other cardiovascular products; C7, beta-blocking agents; C8, calcium antagonists; C9, agents acting on the renin-angiotensin system; C10, lipid-regulating/anti-atheroma preparations; and C11, cardiovascular multi-therapy combination products (EphMRA, 2012).

In this work, the consumption of cardiovascular medications and the behavior of healthcare consumers who take this group of medications in Germany, Great Britain, Sweden, Belgium, and Poland have been estimated on the basis of medication sales from pharmaceutical wholesalers to hospitals and community pharmacies. The period from 2008 to 2012 was analyzed because of the changes that occurred during this period in the pharmaceutical market.

The ratio of sales of cardiovascular Rx medications to cardiovascular OTC medications in community pharmacies and hospitals, the value of sales in Euro per person in each state, and the value of sales in Euro for medication packages to community pharmacies and hospitals were analyzed. A comparison of the number of packages of Rx and OTC medications sold also was made.

Values were calculated for the number of inhabitants, based on data taken from Eurostat. The data for each state (i.e., Germany, Great Britain, Sweden, Belgium, and Poland) refer to January 1st of each year (i.e., 2008, 2009, 2010, 2011, and 2012) or, in some cases, to December 31st of the previous year. The population is based on data from the most recent census, adjusted in compliance with the components of population change since the last census, or is based on population registers (Eurostat, 2014b). Statistical analysis was performed using Statistica 10.0. The results are presented as means and standard deviations.

3.5 Results

Figure 3.1 and table 3.1 show the coefficient values for cardiovascular Rx medication sales to cardiovascular OTC medication sales to hospitals and community pharmacies from pharmaceutical wholesalers in Germany, Great Britain, Sweden, Belgium, and Poland.

Data points in figure 3.1 and table 3.1 reflect the coefficient values for the sales of cardiovascular Rx medications and cardiovascular OTC medications to hospitals and community pharmacies and reveal the differences between the sectors under analysis in most of the states, excluding Great Britain. Changes in the curves were observed for the analyzed period, i.e., 2008 to 2012, with the exception of hospitals and community pharmacies in Great Britain and community pharmacies in Belgium. Generally, the coefficient was less diverse for hospitals than for community pharmacies during the period of analysis.

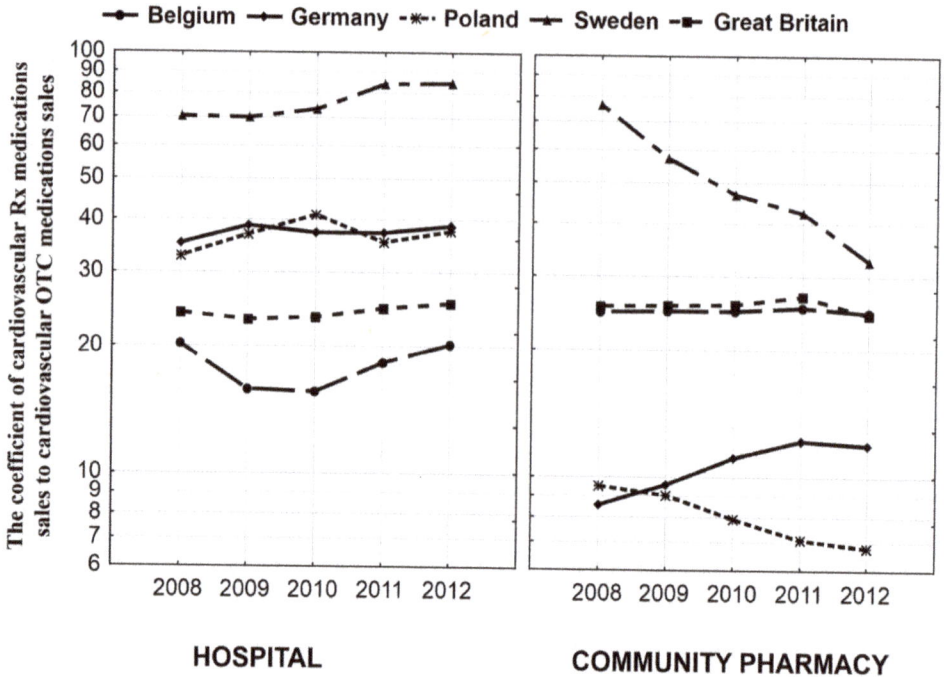

Fig. 3.1: Curves representing the values for the coefficient of cardiovascular Rx medication sales to cardiovascular OTC medication sales to hospitals and community pharmacies from pharmaceutical wholesalers
Source: Authors' calculations based on the data from IMS Healthcare

In the case of Germany, the value of the coefficient was different for hospitals and community pharmacies. These differences are significant. On average, it was at least three times higher for hospitals. Moreover, no significant changes were observed in the period of analysis. For hospitals, the coefficient ranged from 35.10 to 38.70. In the case of community pharmacies, it ranged from 8.60 to 11.90 (Table 3.1).

No significant differences were observed for Great Britain between hospitals and community pharmacies in the entire period of analysis. In the years 2008 to 2012, the coefficient for hospitals ranged from 24.00 to 25.30; whereas, for the community pharmacies, it ranged from 25.40 to 24.40 (Figure 3.1, Table 3.1).

The highest values of the coefficient were observed for Sweden, both for hospitals and community pharmacies (Figure 3.1, Table 3.1). Significant differences were revealed in Sweden for the period of analysis. In hospitals, the coefficient increased from 70.40 to 84.80 in the years 2008 to 2012. However, the opposite took place in community pharmacies. The coefficient value decreased significantly from 76.40 to 32.60 (Figure 3.1, Table 3.1).

Table 3.1: The values of the coefficient of cardiovascular Rx medication sales to cardiovascular OTC medication sales to hospitals and community pharmacies from pharmaceutical wholesalers
Source: Authors' calculations based on the data from IMS Healthcare.

		Year				
State	**Place**	**2008**	**2009**	**2010**	**2011**	**2012**
Germany	Hospital	35.10	38.70	37.20	37.20	38.70
	Community pharmacy	8.60	9.60	11.10	12.20	11.90
Great Britain	Hospital	24.00	23.20	23.50	24.60	25.30
	Community pharmacy	25.40	25.50	25.70	26.90	24.40
Sweden	Hospital	70.40	70.00	73.20	84.20	84.80
	Community pharmacy	76.40	57.20	46.90	42.50	32.60
Belgium	Hospital	20.30	15.80	15.60	18.30	20.30
	Community pharmacy	24.60	24.80	24.80	25.30	24.60
Poland	Hospital	32.80	36.90	41.00	35.40	37.60
	Community pharmacy	9.50	9.00	7.90	7.10	6.80

In Belgium, the coefficient for hospitals reached the lowest value among all the analyzed states. Moreover, it was characterized by a significant volatility. A decrease from 20.30 to 15.60 was observed in the years 2008 to 2010 and, subsequently, an increase to 20.30 in 2012. However, for community pharmacies the ratio was on the same level as in Great Britain (Figure 3.1, Table 3.1).

The data obtained for the Polish pharmaceutical market showed the greatest differences in values between the hospital market and the retail market. However, the structure of the sale of cardiovascular Rx medications and cardiovascular OTC medications for hospitals was on a similar level as Germany. The coefficient for community pharmacies was the lowest among all the analyzed states and decreased from 9.50 to 6.80 in the years from 2008 to 2012 (Figure 3.1, Table 3.1).

Turning to the data presented in figure 3.2 and table 3.2, the analysis of sales of cardiovascular Rx medications and cardiovascular OTC medications to hospitals and community pharmacies in total showed significant differences in the value of sales in Euro *per capita*.

The highest value of sales was observed for Belgium and was second-highest for Germany. Both decreased in the years from 2008 to 2012. Sweden and Great Britain were next highest, characterized in this period by the greatest decrease in sales values per person. On average, the lowest values of sales per person were noted for

Poland. However, that was also the market that underwent growth in the period being analyzed (Figure 3.2, Table 3.2).

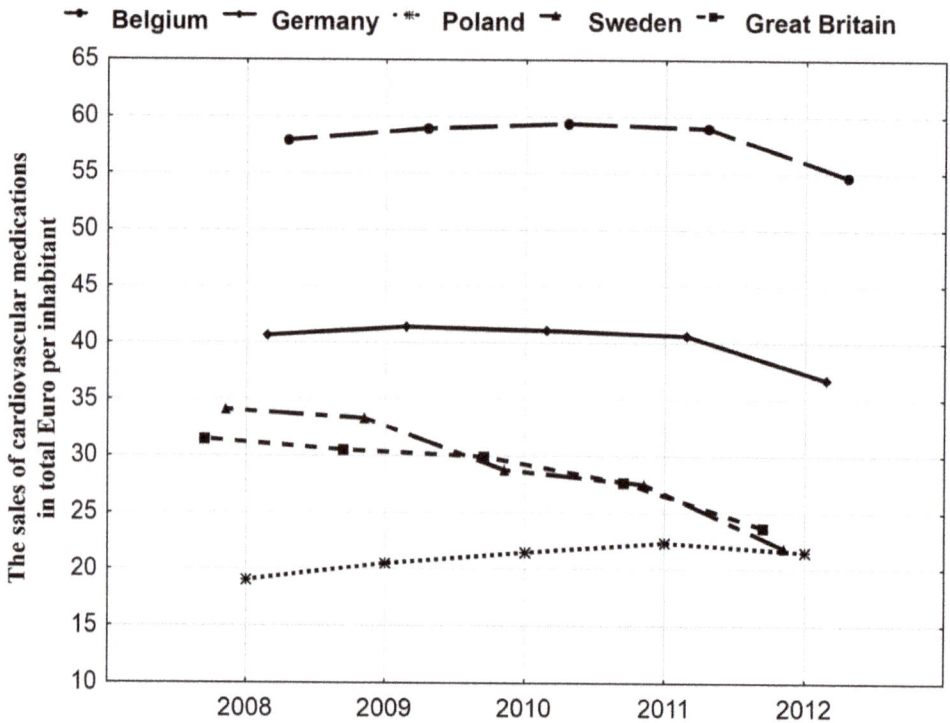

Fig. 3.2: Curves representing the sales to hospitals and community pharmacies of cardiovascular Rx medications and cardiovascular OTC medications in total in Euro per inhabitant
Source: Authors' calculations based on the data from IMS Healthcare

Tab. 3.2: The sales of cardiovascular Rx medications and cardiovascular OTC medications sold to hospitals and community pharmacies in total in Euro per inhabitant
Source: Authors' calculations based on the data from IMS Healthcare

State	2008	2009	2010	2011	2012
Germany	40.65	41.41	41.10	40.64	36.78
Great Britain	31.50	30.51	29.95	27.70	23.73
Sweden	34.10	33.32	28.77	27.51	21.91
Belgium	57.94	58.98	59.43	58.99	54.66
Poland	19.02	20.51	21.50	22.38	21.57

Looking now at the average sales price of cardiovascular Rx medication and cardiovascular OTC medication in Euro per package in hospitals and community pharmacies, the analysis revealed significant differences (Figure 3.3, Table 3.3).

In hospitals, the highest level of mean sales price per package was revealed for Sweden, followed by Great Britain, Poland, Belgium, and Germany in that order. This trend was observed for cardiovascular Rx medications and cardiovascular OTC medications. Moreover, the mean sales price per package was significantly higher for Rx medications in all the analyzed states (Figure 3.3, Table 3.3).

Generally, in Germany, Great Britain, Sweden, Belgium, and Poland, the values for mean sales price per package in the years from 2008 to 2012 in hospitals were relatively stable, both for Rx medications and OTC medications (Figure 3.3, Table 3.3).

At the same time, significant variation in the mean sales price per package was observed for community pharmacies. The analysis of the mean sales price per package of cardiovascular Rx medications also revealed significant differences in comparison to OTC medications in community pharmacies (Figure 3.3, Table 3.3).

For the retail market, the value of the mean sales price of cardiovascular Rx medication packages, from highest to lowest, was observed for Belgium, Sweden, Germany, Great Britain, and Poland. It should be noted that in Belgium, the sales price for Rx medications increased slightly from 19.72 to 20.48 in the period of analysis, i.e., from 2008 to 2012. In 2008, the second-highest result was reached in Sweden. However, Sweden was also the market in which the mean sales price per cardiovascular Rx medication package decreased dramatically, i.e., from 19.21 to 11.65 from 2008 to 2012. In Germany, the mean sales price per Rx package was stable; and the changes were discrete, i.e., from 15.50 to 14.70 in the years from 2008 to 2012 (Figure 3.3, Table 3.3). Significantly lower values were revealed for Great Britain and Poland. Whereas the value in Great Britain significantly decreased from 5.09 to 3.48; in Poland, the value increased slightly from 3.07 to 3.11 (Table 3.3).

The retail market for cardiovascular OTC medication showed significantly divergent sales prices. The highest values were noted, in descending order, for Germany, Belgium, Great Britain, Sweden, and Poland. For Germany, the sales price of OTC medications was stable in the period of analysis. A slight decrease was noted from 12.05 to 11.89. However, a slight increase and a slight fluctuation in sales value per package were observed for Great Britain, i.e., from 5.20 to 5.63 from 2008 to 2012 (Figure 3.3, Table 3.3). In the other states, i.e., Belgium, Sweden, and Poland, a significant increase of sales value per package was observed during this period, from 7.27 to 8.70, 3.89 to 4.39, and 2.78 to 4.57, respectively (Figure 3.3, Table 3.3).

56 —— Artur Turek and Aleksander Owczarek

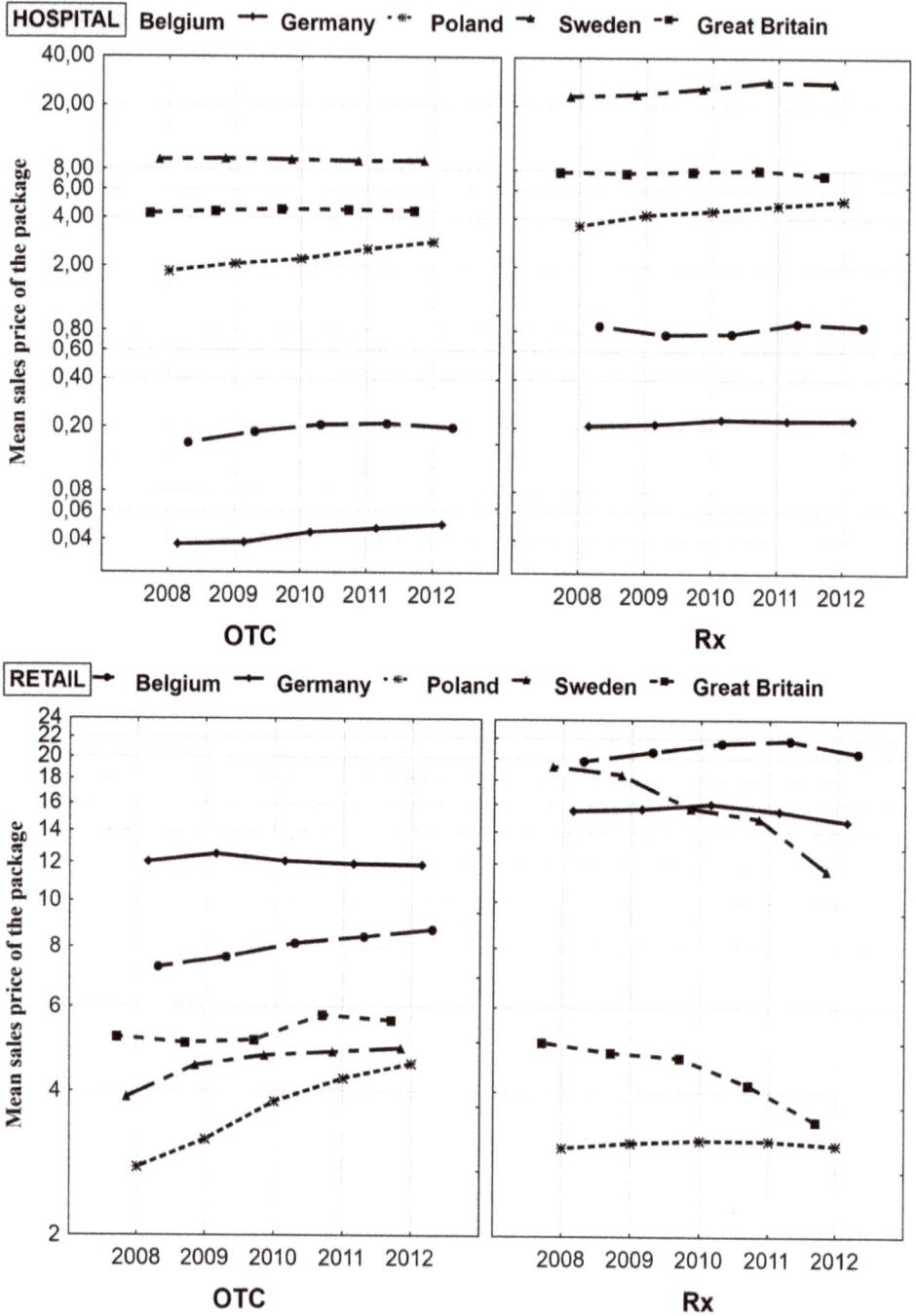

Fig. 3.3: The curves representing the mean sales price per package of cardiovascular Rx medications and cardiovascular OTC medications to hospitals and community pharmacies from pharmaceutical wholesalers

Source: Authors' calculations based on the data from IMS Healthcare

Tab. 3.3: The sales value per unit to hospitals and community pharmacies from pharmaceutical wholesalers
Source: Authors' calculations based on the data from IMS Healthcare

			Year				
State	**Place**	**Medicine**	**2008**	**2009**	**2010**	**2011**	**2012**
Germany	Hospital	OTC	0.04	0.04	0.04	0.05	0.05
Germany	Hospital	Rx	0.21	0.21	0.23	0.22	0.22
Germany	Community pharmacy	OTC	12.05	12.51	12.08	11.92	11.89
Germany	Community pharmacy	Rx	15.50	15.66	16.02	15.47	14.70
Great Britain	Hospital	OTC	4.26	4.41	4.52	4.50	4.45
Great Britain	Hospital	Rx	7.80	7.70	7.90	8.08	7.53
Great Britain	Community pharmacy	OTC	5.20	5.05	5.12	5.78	5.63
Great Britain	Community pharmacy	Rx	5.09	4.85	4.73	4.15	3.48
Sweden	Hospital	OTC	9.18	9.28	9.16	9.00	9.05
Sweden	Hospital	Rx	23.11	23.86	25.90	28.52	28.09
Sweden	Community pharmacy	OTC	3.89	4.53	4.75	4.84	4.93
Sweden	Community pharmacy	Rx	19.21	18.45	15.70	14.95	11.65
Belgium	Hospital	OTC	0.16	0.19	0.21	0.21	0.20
Belgium	Hospital	Rx	0.86	0.77	0.78	0.90	0.86
Belgium	Community pharmacy	OTC	7.27	7.62	8.15	8.42	8.70
Belgium	Community pharmacy	Rx	19.72	20.61	21.47	21.74	20.48
Poland	Hospital	OTC	1.84	2.06	2.21	2.55	2.84
Poland	Hospital	Rx	3.62	4.23	4.50	4.85	5.23
Poland	Community pharmacy	OTC	2.78	3.17	3.81	4.26	4.57
Poland	Community pharmacy	Rx	3.07	3.14	3.18	3.17	3.11

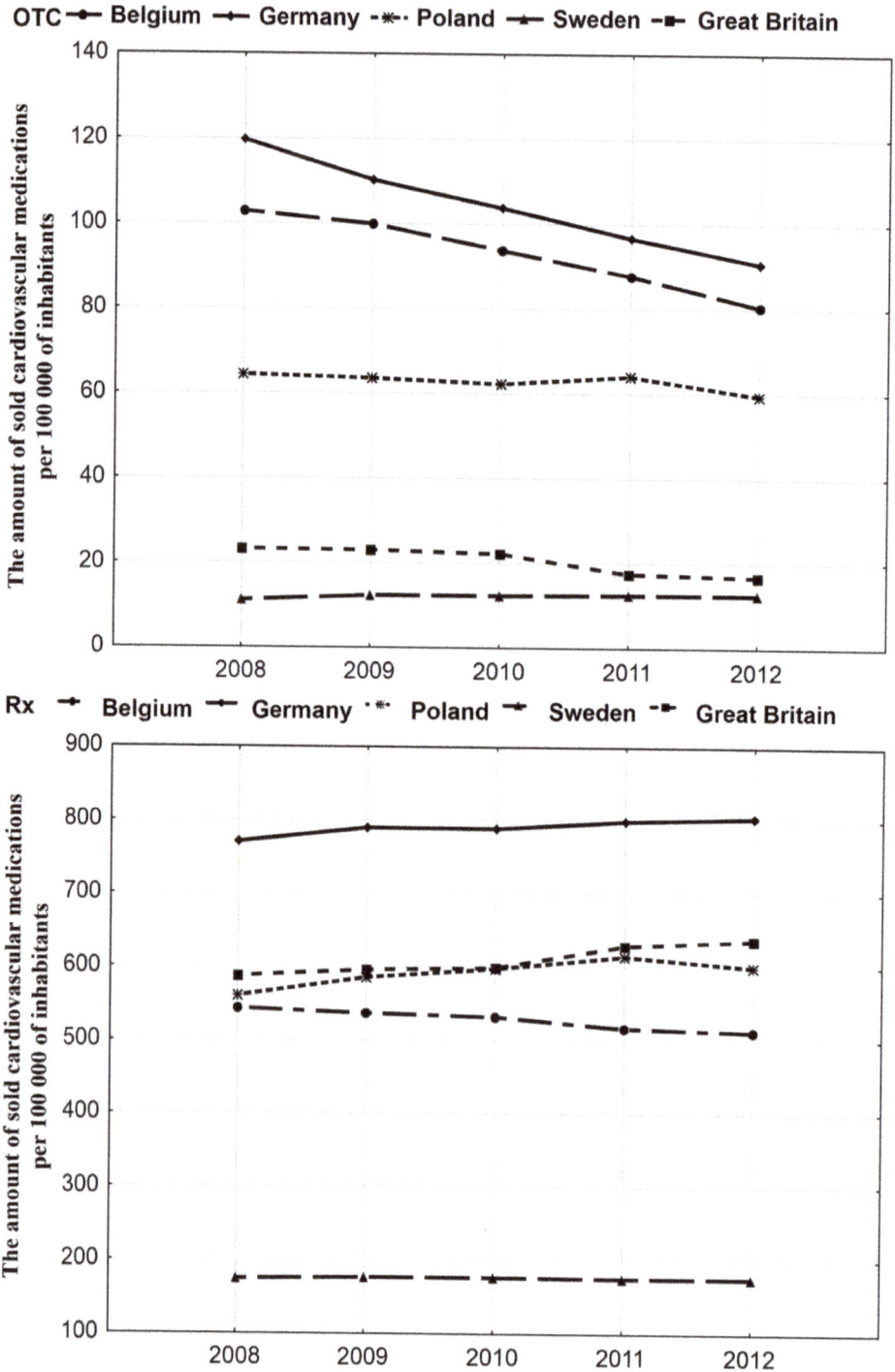

Fig. 3.4: The curves representing the amount of sold cardiovascular Rx medications and sold cardi-ovascular OTC medications per 100,000 inhabitants
Source: Authors' calculations based on the data from IMS Healthcare

Tab. 3.4: The amount of sold packages of cardiovascular Rx medications and cardiovascular OTC medications per 100,000 inhabitants
Source: Authors' calculations based on the data from IMS Healthcare

		Year				
State	**Medicine**	**2008**	**2009**	**2010**	**2011**	**2012**
Germany	OTC	119.70	110.30	103.80	96.70	90.70
Germany	Rx	770.40	788.90	788.60	798.70	803.50
Great Britain	OTC	23.20	23.00	22.10	17.50	16.80
Great Britain	Rx	587.00	595.40	599.00	629.30	636.80
Sweden	OTC	11.10	12.30	12.20	12.50	12.50
Sweden	Rx	174.20	176.00	176.00	175.10	175.10
Belgium	OTC	102.90	99.90	93.80	87.80	80.50
Belgium	Rx	543.40	536.20	531.70	517.00	512.20
Poland	OTC	64.30	63.50	62.30	64.10	59.50
Poland	Rx	560.20	585.30	597.40	614.50	600.40

The analysis of the sale quantities of packages of cardiovascular Rx medications and cardiovascular OTC medications per 100,000 inhabitants from pharmaceutical wholesalers to hospitals and community pharmacies revealed differences in regard to the types of medications, i.e., Rx or OTC (Figure 3.4, Table 3.4).

Analysis of the sales of cardiovascular Rx medications revealed the highest amount in the case of Germany, Great Britain, Poland, Belgium, and Sweden following in that order. Comparing Germany and Sweden, large differences in the sales level of Rx medications were observed, i.e., for Germany, from 770.40 to 803.50; and for Sweden, from 174.20 to 175.10 per 100,000 inhabitants from 2008 to 2012. For Great Britain and Poland, a similar amount of sold packages was noted, i.e., 587.00 to 636.80 and 560.20 to 600.40, respectively, in the period of analysis. Belgium showed lower amounts of sold packages than Great Britain and Poland, i.e., 543.40 to 512.20 from 2008 to 2012 (Figure 3.4, Table 3.4).

An increase in the amount of Rx sold packages was seen in the period of analysis in three states, i.e., Germany, Great Britain, and Poland; while sales in Belgium decreased. Sweden did not reveal any significant changes (Figure 3.4, Table 3.4).

More marked differences were observed for cardiovascular OTC medications. The amount of sold packages was the highest for Germany, Belgium, Poland, and Great Britain; and the lowest was for Sweden. In the period from 2008 to 2012, a decrease was observed in Germany, Great Britain, Belgium, and Poland, i.e., from 119.70 to 90.70, 23.20 to 16.80, 102.90 to 80.50, and 64.30 to 59.50, respectively. An increase was noted only for Sweden, i.e., from 11.10 to 12.50 (Figure 3.4, Table 3.4).

3.6 Discussion

The frequency of cardiovascular disease, the amount of Rx medications and OTC medications being sold, the value of total sales of these medications, and the average price of medication packages may all influence the consumption of cardiovascular medications and the behavior of the health consumers who take them.

From the point of view of consumption and consumer behavior, it is significant where the consumption takes place (i.e., hospital or community pharmacy) and what types of medications are available (Rx or OTC). In this study, the coefficient of cardiovascular Rx medication sales and cardiovascular OTC medication sales to hospitals and community pharmacies from pharmaceutical wholesalers reflects the market share of these categories of cardiovascular medications for inpatient therapy and outpatient therapy (Figure 3.1, Table 3.1).

For purposes of interpretation, it should be noted that if the coefficient increases, the market share of Rx medications increases. In this situation, doctors play the main role. However, if the coefficient decreases, the opposite situation occurs, wherein pharmaceutical recommendation seems to have greater importance.

Significant differences in the values of the coefficients of cardiovascular Rx medication sales to cardiovascular OTC medication sales to hospitals and community pharmacies from pharmaceutical wholesalers were revealed in four of the five states, i.e., Germany, Sweden, Belgium, and Poland. The explanation for this phenomenon should emphasize the following facts. First, this situation is a result of the differences in the systems of medication financing in hospitals and community pharmacies and also in the decision-making process. It is, therefore, obvious that the coefficients would be different. Second, the coefficient values were significantly higher for Germany, Sweden, and Poland in hospitals than in community pharmacies, i.e., in the retail market. It can be noted that cardiovascular Rx medications are consumed more often in hospitals than at home. Taking into account that cardiovascular OTC medications play a supplementary role and/or a preventive role for many cardiovascular diseases, it is understandable that Rx medications were often used in hospitals. Moreover, consumers in hospitals are generally in worse clinical condition than those receiving outpatient treatments. Therefore, the consumption of cardiovascular Rx medication is higher for inpatient treatment. Finally, the values of the coefficient may reflect the efficiency of medical care in the area of cardiovascular diseases and the behavior of the healthcare consumer. However, it is difficult to support this thesis.

In general, cardiovascular medications are of greater importance for older than for younger healthcare consumers. Therefore, a relationship between the median age in the states being analyzed and the sales level may be found. According to Eurostat data for median age in 2010, the highest is German (44.20), then Swedish (40.70), Belgian (40.90), British (39.60), and Polish (37.70) (Eurostat, 2012). However, it seems more important to note that the share of the population aged 80 or over in 2010 was 5.30 percent for Sweden, 5.10 percent for Germany, 4.90 percent for Belgium, 4.60 percent for Great Britain, and 3.30 percent for Poland (Eurostat, 2012). These data on age partially correspond to the obtained results. The oldest consumers from all the analyzed states live in Sweden, and the highest sales of cardiovascular Rx medication occur in Sweden. However, according to Eurostat data for 2009, Sweden has the lowest number of hospital beds per 100,000 inhabitants (277.10), which may indicate the efficiency of medical care in the field of cardiology. The same relationship between the coefficient value and the share of the population aged 80 or over was visible for Germany and Great Britain in hospitals.

However, the opposite situation was observed for Belgian hospitals. On the basis of the data presented, Belgium can be presumed to be an example of correct measures to promote health and provide efficient healthcare. This thesis is confirmed by epidemiological and demographic data. First, it should be pointed out that Belgium showed a relatively low standardized death rate in 2010 for circulatory disease, despite a relatively high share of the population aged 80 or over compared to the other states being analyzed. Moreover, the coefficient value was lowest for Belgium compared to all the states in hospitals, which indicates a relatively good clinical state for the hospitalized healthcare consumers.

An interesting situation was noted for Poland in hospitals. The value of the coefficient was on the same level in the case of Poland and Germany. However, for Poland the share of the population aged 80 or over was about 35 percent lower. This smaller number of people over 80 may be related to low-priced procedures in cardiology and/or poor medical care. It should be noted that consumers in Poland encounter a limited availability of medical visits (CBOS, 2008; CBOS, 2010). This fact is accompanied by the highest standardized death rate in 2010 for circulatory disease and heart disease in Poland compared to all the other analyzed states (Eurostat, 2010).

In the period from 2008 to 2012, changes in the value of the coefficient were noted for hospital treatment. Taking into account the changes that took place in the retail market, it may be said that the market share of cardiovascular Rx medications and cardiovascular OTC medications is stable. It may also be stated that this is a result of the decision-making process.

Undoubtedly, the changes during the period of analysis, i.e., 2008 to 2012, concerning the values of the coefficient correspond to changes in the market, which were conspicuously visible in the retail market – i.e., in community pharmacies, where healthcare consumers make decisions about treatment and the purchase of medications. Medication use depends entirely on consumer decisions. Consumers often stop buying Rx medications for financial reasons. Moreover, Rx medications are often supplemented by or replaced by OTC medications (Cohen, 2003: 370; Mahecha, 2007: 380; Pawaskar and Balkrishnan, 2007: 42; Hemwall, 2010: 267; Faerber and Kreling, 2012: 66).

It should be noted that in community pharmacies, healthcare consumers exert real influence on the purchase process. A high coefficient value was noted for Sweden in the retail market and next for Great Britain and Belgium. However, the values for Great Britain and Belgian markets were similar and did not reveal any significant changes. A relatively low value was observed for Germany and Poland.

It should be pointed out that consumption of Rx medication is the highest in Sweden and the lowest in Poland (Figure 3.1, Table 3.1). This fact may be connected with the number of practicing physicians, highest in 2009 in Sweden and lowest in Poland of all those analyzed, i.e., 371.50 and 217.00 per 100,000 inhabitants, respectively.

It has already been emphasized that in the case of the hospital market, i.e., inpatient treatment, a clear trend was not visible during the analyzed period (2008 to 2012). For the retail market in community pharmacies, i.e. outpatient treatment, trends are clearly visible for Sweden, Germany, and Poland. The changes in the values of the coefficient might reflect the changes in the retail market described above. The observed increase in the coefficient value in Germany in the years from 2008 to 2012 might result from changes in legislation, which introduced a reduction of the fixed fee for pharmacies and a reduction of the wholesale margin for Rx medications.

However, the highest decrease of a coefficient was noted in Sweden. In 2009, the privatization of community pharmacies took place. Following that, the number of community pharmacies increased by 20 percent. Hours of operation were increased and a decrease in prices took place. The increase in the market share of OTC medications undoubtedly resulted from the increased availability of OTC medications in community pharmacies (Anell et al., 2012: 1; Läkemedelsverket, 2014). Therefore, the increase of OTC medications in market share can be considered to be correct (Figure 3.1, Table 3.1).

In the years from 2008 to 2012, a decrease in the coefficient was also noted for Poland. However, the decrease possessed a less dynamic character than in Sweden. This decrease resulted from the introduction of fixed margins and prices in the retail market for reimbursed Rx medications based on legislative acts (Zimmermann, 2013: 339). According to the authors of the legislative act, the prices for reimbursed Rx medications in the community pharmacies needed to be lower. In practice, the lack of a discount at the respective stages of the distribution channel resulted in an increase in the final price in community pharmacies, which might result in an increase in the sales of cardiovascular OTC medications. On the other hand, the observed effect in Poland might also result from the growing needs of the broadly understood notion of health and the limited availability of medical visits (CBOS, 2010). Therefore, the substitution of OTC medications for Rx medications might take place.

The analysis of the sales of cardiovascular Rx medications and cardiovascular OTC medications in total to the hospitals and community pharmacies from pharmaceutical wholesalers in Euro per inhabitant (Figure 3.2, Table 3.2) indirectly shows the average total cost of inpatient and outpatient therapy per healthcare consumer.

This parameter may estimate the expenses incurred by the reimbursement system for cardiovascular medications, access to medical care, and the state of health.

Similar values were noted for Sweden and Great Britain., i.e., the states representing the tax model. However, significant differences in the values were observed between Belgium, Germany, Sweden, and Great Britain (treated as one group) and Poland. These differences probably reflect the insurance model. It is difficult to say clearly which factors determined the differences. However, attention should be paid to the following facts: (i) Belgium possesses an average value for some parameters, i.e., standardized death rate for circulatory disease and heart disease in 2010, the share of population aged 80 or over in 2010 (Eurostat, 2010), and the number of practicing physicians and hospital beds in 2009 (Eurostat, 2012); (ii) the highest median age in 2010 was seen in Germany as well as the highest number of hospital beds in 2009 (Eurostat, 2012); (iii) in 2009, Great Britain and Sweden had the lowest number of hospital beds (Eurostat, 2012); (iv) in 2010 in Poland, the standardized death rate for circulatory disease and heart disease was the highest (Eurostat, 2010); in 2009, the number of practicing physicians was lowest (Eurostat, 2012); and the value of sold cardiovascular medication in Euro per inhabitant was lowest; and (v) in the case of all states excluding Poland, the trend in the value of cardiovascular medication sales in Euro per inhabitant was downward.

Against this background, it can be assumed that medical care is being optimized, even though the population is aging. In addition, the insurance system in Germany, Great Britain, Sweden, and Belgium may be more effective than in Poland.

The analysis of sale values of cardiovascular Rx medications and cardiovascular OTC medications to hospitals and community pharmacies from pharmaceutical wholesalers (Figure 3.3, Table 3.3) yielded the mean sales price in Euro per package in the states being analyzed. This parameter points to what price per package is acceptable in the hospital and non-hospital sectors.

It should be pointed out that price is an integral part of the marketing mix. Smith (2009: 3) has noted that necessary medications will be purchased regardless of price. Therefore, in the case of medication, price should have secondary importance. However, the authors' own observations of the European market indicate that medications are overly expensive. In turn, Smith (2009: 3) has emphasized too that medication prices are regularly criticized publicly. This is hard to understand, given the fact that health is of the highest value.

The mean price of cardiovascular medications in the hospital and retail market reflects supply and demand. It should be emphasized that the amount of cardiovascular medicinal products for inpatient and outpatient therapy continues to increase. On the other hand, demand, in the case of medications, depends on age, morbidity, funding of healthcare, access to medical care, and many other factors. In this study, significant differences were found in the mean sale prices between hospitals and community pharmacies for cardiovascular medications, and also between cardiovascular Rx medications and cardiovascular OTC medications.

However, it should be noted that the market for hospitals was less varied than the market for community pharmacies. For hospitals, certain regularities were observed in the period of analysis (2008 to 2012). For example, the following regularities may be noted: (i) the same trend was observed in the value of mean sale prices for Rx medication and OTC medication packages for each state, i.e., the highest prices were revealed for Sweden, Great Britain, Poland, Belgium, and Germany, respectively; (ii) in each state, there was a higher price for Rx medications than OTC medications; (iii) there was a relatively low volatility in prices for Rx medicines and OTC medicines; and (iv) none of the sectors revealed clear upward and downward trends (Figure 3.3, Table 3.3).

It is interesting that the highest values were noted for states with a tax model of insurance, i.e., Sweden and Great Britain. It should be emphasized that the value levels are more dependent on macroeconomic data than on consumer and consumption determinants. This is so because in the hospital sector, consumers are passive participants in the decision-making process. The highest values in Sweden may result from the fact that in Sweden in 2010, the highest employment rate was noted in the age group 15 to 64 years of age and the lowest value for the population at-risk of poverty or social exclusion. Of all the states, Sweden also had the highest value, in 2010, for gross domestic product *per capita* (Eurostat, 2012). Moreover, analyzing healthcare expenditures by provider in 2009, a more or less equal distribution between hospitals and ambulatory healthcare may be noted for Germany, Belgium, and Poland; only in Sweden were expenditures more than 100 percent higher for hospitals (Eurostat, 2012). For other states, it is difficult to find analogies with macroeconomic data.

In hospitals, a relatively low volatility of mean sale prices for cardiovascular Rx medications and cardiovascular OTC medicines and the lack of a clear trend may point to the fact that the hospital sector is not competitive. The prices are acceptable to the hospital sector. The results may indicate also that the behavior of healthcare consumers and other market participants did not play a significant role in the forming of prices for cardiovascular medications in hospitals in the period of analysis. The prices for cardiovascular Rx medications are regulated by governmental laws. Orders for hospitals are held on the basis of public procurement for state entities.

However, a significant variation in mean sale prices was observed for cardiovascular medications for community pharmacies. In the area of Rx medications, the prices are regulated by government with respect to the level of reimbursement. The prices of OTC medications are regulated in the retail market. Consumers make adaptations when they consider the price level to be excessive. This leads to significant differences between the prices of Rx medications and OTC medications.

Various trends were also noted across states for the values for Rx medications and OTC medications. They result from different legislative acts in the respective states and different sensitivity to price by consumers. The Polish market showed the lowest value, both for OTC medicines and Rx medicines. The low price may stem from the fact that Polish consumers are the most sensitive to price. It also reflects macroeconomic and epidemiologic data. In 2010, the consumption expenditure of households *per capita* was the lowest for Poland, i.e., 8600. Moreover, in Poland, the real adjusted gross disposable income of households *per capita* in 2010 was approximately 50 percent lower than in Germany (Eurostat, 2014a). It may be pointed out that in 2010, the standardized death rate for circulatory disease and heart disease showed the highest value in Poland (Eurostat, 2010). In the same year in Poland, the employment rate in the group from 15 to 64 years of age was the lowest. Therefore, these data may influence the values for Rx medications and OTC medications.

Based on the available macroeconomic data, it is difficult to explain clearly what factors shape the average price per package of cardiovascular Rx medications in Germany, Great Britain, Sweden, and Belgium. Undoubtedly, the prices are acceptable to both legislators and consumers. It should be noted that in 2010, the adjusted gross disposable income of households *per capita* and the employment rate were relatively high in these states in comparison to Poland (Eurostat, 2010).

From 2008 to 2012, there was a decrease in the mean sales price for Rx medications per package in Germany, Great Britain, and Sweden in the retail market. However, in Poland and Belgium, an increase in the mean sales price was noted (Figure 3.3, Table 3.3). In the case of Rx medications, government acts exert a significant influence on prices.

On the other hand, consumers have a significant influence on OTC medication prices. First of all, consumers demand a decrease in prices. Only in the case of Germany was a decrease in the mean sales price of cardiovascular OTC medications noted, and this decrease cannot be defined as significant. Other retail markets were characterized by an increase, which may be linked to the demand for this group of medications in the given insurance model. The increase is significantly visible for Sweden and Poland, where the highest increase was observed (Figure 3.3, Table 3.3).

In 2009 in Sweden, the privatization of community pharmacies took place, improving access to medications (Anell et al., 2012: 1; Läkemedelsverket, 2014). It should also be emphasized that Poland was the sixth largest medication market in Europe (URPL, 2010). The expenses of a typical Pole increased from PLN 5 in 1995 to PLN 29 in 2009 (Skrzypczak, 2011). In this aspect, the increase of mean sale price of cardiovascular OTC medications may be connected with the increase of demand.

Regarding medication prices, the large differences in their values across the states being analyzed may lead to a balanced price Europe-wide. The reason is the importation of patented or trademarked products from countries where they are already marketed (WHO, 2014). This phenomenon leads to negative results in the area of consumption because a deficit of medications with a lower price may occur. Recently, this has been the case with low molecular weight heparyn (MHRA, 2008).

The final answer concerning the consumption of cardiovascular Rx medications and cardiovascular OTC medications relies on the analysis of the amount of packages sold by wholesalers per 100,000 inhabitants. The consumption level may be estimated directly on the basis of this parameter. Both for cardiovascular Rx medications and cardiovascular OTC medications, significant differences among the states being analyzed were observed; however, in the case of OTC medications, these differences were more marked, probably because healthcare consumers have stronger influence in this part of the market (Figure 3.4, Table 3.4).

The amount of sold cardiovascular Rx medications per 100,000 inhabitants was significantly higher than cardiovascular OTC medications for each of the states being analyzed (Figure 3.4, Table 3.4), which demonstrates that medical care fulfills its role in all insurance models in each of the analyzed states. It can be said that healthcare consumers choose medical visits and purchases of prescribed medications. This does not mean that doctors do not prescribe OTC medications. However, the consumption of cardiovascular Rx medication plays a leading role. In the case of cardiac problems, it is natural to pursue medical care and use Rx medications. This only shows healthcare consumers' awareness.

The analysis of the data may indirectly point to the frequency of cardiovascular diseases. According to this thesis, Swedes get sick the least frequently with cardiovascular diseases. This may be concluded because the amount of Rx medicines and OTC medicines was the lowest in Sweden. The opposite effect was noted for Germany. However, it is not appropriate to announce that Germans are in a worse health condition. This thesis is not confirmed by the value of the standardized death rate for Germany, which was one of the lowest in comparison to Poland (Eurostat, 2010).

In the period of analysis, i.e., 2008 to 2012, in the case of Germany, Great Britain, Belgium, and Poland, a decrease in the amount of cardiovascular OTC medications was observed. However, non-significant trends were visible for cardiovascular Rx medications. From a medical point of view, this situation may be the result of a relatively fixed number of medical cases (Figure 3.4, Table 3.4). It can also be said that a switch from cardiovascular Rx medications to cardiovascular OTC medications did not take place, although some contain the same active substance.

Every now and then, the issue of pharmaceutical lobbying is raised. However, in the analyzed data, it is difficult to find the influence of lobbying on the amount of packages being sold. Moreover, the effect of the introduction of generic medication on potential savings has not been captured.

Conclusions

Given this analysis, it is difficult to state exactly how the insurance model has influenced the consumption of cardiovascular medications and the behavior of healthcare consumers. Undoubtedly, in each insurance model, two areas of consumption may be distinguished: hospitals for inpatient consumers and home for outpatient consumers, i.e., the retail market (community pharmacy). The consumption setting of cardiovascular medications is significant due to the decision-making process. In hospitals, healthcare consumers are passive participants in the market; they do not make decisions because consumers do not choose the method of treatment, purchase, and consumption. At home, consumers do not choose the type of treatment in the case of Rx medications either, but they make decisions about their purchase and consumption. It should be emphasized that the efficiency of the purchasing process results directly from the efficiency of the reimbursement system for reimbursed medications. However, OTC medications in cardiology are used more for the prevention of heart disorders and diseases to supplement pharmacologic therapy. The results did not point clearly to the replacement of Rx medications with OTC medications. Use of OTC medications also reflects the consumer's awareness of diseases. Undoubtedly, consumption increases with an increase of awareness. Cardiovascular OTC medication is an area of the market where health consumers make decisions about the method of treatment, purchase, and consumption.

The level of sales of cardiovascular medications may give information about life expectancy, life style, morbidity, income, effectiveness of the reimbursement system, and effectiveness of healthcare. The results of the study point to differences in the data, i.e., in the amount of Rx medication sales and OTC medication sales, the value for total sales of medications, the average price of a medication package, and the amount of sold medication packages per a given number of inhabitants for states with different insurance models. The findings may reflect the basic differences resulting from the insurance model. The consumption of cardiovascular medications by relevant healthcare consumers depends rather on the type (i.e., Rx and OTC medications) and the setting of consumption. When analyzing the results, the influence of macroeconomics and epidemiology was also taken into consideration.

Acknowledgments

The authors thank IMS Healthcare for providing data.

References

Anell, A., Glenngård, A.H. and Merkur, S., 2012. Sweden health system review. *Health Systems in Transition*, 14 (5): 1–159.

Cameron, A., Ewen, M., Ross-Degnan, D., Ball, D. and Laing, R., 2009. Medicine prices, availability, and affordability in 36 developing and middle-income countries: a secondary analysis. *Lancet*, 373 (9659): 240–249.

Cameron, A., Mantel-Teeuwisse, A.K., Leufkens, H.G. and Laing, R.O., 2012. Switching from originator brand medicines to generic equivalents in selected developing countries: how much could be saved? *Value Health*, 15 (5): 664–673.

CBOS, (Centrum Badań Opinii Społecznej), 2008. *Komunikat z badań. Warunki życiowe społeczeństwa polskiego: problemy i strategie. Korzystanie ze świadczeń zdrowotnych.* BS/32/2008. Warszawa: Fundacja Centrum Badania Opinii Społecznej.

CBOS, (Centrum Badań Opinii Społecznej), 2010. *Opinie o opiece zdrowotnej.* BS/24/2010. Warszawa: Fundacja Centrum Badania Opinii Społecznej.

Cohen, J., 2003. Switching omeprazole in Sweden and the United States. *American Journal of Therapeutics*, 10 (5): 370–376.

EphMRA, (European Pharmaceutical Marketing Research Association), 2012. *EphMRA Anatomical Classification Guidelines.* Retrieved December 30, 2013 from: http://www.ephmra.org/pdf/ATCGuidelines2012Final%20V2%20revised.pdf.

Eurostat, 2010. *Causes of death – standardised death rate, 2010 (1) (per 100 000 inhabitants).* Retrieved March 31, 2014 from: http://epp.eurostat.ec.europa.eu/statistics_explained/index.php?title=File:Causes_of_death_-_standardised_death_rate,_2010_%281%29_%28per_100_000_inhabitants%29.png& filetimestamp=20121022145128.

Eurostat, 2012. Eurostat yearbook 2012. *General and regional statistics.* Luxembourg: Publications Office of the European Union.

Eurostat, 2013. *Causes of death statistics.* Retrieved March 31, 2014 from: http://epp.eurostat.ec.europa.eu/statistics_explained/index.php/Causes_of_death_statistics #Diseases_of_the_circulatory_system.

Eurostat, 2014a. Real adjusted gross disposable income of households per capita. Retrieved March 31, 2014 from: http://epp.eurostat.ec.europa.eu/tgm/table.do?tab=table&plugin=0& language=en&pcode=tec00113.

Eurostat, 2014b. Retrieved March 31, 2014 from: http://epp.eurostat.ec.europa.eu/portal/page/portal/population/data/main_tables.

Faerber, A.E. and Kreling D.H., 2012. Now you see it. Now you don't: fair balance and adequate provision in advertisements for drugs before and after the switch from prescription to over-the-counter. *Health Communication*, 27 (1): 66–74.

Holdford, D., 2007. *Marketing for pharmacists.* Washington DC: American Pharmacists Association.

Hemwall, E.L., 2010. Increasing access to nonprescription medications: a global public health challenge and opportunity. *Clinical Pharmacology and Therapeutics*, 87 (3): 267–269.

IMI_EFPIA, 2012. *Pharmacoepidemiological research on outcomes of therapeutics by a European Consortium. Drug consumption databases in Europe.* Retrieved May 30, 2014 from: http://www.imi-protect.eu/documents/DUinventory_2012_COUNTRIES.pdf.

Läkemedelsverket, Medical Products Agency, 2014. *The Swedish pharmacy market.* Retrieved May 30, 2014 from: http://www.lakemedelsverket.se/english/overview/About-MPA/pharmacy-market/.

Mahecha, L.A., 2006. Rx-to-OTC switches: trends and factors underlying success. *Nature Reviews. Drug Discovery*, 5 (5): 380–385.

Medicines and Healthcare Products Regulatory Agency (MHRA), 2008. *Class 4 Drug Alert (Caution in Use): Parallel imports of low molecular weight heparin – Enoxaparin sodium (Clexane) pre-filled syringes.* Retrieved May 30, 2014 from: http://www.mhra.gov.uk/Publications/ Safetywarnings/DrugAlerts/CON015377.

Millier, A., Cohen, J. and Toumi, M., 2013. Economic impact of a triptan Rx-To-OTC switch in six EU countries. *PLoS One*, 8 (12): e84088.

Ognyanova, A., Zentner, A. and Busse, R., 2011. Pharmaceutical reform 2010 in Germany: striking a balance between innovation and affordability. *Eurohealth*, 17 (1): 11–13.

Paris, V. and Docteur, E., 2008. *Pharmaceutical pricing and reimbursement policies in Germany. OECD Health Working Papers No. 39*, Paris: OECD Publishing. Retrieved December 30, 2013

from: http://www.oecd-ilibrary.org/docserver/download/5ksqczrw7jjj.pdf?expires=
1368520541&id=id&accname=guest&checksum=1C5E6F5A35C13B6C3A5E4960A44F30EA.

Pawaskar, M.D. and Balkrishnan, R., 2007. Switching from prescription to over-the counter medications: a consumer and managed care perspective. *Managed Care Interface*, 20 (1): 42–47.

Skrzypczak, Z., 2011. *Wydatki polskich konsumentów na zakup leków*. Rzeczpospolita. Retrieved
December 30, 2013 from: http://www.rp.pl/artykul/639301.html.

Smith, M., 2009. General environment. In: Smith, M.C., Kolassa, E.M., Perkins, G. and Siecker, B.
(Ed.) *Pharmaceutical marketing. Practice Environment and Practice*: 17–69, New York: Informa
Healthcare.

Smith, M., 2009. General principles. In: Smith, M.C., Kolassa, E.M., Perkins, G. and Siecker, B. (Ed.)
Pharmaceutical marketing. Practice Environment and Practice: 3–15, New York: Informa
Healthcare.

Turek, A. and Owczarek, A., 2014. Determinant of consumption behavior of over-the-counter
mecications – The case of painkillers and anti-inflammatory medications. *Journal of Economics
and Management*, 2014, 15: 25–59.

URPL, (Urząd Rejestracji Produktów Leczniczych Wyrobów Medycznych i Produktów Biobójczych),
2010. *Ogólnopolska Kampania "Lek bezpieczny"*. Retrieved May 30, 2014 from:
http://www.urpl.gov.pl/lek-bezpieczny.

Vogler, S., Habl, C., Bogut, M. and Voncina, L., 2011a. Comparing pharmaceutical pricing and reimbursement policies in Croatia to the European Union Member States. *Croatian Medical Journal*,
52 (2): 183–197.

Vogler, S., Zimmermann, N., Leopold, C. and de Joncheere, K., 2011b. Pharmaceutical policies in European countries in response to the global financial crisis. *Southern Med Review*, 4 (2): 69–79.

Ward, T. and Ozdemir, E., 2012. *Social situation observatory income distribution and living conditions. Disparities in access to essential services. Applica (BE), European Centre for social welfare policy and research*. ISER – University of Essex (UK) and Tarki (HU).

WHO, (World Health Organization), 2013. *The top 10 causes of death*. Retrieved December 30, 2013
from: http://who.int/mediacentre/factsheets/fs310/en/.

WHO, (World Health Organization), 2014. *Trade, foreign policy, diplomacy and health. Parallel
imports*. Retrieved May 30, 2014 from: http://www.who.int/trade/glossary/story070/en/.

WHOCC, (World Health Organization Collaborating Centre for Drug Statistics Methodology), 2014.
History. Retrieved May 30, 2014 from: http://www.whocc.no/atc_ddd_methodology/history/.

Zimmermann, A., 2013. Restrictions on the reimbursement policy with regard to retail marketing of
medical products in Poland. *Acta Poloniae Pharmaceutica*, 70, 339–343.

Agnieszka Hat

4 New Trends in Consumer Behavior in the European Healthcare Market

Abstract This chapter reviews the consumer behavior trends in the European healthcare market, paying special attention to five particular European countries: Germany, Great Britain, Sweden, Belgium, and Poland.[1] Taking into account consumers' actions and changes in their attitudes as well as some of the macro- and microeconomic factors underlying these actions, the author presents general conclusions regarding the trends, which includes identifying the evolution of informed and active players in the European healthcare market in the form of a Doctor Consumer.

Keywords: Consumer behavior trend, Healthcare, European market, Doctor Consumer

4.1 Introduction

The new face of the market that has emerged as a result of globalization and general technological advances has had a huge influence on changes in consumer behavior in the European healthcare market. The main goal of this chapter is to present how these changes have taken the form of consumer behavior trends, with a special focus on those trends that are the most specific to the healthcare market. Although the countries being analyzed (Germany, Great Britain, Sweden, Belgium, and Poland) represent different healthcare models, still consumers have experienced similar psycho and social changes in the society and also have faced relatively similar internal and external forces driving changes in the healthcare system. That is the reason, for the purposes of the following thesis, that a range of general consumer behavior trends possible to observe in the European healthcare market has been presented.

4.2 Trends in consumer behavior – notion, types, and characteristics

Globalization of the economy, internationalization of business activities, constant development of technology, and general advances of civilization are just a few of the characteristics of the contemporary turbulent environment. All of the changes

---

1 Project financed with the resources from the NCN (National Science Centre). Decision number: DEC-2011/03/N/HS4/00611. Project supervisor: Agnieszka Hat.

have just recently occurred in the market; and they have not left consumer behavior unchanged. They have stimulated changes in consumption and in consumer behavior for a longer period of time so they have set a trend.

Originally, the word 'trend' was derived from Old English and meant 'to turn', so literally it simply means 'turn' as in 'curve'. In statistics, the word 'trend' is used to define the direction of a curve, while in culture, art, or design, trend does not mean something that can be easily measured as it does in statistics. Sociologists, in turn, perceive 'trend' as 'not something that has happened, but rather a prediction of something that is going to happen in a certain way – specifically something that will be accepted by the average person' (Vejlgaard 2008: 6–8). H. Vejlgaard, the author of *"Anatomy of a Trend"*, defines 'trend' as a process of change that can be considered from the psychological, sociological, and economic perspective (Tkaczyk 2012: 126). Others describe it as 'the direction in which something (and that something can be anything) tends to move and which has a consequential impact on the culture, society, or business sector through which it moves' (Raymond 2010: 14). Raymond elaborates by saying that 'trends are a fundamental part of our emotional, physical, and psychological landscape, and by detecting, mapping, and using them to anticipate what is new and next in the world we live in we are contributing in no small way to better understanding the underlying ideas and principles that drive and motivate us as people' (2010: 15).

But regardless of the definition of 'trend' and what context the authors are using the word in, the concept of change is always the crucial part of the definition. There are many types of changes that characterize trends: shifts in politics, economy, technology, law, society, or culture. Depending on the type of change and its character, trends may be considered short- or long-term as well as of a local or global scope. Finally, no matter what field the trend is occurring in, whether it is art or the economy, its common characteristic is co-existence (inter-connection) and divergence (trends creating counter-trends) (Tkaczyk 2012: 126).

In terms of consumers, these changes, if longer, are defined as **consumer behavior trends**. Euromonitor defines them as 'directional tendencies in lifestyle, which may be obvious or imperceptible', and emphasizes the interaction between consumers and trends:

- the lives, lifestyles, and purchasing of consumers are changed by politics, wars, religion, economics, technology, disease, culture, media, and ideas;
- trends are always inter-connected;
- trends often create counter-trends; and
- changes in consumer mindsets create their own trends (2005).

S. Smyczek, in turn, pays attention to the fact that they do not consist only in the consumption of new products, services, or modifications to existing goods but also in considerable changes in the level at which needs are satisfied and in numerous consumer decisions in the market and households. He says 'consumer behavior trends intensify in some consumer groups, penetrate other groups, or finally are subject to modifications and disappear with time' (2012: 256). A. Dąbrowska concludes, when defining consumer behavior trends, that the concept of behavior change is strictly bound with a number of underlying driving factors (2006: 178) that can be understood as a number of processes, phenomena, subjects, and so on that determine the contemporary consumer's behavior. These factors can be either unknown or familiar but change the direction or the intensity scale of the consumer's behavior. They are as follows:

- economic factors (personal income, level of prices, prices of goods vs prices of services, available goods),
- social-demographic factors (sex, place of living, life expectancy, birth rate, mobility, aging of society),
- cultural factors (habits, traditions, change in value systems, consumer education, focus on quality of life),
- technological factors (development of communication means, development of biotechnology),
- political factors (legal changes, government activities), and
- psychological factors (consumer motivation, emotions, learning, attitudes, lifestyle) (Dąbrowska 2006: 178).

Finally, Cz. Bywalec explains that consumer behavior trends can be considered to be ongoing processes in contemporary economies that are so extensive and noticeable that they have been granted the name 'new consumption'. 'New' means different than the 'old one' in diffusion of new goods consumption and modification of the old ones as well as changes in the needs hierarchy; the ways and means of needs satisfaction; and last, but not least, the criteria of customer choice. Finally, it is worth mentioning that the life-cycle of these trends escalate in some environments; penetrate into others; undergo some modifications; and, as time passes by, fade away (Smyczek & Sowa 2005: 222). That is why, when defining a consumer behavior trend or new consumption (as it has just been called), it is not possible to indicate where a new one has its beginning and an old one ends.

Still, there are several new trends currently; and the most distinctive trends in consumer behavior that can be differentiated and named are the following: globalization, ethnocentrism, homogenization and heterogenization, ecologization, ethical consumption, home consumption, virtualization, and prosumption (Bywalec 2002: 137). **Globalization** of consumption is one of the factors that stimulates changes in consumption and consumer behavior and, at the same time, sets new trends for them (Smyczek 2012: 256–257). Its main characteristics are intermingling of consumption patterns observed on an international scale, spreading of these patterns, and creation of a global consumption culture, which in turn leads to the creation of global sectors that are not based on location but rather on values, attitudes, and approach to objects and brands (Smyczek 2012: 256–257). The main advantage of this phenomenon is obvious – the objects, the way of using them, the services – all become widely available and universal, regardless of region, culture, language, and so forth.

A trend that is contrary to globalization of consumption is **ethnocentrism.** Consumer ethnocentrism can be defined as a consumer's preference for domestically manufactured products or, conversely, as a bias against imported products (Shimp and Sharma 1987: 280–289). It involves transferring a feeling of ethnocentrism, that one's own population group is superior to other groups, into economic actions, such as purchasing or boycotting foreign products. In their study, Shimp and Sharma found that consumers with a higher level of consumer ethnocentrism evaluated imported products according to their perceived effect on the economy. These consumers considered purchasing imported products to be unpatriotic because it results in a loss of domestic jobs and causes harm to the domestic economy. On the other hand, consumers exhibiting low levels of ethnocentrism tended to evaluate imported products using product attributes rather than the country of origin of the product (1987: 280–289). Consumer ethnocentrism towards services can be defined as the beliefs held by consumers about the appropriateness of making use of services provided by foreign institutions. Consumers with ethnocentric tendencies believe that the use of services that are provided by foreign companies will be harmful to the domestic economy and can negatively affect their own personal well-being, e.g., in terms of unemployment. Such an opinion leads to systematic preferences for domestic services and rejection of foreign ones.

Homogenization of consumption is simply an assimilation of consumer behaviors. Its main characteristic is the shifting and blurring of differences among life phases, elderly people becoming economically emancipated, and life styles of various age and social groups becoming similar. One of the essential factors that stimulates homogenization of consumption is a longer lifespan, i.e., when particular phases of life are longer and differences among them become blurred. Nowadays, when medicine benefits from technological advances and, as a result, more and more people have access to healthcare, they are still in good health when they retire and are able to live an active life (Smyczek 2012: 260). However, the current market faces the opposite trend toward homogenization as well, i.e., a diversification of consumption or differentiation of consumer behaviors, called **heterogenization.** As discussed above, common characteristics of trends are co-existence (interconnection) and divergence (trends creating counter-trends). In the case of heterogenization, the trend is fostered by other trends, such as ethnocentrism, individualization, or virtualization (spread of the Internet) (Bywalec 2007: 139).

Another trend that can be observed in the market is a growing interest among consumers in environmental protection and, as a result, changes in their consumption choices, manifested in excluding brands of manufacturers that do not pay enough attention to the care of the environment, modification of consumption to reduce possible negative influences, or simply making rational decisions in the market that combine care for health and care for the environment (Smyczek 2012:

261–262). Since taking care of the environment is not possible without the cooperation of all the market players, such an attitude is also desirable and more frequent
among manufacturers, state bodies, and local authorities, providing more opportunities for consumers to be eco-friendly. This **ecological consumption** trend is strictly connected to what is widely called ethical consumer behavior. Although **ethical
consumption** has a very broad meaning, in general terms, it is mainly concerned
with obtaining and using goods in a way that conforms to the basic rules of modern
ethics (Smyczek 2012: 269) i.e., refusing to consume goods produced with forced
labor or goods coming from manufacturers displaying unethical behavior and so on.

Finally, with broader access to the Internet and growing possibilities for self-
service, thanks to technological advances, several consumer behavior trends are occurring in the contemporary market and inter-connect with one another. **Virtualization**, as a direct consequence of Internet access benefits, is, in general terms, satisfying consumer needs by means of electronic media. Since it is possible for consumers
to satisfy their needs by means of the Internet, there is a visible shift from public institutions to home (**home consumption**) to satisfy, for example, educational or medical
needs at any convenient time. What is more, with households becoming equipped
with more electronic devices and consumers being equipped with greater knowledge
(thanks to broader access to information and the spread of education), consumers are
able to play at least a partial role as producer and be incorporated in the process of
goods or services 'production'. It may be noted mainly in an increase of self-service in
the process of customer service and an increase in so-called do-it-yourself activities
(self-service in department stores, solving technical problems by phone, or serving as
a bank teller at the ATM machine) (Rupik 2010: 322–323).

Taking into account all of the briefly discussed general consumer behavior trends
visible in the market nowadays, it may be concluded that either they are not unified
and very often oppose one another or, conversely, they are synergetic. However, the
consumer behavior trends described above cannot be taken for granted in terms of
every type of market or every country area. The intensity of these trends may be lower
or completely different interconnections may be observed in the case of any particular
market type being analyzed. Since the function of this chapter is to discuss consumer
behavior trends in the healthcare market in particular European countries, it is advisable now to focus on the trends in consumer behavior mentioned above and apply them
to the area of healthcare, taking into consideration the specificity of this market.

4.3 Consumer behavior trends on the European healthcare
market

Health is one of the most important values in human life – a basis of a person's existence. Health is a specific good, of a utilitarian value, but not exchangeable; there
is no market where health can be purchased. In the healthcare market, the only

goods that can be acquired are services and products that can improve or maintain one's current health condition. Healthcare services, besides the attributes character-istic of all service types, have their own set of attributes that concern only health matters and care (Janoś-Kresło 2007: 31–32). Some of these specific attributes are the following: there is asymmetry of information (the patient lacks information concern-ing health, illness), the healthcare service is loaded with uncertainty, healthcare services are individualized (requiring contact with a service provider), and patients are in a passive position (subordinate to the service provider with reduced freedom of choice) (Rudawska 2009: 247).

Changes in healthcare consumer behavior are the result of a complex set of factors that act with different intensities. Some of these factors are related to macroeconomic policy set by health legislation or corporate strategies that limit or expand consumer access to certain services. On the other hand, there are a number of cultural factors – social, personal, and psychological factors – that determine the behavior of healthcare consumers. These cultural factors are connected with creating new health needs, which are the result of increasing longevity and education levels, the increasing im-portance and availability of information transfer, and changes in cultural patterns (Rudawska 2007: 20). It may be assumed, that patients' preferences have matured over recent years. They are focusing more attention on personalized medicine and play an active role in the care they receive (Meissner 2013). Patients' behavior has changed, among others, in their relations with medical entities, which can be active or passive; in the channels of medical service usage, which can be a PC, mobile electron-ics, or phone; in their contact with a medical entity, which may be direct contact, virtual contact, or mixed; and in a reduction of uncertainty in virtual environments, avoiding uncertainty and seeking information, marketing communication, and rec-ommendations) (Matysiewicz & Smyczek 2012: 122). In addition, consumer behavior is the result of various **stakeholders**, such as doctors, who recommend or prescribe consumption or use of services, and trusted advisors, like family members or opinion leaders, who by their social position influence the behavior of consumers. Public health initiatives at national and international levels also influence consumer behav-ior by means of promotion or disease prevention.

Taking into consideration European countries, especially those integrated un-der the European Union name, and widely discussed processes of globalization and integration, the underlying driving factors of consumer behavior change can be perceived in a holistic way. The attitude toward globalization changed at the begin-ning of the twenty-first century. It is no longer considered solely on the macro level of influence but also meso- and micro-levels are taken into account. It is crucial to keep in mind that globalization not only concerns economic matters but it also con-cerns the flow of the cultural values. Both globalization and integration have con-tributed to the development of the European culture of consumption, which is char-acterized by processes and phenomena common to all the European countries and developed irrespective of cultural differences. As a result, the diffusion of changes in consumer behavior patterns can be observed as well as the segments of European consumers sharing similar values, lifestyles, and behaviors (Kieżel 2010: 91–93). Vejlgaard emphasizes that 'if a new innovative style is visible in two (or more) industries at the same time, it is likely to be a trend' (2008: 27). Keeping this idea in mind, for the purposes of the following analysis, when the observed new trends in consumer behavior are identical for all of the countries being analyzed, they will be considered and described jointly; but particular attention will also be paid to any discrepancies that are occurring.

Taking into account the European countries being analyzed (Germany, Great Britain, Sweden, Belgium, and Poland) as well as the general consumer behavior trends discussed above (i.e., globalization, ethnocentrism, homogenization and heterogenization, ecologization, ethical consumption, home consumption, virtualization, and prosumption), it is possible to single out those occurring 'in all their glory' or at least partially in the healthcare market.

4.3.1 Globalization of consumption in the healthcare industry

Since globalization of consumption is one of the trends that stimulates changes in consumption and consumer behavior and, at the same time, sets new trends for them, in the healthcare market it is possible to observe several consumption patterns on a European scale that have led to the creation of a global consumption pattern. In the European countries being analyzed, the pattern is mainly manifested in a global consumer that is better informed and aware as well as consumer lifestyle changes in the area of healthcare.

The need of consumers to be better informed in the healthcare industry is a consequence of a shift from a physician-centered paradigm to a patient-centered paradigm. Under this new paradigm, patients, instead of being passive recipients of services from healthcare providers, have started to play a more active role in preventing diseases, collaborating with providers to make treatment decisions, and managing their own health and diseases (Anderson & Funnell 2005: 153–155; Lewise, Chang, & Friedman, 2005: 1–7). Patients have become able to actively seek information and, moreover, effectively process information and make decisions (Zhang 2011: 1). They feel empowered to make their own healthcare decisions, without the mediation of a medical professional. Moreover, they take an active role in obtaining medical information from so-called trusted advisors: family and friends (their personal recommendations are a trusted source for medical information), chemists/pharmacists (some consumers perceive them as medical professionals equal to doctors), blogger moms (trusted sources of information, especially concerning child-specific products), and website reviews (online shopping sites that allow consumers to rate both individual products and online retailers – not so much trusted because some manufacturers use company employees to post positive reviews) (Euromonitor 2013: 8).

The global trend of better informed healthcare consumers would not have occurred without healthcare companies, which are not idle either. Advertisements, patient brochures, toll-free numbers, and websites are used to inform and educate patients about their product offerings (discounts/coupons), medical conditions, or public health threats. Typical retailer websites selling OTC medicines, i.e., Amazon (global), Apotheke.de (Germany), and Tesco (Great Britain), allow consumers to search for products, review products, receive 'online only' sales promotions, create shopping lists with reminders, read product recall announcements, and connect with fellow consumers (Euromonitor 2010: 10).

Contemporary consumers also take advantage of broad access to health information via computers and mobile phones. They use social media in order to be 'up-to-date' with health as well as take part in online marketing campaigns and mobile apps to foster relationships with their customers. What is more, consumers like being fans – a part of a special global community with access to unique offers or media content. This is the reason companies create an online space for their consumers and, in return, are rewarded with the ability to receive quick-response surveys, collect valuable demographic information, and track purchasing patterns. Besides the most powerful and world renowned social medium, Facebook, in Europe, microsites are another popular way of providing information for consumers. These are sections of websites devoted to one topic, usually informational or retail-focused, e.g., Tesco (Great Britain) offers a Diet Club, where people receive meals, personalized fitness plans, and a diet mentor for a fee (Euromonitor 2013: 10). Another example of social media healthcare information phenomena is iWantGreatCare. Anyone with access to the Internet is able to read anonymous patients' reviews of individual doctors in Great Britain, searchable by name, location, and specialty. iWantGreatCare is a compilation and sharing of facts and opinions by patients equipped with new techniques for sharing multimedia data (Cross 2008: 203).

However, when taking into account the trustworthiness of health information, European consumers still have more belief in trusted advisors than online sources. In the Deloitte Survey of Healthcare Consumers, the Internet was not well regarded as a trustworthy source of information by most consumers in most countries. (When asked: *If you wanted information about the most effective and safe treatment(s) for a certain health condition, how much trust would you have in "third-party" sources to provide reliable information?*, consumers showed concern that Internet-based information might put privacy and security of personal health or medical information at risk: 23% in Belgium, 27% in the UK, and 50% in Germany) (Deloitte 2011: 4).

Another consumption pattern that manifests the globalization of consumption and has spread on the European level is a global lifestyle change among consumers in the area of health. Most industrial European countries are facing substantial changes in their demographics, with a growing share of aged citizens within their population. Since the level of healthcare services claimed is proportionate to the age of an individual, overall demand and expenditure for the population as a whole can be expected to rise in the years to come (Berger 2007: 7). The UN's World Population Prospects report projects that the proportion of Europeans aged 65 years and older will grow from 16% in 2000 to 24% by 2030 (The Economist 2011: 6). With birth rates slow and life expectancy continuing to rise, individuals aged 65 and older are claiming greater representation in the overall population.

However, in recent years, health has become a topic of growing significance across the European population, regardless of age. Both aging populations and the new urbanites (young consumers who have moved from rural to urban areas) have increased interest in preventative medicinal products: vitamins, dietary supplements, and herbal/traditional products are the typical beneficiaries of this trend. With hectic work schedules and demanding careers, there is a focus on being healthy and fit and reducing the chance of minor illnesses, such as flus, colds, and headaches (Euromonitor 2010: 34). Therefore, a new European healthcare market – a preventive market – has appeared, i.e., a 'secondary healthcare market' as opposed to the primary market of statutory health insurance. For example, in Germany in 2007 alone, the secondary healthcare market had already achieved an annual volume of EUR 60 billion – or 2.5% of the German GDP – and demonstrated annual growth of 6% since the year 2000 (spending on medical checkups, alternative medicine, wellness, sports, and health food) (Berger 2007: 22–23). The preventive trend is nothing more than treating yourself like a doctor, who provides a diagnosis of potential health dangers and chooses the most effective medicinal preventive products. One of the main reasons for this type of consumer behavior is the fact that self-care is simply more convenient. Many consumers in countries like Poland find waiting for a doctor's appointment to be too time consuming and, as a result, prefer to consult a pharmacist about OTC treatment options or a medical website or a mobile device offering interactive applications and self-diagnosis.

The more **preventive lifestyle** of European consumers is boosted by public health initiatives encouraging consumers to adopt healthier lifestyles, spending more on preventive health products and at the same time reducing the cost burden of the healthcare system. In Great Britain, the Department of Health manages the campaign '5 A Day' to promote healthy diets, along with the new 'Let's Get Moving' public health campaign to motivate people to increase physical activity. The most popular public health initiative in Poland is the '5 a day portions of fruit, vegetables, or juice' campaign, which aims at providing knowledge and raising the awareness of Poles about the healthy effects of eating vegetables and fruit as well as drinking juice five times a day. The research shows that in 2012, only 7% consumed the recommended five a day portions; so there is a lot to be done to raise the awareness of consumers (5 porcji warzyw, owoców lub soku 2013). The campaign is supervised by the Polish Association of Juice Producers (KUPS), the Agriculture Agency, and European Union funds.

Besides general health campaigns, many European public health campaign initiatives include scheduled campaigns addressing different issues, such as heart health, cancer prevention, flu awareness, HIV/AIDS prevention, and many others; but still the main focus is placed on two main areas: smoking and obesity. To give an example, in Poland, recent bans on smoking in public places in many countries are forcing people to rethink their smoking habits and aim to reduce the number of smokers. The growing number of preventive behaviors is also fostered by efforts other than legislative actions, namely, the use of celebrities and social networking websites (Euromonitor 2010: 20). For example, in Great Britain, the government used pictures of celebrities to introduce health campaigns in 2009 and presented the 'Change4Life' social network campaign to help reduce obesity rates (Change 4 Life 2013).

As a result, consumers have become better educated about the causes of common diseases; and most European consumers believe that preventive medicine in the form of self-medication, protection against stress, and healthy lifestyles can prevent or delay serious illness or significant health problems.

4.3.2 Ethical consumption in the healthcare industry

Ethical consumption involves mainly the consumer attitude towards money as well as what kind of purpose money should be used for. That is the reason that the growing number of consumers with economic concerns is for sure clear evidence of the development of ethical consumption.

Shrinking personal household budgets have led to greater scrutiny of healthcare expenses. While governments are launching public health initiatives, individual consumers are seeking lower cost products to reduce expenses. However, they are still aware that economic conditions remain uncertain; and they still need to stay healthy so they can work and cannot afford to be ill (Euromonitor 2010: 22). This explains why consumers make decisions to spend more wisely and only on necessary products even in the healthcare market. Considering the instability in employment and the need to remain healthy in order to work, consumers search for products that ensure their general health and stamina. Consequently, they purchase products that can treat multiple symptoms, maximizing their spending in his way. Since they have no time to be ill, they have become more confident about self-medication; and when feeling sick or injured, in order to quickly treat medical conditions, they use products that provide immediate relief (Euromonitor 2010: 30).

As consumer expenditures for frequently used products, including medicines, have come under pressure, consumers have turned to private labels to manage their shrinking wallets. While private label products have generally performed well in other fast-moving consumer goods markets, such as packaged food, this was not the case in consumer health before 2008. Since then, the European private label medicines have taken a great share from brand name products. What is more, the growth of private label medicines is expected to outpace the growth of branded products because of their higher profit margin for retailers. As for the consumer perception of private labels in Eastern European countries[2], consumers generally do not trust private label products, which historically have been considered low-quality products. However, in Western Europe[3], the perception is completely different, e.g., in Great Britain, the trust is apparent; and private labels together comprised 32% of the value of total consumer health retail sales in 2009 (Euromonitor 2010: 39).In other countries as well, such as the Netherlands and Germany, the success of generics is obvious. However, the Western European countries are not identical in this case – Belgians remain loyal to established brands and have proven reluctant to choose lesser-known products (Consumer health in Belgium 2012: 26). What is interesting for serious healthcare concerns, such as H1N1 flu, is that consumers still choose branded OTC products because of general trust in the safety and quality of the products.

4.3.3 Ecologization of consumption in the healthcare industry

As mentioned above, a trend originating directly in the idea of ethical consumption is ecologization of consumption – a trend that concerns a growing interest of consumers in environmental protection, modification of consumption choices manifested by excluding some brands or manufacturers, and simply making rational decisions in the market that combine care for health and care for the environment. In the case of the healthcare market, this trend is mainly manifested when consumers modify their purchasing choices (i.e., exclusion of chemists) and distribution channels of OTC expand into modern grocery channels, such as hypermarkets, supermarkets, and discount stores, as well as drugstore chains. In the end, this leads to self-medication by consumers. This shift is mainly a result of chains offering lower prices due to bulk purchasing, giving consumers more opportunities to purchase products at their convenience, and introducing more products to consumers, e.g., via such chain retailers as Carrefour or Tesco, which expanded their range of both branded and private label consumer health products (Euromonitor 2010: 24). To give an example, in 2009, Swedish pharmacy legislation was reformed, ending the forty-year state monopoly of Apoteket AB and allowing for a range of OTC products to be sold outside pharmacies. The purpose of the reform was to increase competition and the availability of OTC medicines as well as to reduce prices for consumers (Euromonitor 2013: 26). Grocery retailers were the first to start selling OTC; and more and more of them (mainly mass-market retailers such as Migros, Manor, and Coop)

---

2 Euromonitor Eastern Europe definition includes countries such as: Belarus, Bosnia-Herzegovina, Bulgaria, Croatia, Czech Republic, Estonia, Georgia, Hungary, Latvia, Lithuania, Macedonia, Poland, Romania, Russia, Serbia and Montenegro, Slovakia, Slovenia, Ukraine.
3 Euromonitor Western Europe definition includes countries such as: Austria, Belgium, Denmark, Finland, France, Germany, Greece, Ireland, Italy, Netherlands, Norway, Portugal, Spain, Sweden, Switzerland, Turkey, United Kingdom.

are interested in putting them on the general sale list (Euromonitor 2013: 28). There are even some European-wide drugstore chains like Schlecker AG, the fourth largest company in the world (!) in 2009, with a share of 2.3% or more locally, and the leading retailer in Great Britain, Alliance Boots, operating more than 3,200 health and beauty retail stores in 2009 (Owning health 2010: 31).

However, the trend is not identical in all the European countries being analyzed; and in some of them, consumers do not have a straightforward anti-chemist attitude. In countries such as Belgium, where OTC products can only be sold through chemists/pharmacies, people are not accustomed to purchasing medicines in chain stores; and self-medicating and self-service is forbidden in pharmacies for nonprescription medicines, based on the Code of Ethics issued by the Ordre des Pharmaciens. As a result, the vast majority of such products are still purchased at the counter in pharmacies in Belgium. Consequently, free selection by consumers is impossible, as pharmacists remain strategic intermediaries in the sale of consumer health products (Consumer health in Belgium 2012: 24).

Making rational decisions in the area of new channels of distribution is not the only symptom of ecologization of consumption that has appeared in the healthcare market. While health awareness is one of the main drivers in consumer markets, there are virtually no products that can be marketed without addressing health concerns. These concerns are also present in the food market, with all its functional foods and organic foods that have undeniable health benefits. And the trend is being boosted by government campaigns against obesity, smoking, sugar, salt, and fat consumption, as well as consumer concerns about over-ingesting chemicals or other contaminants. All of this creates marketing opportunities for herbal products or functional food with natural ingredients (Euromonitor 2010: 30). The growth trend for organic foods shows that increasing numbers of consumers are eager to buy organic foods, despite the higher prices, because consumers fear the effects of chemicals. For example, the British market for organic food is growing at twice the rate of the general grocery market; sales from direct sources rose by 16% to £108 million in 2004, and sales from supermarkets fell by 1%. This shows that customers increasingly prefer purchasing from direct sources, such as a farmers' market. These changes may also have been affected by the marketing campaigns presenting celebrities, such as Jamie Oliver, encouraging improvement of school lunches, which appears also to be affecting adult eating habits. According to a survey for PruHealth by YouGov, more than a quarter of adults think more about the meals they prepare at home as a direct result of Channel 4's Jamie's School Dinners (PruHealth with Vitality 2013).

4.3.4 Home consumption and prosumption in the healthcare industry

Since it is possible for consumers to satisfy their healthcare needs in the form of self-care by means of the Internet, the broader range of knowledge consumers possess and the possibility of free choice of purchasing options has resulted in a visible shift from public institutions to home, resulting in home consumption. Moreover, with all the support consumers are equipped with and households having more electronic devices, more and more European consumers are able to enter into the process of production and have at least a partial role of producer in the healthcare market, which has its effect in self-care mainly and reducing contacts with a GP. The trend of access to healthcare from the consumers' own home is mainly possible by means of intelligent assistive technology. (Technology as a force will be discussed later.) Home care offers general sustainability advantages, including reduced admissions; readmissions; length of stay when people are admitted; patient travel; and other clinical, social, and economic benefits (Jeffrey 2011: 1).

Home consumption in the healthcare industry is strictly connected with taking full control of one's own health and making self-care the first choice when suffering from minor ailments. For example, in Germany, according to a TNS Healthcare survey conducted in 2008, a number of GPs (82%) emphasize that self-medication plays an important role in treating mild to medium symptoms; up to 14% of the prescriptions they write are for Rx-only drugs (prescription only) in cases where an OTC alternative is available. This provides evidence that there is a significant area of possible consumer decisions on self-medicating, especially when it is fostered by encouragement from governments as in the case of the British National Pandemic Flu Service (launched in 2009). This consisted of an online and phone self-care service for people to check symptoms and access advice and treatment. Patients diagnosed with a virus were allocated a unique number, giving them access to antivirals if necessary, and told where their nearest antiviral collection point was (Owning health 2010: 24).

Both various external institution campaigns as well as greater consumer knowledge support and enable self-medication, helping at the same time to ease the burden on the National Health Service caused by the so-called 'worried well' consumers – those who frequently visit GPs for minor ailments, from back pain to colds and coughs.

4.3.5 Virtualization of consumption in the healthcare industry

The trend toward virtualization of consumption in the healthcare market somehow comprises almost all of the forces mentioned above and their tangible results in the form of consumer behavior. Online sales of medication, DIY doctors, and social media would not have existed had it not been for technological advances. In the last decade, the number of Internet users worldwide has dramatically increased. People are using the Internet for various health-related purposes; and, as a result, it has a major impact on the way consumers deal with health issues (The European eHealth Consumer Trends Survey 2007). On the one hand, there is this defined and growing eHealth market, described mainly as the use of information and communication technologies (ICT) for health, including treating patients, conducting research, educating the health workforce, tracking diseases, and monitoring public health. On the other hand, there is a wide range of casual and uncontrolled consumer actions taken on the Internet to self-diagnose, gain information on medical products and services, interact with other sufferers by means of social media, compare prices of health products and treatments, and purchase both prescription and nonprescription medicines. Still, these activities result mainly in making consumers more informed while their relationships with doctors become more equal and sometimes even less trustful (Owning health 2010: 48). The potential of using the Internet in healthcare seems promising, given the large group of people that can be reached with this source of information rapidly and at a low cost.

However, more and more frequently, information is not enough; and consumers demand an even greater dose of 'power' in self-treatment or support for regular treatment. Mobile health, also referred to as mHealth is a delivery of platforms and applications (apps) via mobile devices, giving access to medical care in a relatively inexpensive and efficient way. With the globalization of digital technology and wide Internet access, there are thousands of health and wellness applications available for upload in mobile devices. The European Union, being aware of the growing importance of mobile technology, put forth an international effort to help European governments adopt mobile technology in general (MobiWebApp project – European Union Seventh Framework Programme – FP7/2010–2012); but some of the initiatives include improved communications between governments and their citizens related to public health.

Conclusions

Observation of consumers, their actions and changes in attitudes in the European healthcare market, as well as some of the underlying macro- and microeconomic factors that affect consumer activities lead to some general conclusions concerning noteworthy trends in European consumer behavior. Contemporary European consumers, while present in the healthcare market, are full of fear as a result of an unpredictable world and witnessing extensive demographic changes. They pursue a state of inner peace. For this reason, they opt for consumption of a safer lifestyle; concern for the environment and health matters; obtaining greater amounts of specific knowledge; taking advantage of technology advances in the area of health; and, finally, taking greater responsibility for themselves.

Taking into account the general consumer behavior trends in the European healthcare market and the determinants that do not leave consumers unchanged, it is possible to draw the conclusion that the specific consumer behavior trend emerging from the foregoing discussion is the trend of Doctor Consumer.

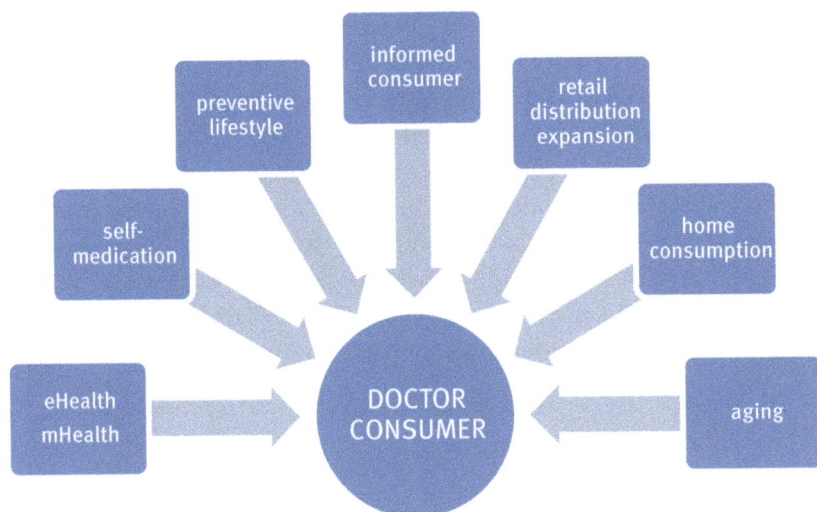

Fig. 4.1: The Doctor Consumer trend
Source: *Adapted from author's elaboration*

As presented in figure 4.1, Doctor Consumer is a specific consumer behavior trend that has emerged as a result of the observed interconnections among the general consumer behavior trends described above as well as additional external determinants that exist in all of the countries being analyzed.

Doctor Consumers are, first of all, empowered consumer/patients that have high expectations regarding their own involvement and engagement with healthcare. Doctor Consumers are increasingly interested in actively participating and managing their own health through shared decision making; becoming more educated and responsible; and, finally, being able to self-medicate. For this reason, they are interested in the opportunities that technology presents for healthcare information, management, and monitoring. Being informed is a key driver for consumers since it gives them the sense of an equal relationship with service providers (health professionals) as well as a sense of empowerment to make choices about medication, prevention, and intervention, taking into account their unique circumstances and preferences. The sense of empowerment results from some factors that 'feed' their desire for control:

- advances in communications and information technology that are constantly reducing the cost of information (eHealth, mHealth);
- availability of more information from trusted advisors and other expanded sources of information that consumers are precisely aware of (better informed consumer); and
- direct access to products in the market – no need to contact professional intermediaries (retail distribution expansion, self-care, home consumption).

When considering the changes in consumer behavior in the European countries being analyzed (Germany, Great Britain, Sweden, Belgium, and Poland), it may be concluded that all of these factors are universal factors – i.e., they influence the behavior of European consumers in a similar way – however, it is also important to remember that the consequences of these factors may be influenced by different local perspectives (different preparation levels of the economies of European countries and differences in the local healthcare industry). However, for the purposes of this thesis, the foregoing discussion leads to the general conclusion that all of these factors have resulted in significant changes in the nature of Euro-consumers, from uninformed and passive to informed and active players in the European healthcare market.

References

5 porcji warzyw, owoców lub soku, 2013. Homepage – About action. Retrieved June 23, 2013 from: http://www.5porcji.pl

Anderson, R. M. & Funnell, M. M., 2005. Patient empowerment: reflections on the challenge of fostering the adoption of a new paradigm. Patient Education and Counseling, 57 (2).

Bywalec, Cz., 2007. Konsumpcja w teorii i praktyce, Wydawnictwo Naukowe PWN, Warszawa.

Change 4 Life, 2013. Homepage – About Change 4 Life. Retrieved June 23, 2013 from: http://www.nhs.uk/change4life/Pages/change-for-life.aspx

Consumer Health Information Searching Process in Real Life Settings Yan Zhang School of Information University of Texas at Austin, 2012. *ASIST 2012*, October 28–31, Baltimore, MD, USA.

Cross, M., 2008. How the internet is changing healthcare, BMJ, Volume 337.

Dąbrowska, A., 2006. Przemiany w strukturze konsumpcji i ich uwarunkowania. In: Janoś-Kresło M., & Mróz B. (Ed.) *Konsument i konsumpcja we współczesnej gospodarce*, SGH, Warszawa.

Daszkowska, M., 1998. Usługi. Produkcja, rynek, marketing, Wydawnictwo Naukowe PWN, Warszawa.

Deloitte Center for Health Solutions, 2011. Survey of Healthcare Consumers Global Report. Key Findings, Strategic Implications. Retrieved June 23, 2013 from: https://www.deloitte.com/assets/Dcom-UnitedStates/Local%20Assets/Documents/US_CHS_2011ConsumerSurveyGlobal_062111.pdf

Euromonitor International, 2011. Health On The Go: A Review of Mobile Applications. Retrieved June 23, 2013 from: http://blog.euromonitor.com/2011/10/health-on-the-go-a-review-of-mobile-applications.html

Euromonitor International. Strategy Briefing November 2005. Forty Key Trends for the Next Decade: 20 Key Global Trends and 20 Key Consumer Trends 2005–2015. Retrieved June 23, 2013 from: http://www.researchandmarkets.com/reports/313019/forty_key_trends_for_the_next_decade_20_key

Euromonitor International: Strategy Briefing, 2010. Owning Health: The Move Towards Self-care and Implications for Marketers. Retrieved June 23, 2013 from: http://www.euromonitor.com/owning-health-the-move-towards-self-care-and-implications-for-marketers/report

Euromonitor, 2010. The Power of the Consumer: How the Consumer Health Industry Can Succeed with the Next Generation of Consumers. Retrieved June 23, 2013 from: http://www.euromonitor.com/the-power-of-the-consumer-how-the-consumer-health-industry-can-succeed-with-the-next-generation-of-consumers/report

Euromonitor, 2013. Consumer health trends, developments and prospects. Retrieved June 23, 2013 from: http://www.euromonitor.com/consumer-health-trends-developments-and-prospects-2013/report

Evans, R. G., 1984. Strained Mercy: The Economics of Canadian Healthcare, Buttersworth, Toronto.

Flejterski S., (Ed.), 2005. Współczesna ekonomika usług, Wydawnictwo Naukowe PWN, Warszawa.

Hollensen, S., 2010. Global marketing: a decision oriented approach. Harlow: Pearson Eduacation.

Janoś-Kresło, M., 2007. Zachowania konsumentów na rynku usług opieki zdrowotnej w wybranych krajach Europy Środkowo-Wschodniej (w świetle wyników badań empirycznych), Studia i Prace Kolegium Zarządzania i Finansów. Zeszyt Naukowy 85, SGH Warszawa.

Jeffrey S., Mustafa, A. & Ying S., 2011. Consumer managed home healthcare for the next decade, The 11th International Conference on Electronic Business, Bangkok, Thailand.

Kieżel, E. and Mazurek-Łopacińska K., 2001. Polscy konsumenci w drodze do UE. In: Kędzior Z., Karcz K. (Ed.) Zachowania podmiotów rynkowych w Polsce a proces integracji europejskiej, Akademia Ekonomiczna, Katowice.

Kieżel, E. and Zorska A., 1998. Ku globalizacji. Przemiany w korporacjach transnarodowych i w gospodarce światowej, Wydawnictwo Naukowe PWN, Warszawa.

Kieżel, E., 2010. Konsument i jego zachowania na rynku europejskim, PWE Warszawa.

Lewise, D., Chang, B.L. & Friedman, C.P., 2005. Consumer health informatics. In: Lewise, D. (Ed.) Consumer Health Informatics: Informing Consumers and Improving Healthcare: 1–7, Springer.

Lober, W.B. & Flowers, J.L., 2011. Consumer Empowerment in healthcare amid the Internet and social media, Seminars in Oncology Nursing, Vol 27, No 3 (August).

Matysiewicz, J. & Smyczek, S., 2012. Modele relacji jednostek medycznych z pacjentami w otoczeniu wirtualnym, Placet, Warszawa.

Medical Device and Diagnostic Industry, 2013. Meissner, A. The Global healthcare Industry in the year 2020, Retrieved June 23, 2013 from: http://www.mddionline.com/article/global-healthcare-industry-year-2020

PruHealth with Vitality, 2013. Homepage – Advisers. Retrieved June 23, 2013 from: http://www.pruhealth.co.uk

Raumond, M., 2010. Trend Forecasters Toolbook. Laurence King Publishing.

Roland Berger Strategy Consultants, 2007. Trends in European healthcare How to create value in a dynamic environment. Retrieved June 23, 2013 from: http://www.rolandberger.com/media/pdf/rb_press/RB_Trends_in_European_healthcare_20070901.pdf

Rudawska, I. & Soboń M., 2009. Przedsiębiorstwo i klient w gospodarce opartej na usługach, Difin, Warszawa.

Rudawska, I., 2007. Opieka zdrowotna, aspekty rynkowe i marketingowe, Wydawnictwo Naukowe PWN, Warszawa.

Rupik, K., 2008. Prosument w procesie planowania marketingowego, W: Zeszyty Naukowe Uniwersytetu Szczecińskiego. Relacyjne aspekty zachowań konsumenckich. Wydawnictwo Naukowe Uniwersytetu Szczecińskiego, Szczecin.

Shimp, T & Sharma, S., 1987. Consumers ethnocentrism – Construction and Validation of the CETSCALE. Journal of Marketing Research, Vol. 8.

Smyczek, S. & Sowa, E., 2005. Konsument na rynku. Zachowania, modele, aplikacje. Difin.

Smyczek, S., 2012. Consumer behaviour on international market. Placet.

The Economist Intelligence Unit Limited, 2011. The future of healthcare in Europe A report from the Economist Intelligence Unit. Retrieved June 23, 2013 from: http://www.janssen-emea.com/sites/default/files/The%20Future%20Of%20Healthcare%20in%20Europe.pdf

The Polish Association of Juice Producers (KUPS) 2013. Homepage – About KUPS. Retrieved June 23 from: http://www.kups.org.pl/konsumenci

Tkaczyk, J., 2012. Trendy konsumenckie i ich implikacje marketingowe: Handel wewnętrzny, Konsumpcja i konsument – nowe trendy.

Vejlgaard, H., 2008. Anatomy of A Trend. McGraw- Hill Books.

WHO European survey on E-health Consumer Trends, 2008. Project report eHealth Trends across Europe 2005–2007, Andreassen, H. K., Sørensen, T., Kummervold, P. Retrieved June 23, 2013 from: http://www.jmir.org/2008/4/e42/

Wróbel, A., 2009. Międzynarodowa wymiana usług, Wydawnictwo Naukowe SCHOLAR, Warszawa.

Zorska, A., 2003. Globalizacja a konwergencja. Szanse a zagrożenia w procesie doganiania. In: Zdanowski, J. (Ed.) *Globalizacja a tożsamość*, Wydawnictwo Naukowe ASKON, Warszawa.

Sławomir Smyczek

5 Relationship Marketing Performance of Medical Facilities

Abstract Relationships between medical facilities and patients present a very dynamic, yet not entirely recognized category. As a result, the literature lacks a complex and clear way of showing this phenomenon, which could allow assessment of activities related to relationship marketing. Contemporary research into the relationships between market subjects is certain to contribute to better knowledge about these relationships and better understanding of particular aspects of the relationships, including factors that affect whether subjects enter into relationships or affect the length and strength of relationships between medical facilities and patients. This chapter evaluates the effectiveness of relationship marketing, describes the dimensions and strength of relationships between medical facilities and patients, and presents a model showing the performance of medical facilities acting in the European market in the area of the relationships between medical facilities and patients.

Keywords: relationship marketing, dimensions of relationship, strength of relationship, model of relationship, healthcare market

5.1 Introduction

The following chapter describes the nature and stages of the development of relationship marketing in the healthcare services sector, especially processes of formation, management, result assessment, and evolution. Our empirical study focuses on the dimensions and strength of relationships between medical facilities and patients and presents a model that shows the performance of medical facilities acting in the European market in the area of long-lasting relationships with their patients. The chapter presents the results of surveys of different types of medical facilitates. The field research was conducted in 2013 in five European countries that represent different models of the healthcare system.

5.2 The nature and stages of relationship marketing in the healthcare services

The issue of **relationship marketing** in the context of the services sector was first raised by L.L. Berry, who stressed the importance of development of customer relationships as a process, and who underlined the need of extending the value of this relationship (cross-selling) in service companies of a diverse assortment (Berry and

Parasuraman, 1991). C. Gronroos (1994: 9–29), in turn, has approached customer relationships in a more detailed way, preserving its more universal character, and has claimed that this paradigm of marketing has a wider application in the market of services, including professional ones such as medical services. The concept of marketing comprises the following elements:

(1) real partnership between related entities, partnership not only confined to its formal and legal aspects;

(2) the partnership comprises not only "external" participants of the relationship, but also internal ones, within the company;

(3) marketing consists of positive assessments, in the longer term, of feelings (satisfaction) experienced by a trading partner that exceed the values offered by rival companies;

(4) this process occurs through relationship portfolios, where values and feelings are co-created and exchanged by partners;

(5) successful development of these relations is possible thanks to mutual trust and fulfillment of the promises made by partners, as well as thanks to dynamic marketing; and

(6) a network of partners, and the bonds existing between them, form an organization without distinct borders (Zabinski, 2000: 26).

It is worth adding that C. Gronroos (1994: 9–29) puts great emphasis on trust between partners in the concept of marketing relationships in service companies. M. Rydel and C. Ronkowski, in turn, point to the partnership as the target of the market relationships of a service company. Partner relationships comprise not only the consumer but also other market players that remain in some relationship with a service company (Egan, 2008).

Relationship marketing should be approached both in a static and dynamic way. The dynamic approach reflects the commonly accepted thesis that the relationship between customer loyalty and company profitability is noticeable in the long run. Development of a relationship with customers is influenced by effective activities undertaken by a service company with respect to its own employees. It is also necessary to take into consideration the fact that inclusion of individualized offer into relationship marketing requires some preliminary analyses of customer relationships in terms of their profitability value for the company (Zabinski, 2001: 45–57).

Employment of the relationship marketing concept in healthcare companies is completed through four stages or sub-processes (Sheth and Parvatiyar, 2000: 15–26):

(a) formation,

(b) management,

(c) result assessment, and

(d) evolution.

Formation comprises decisions regarding the following areas: definition of activity goals, activity partners, and activity programs (schemes). The stage of management is an indispensable continuation of implementation of a marketing relationship. In the healthcare services market, the asymmetry between partners is most vividly demonstrated and clearly present; yet relationships can be developed despite a passive attitude on the part of consumers (Arnould et al., 2004). During the management stage, the following sub-processes take place: role definition, communication, bond development, mutual planning, assurances of operational consistency, motivating, staff training, and monitoring. The stage of result assessment is of key importance as it allows corrections with respect to defined goals, programs, and management of the relationship marketing process. Evaluation of effectiveness of undertaken activities cannot be rendered exclusively by means of traditional measures such as participation in the market or volume of sales because, due to their one-sidedness, they do not take into account the specific goals of a marketing relationship. Evaluation of relationship marketing effectiveness should, above all, comprise dimensions of the relationship, determination of the strength of the current relationship between the consumer and the company and, in addition, a definition of the conditions of the company's engagement in definite market relationships. The stage of evolution usually begins when definite relationships with customers already exist or a relationship marketing program has been in operation for a longer time. The process of evolution can be planned only patially as it develops under the influence of factors that are independent of the program designer (Glowik and Smyczek, 2011). Great satisfaction with the relationship experienced both by the customer and the company often leads to transformation of this relationship.

5.3 Quality evaluation of relationships between medical facilities and patients in the European healthcare services market

Relationships between medical facilities and patients present a very dynamic, yet, not entirely recognized topic. For this reason, the subject literature lacks a model that could in a complex and clear way show this phenomenon and that could allow assessment of activities related to relationship marketing. Contemporary research into relationships between market subjects is certain to contribute to better knowledge about these relationships and a better understanding of particular aspects of the relationships, including factors that influence entering into them or that influence the length and strength of relationships (Mitrega, 2005: 24). With respect to evaluating the effectiveness of relationship marketing, it is advisable to identify the dimensions and strength of relationships between patients and medical facilities in the healthcare services market, and next, to try to build a model of long-lasting relationships with patients.

In order to reach this goal, research was carried out on samples of managers of healthcare facilities from five European countries. The study of the German, British, Swedish, Belgium, and Polish markets was conducted by means of a survey questionnaire of a group of 250 healthcare facilities in each country. The procedure of quota selection was employed to select a sample of medical facilities. Quota used in the study included the size of a medical facility measured by the number of employees and range of its activity. After completion of the study, data were checked, systematized, counted, described, and analyzed with respect to their quality and quantity. The study was carried out in 2013. The average questionnaire response rate equaled 71%; but after verification of the material, 58.6% questionnaires were approved for further analysis. The choice of the countries was deliberate and based on the different models of healthcare system organization represented by the selected countries.

The process of development of a relationship model between medical facilities and patients consisted of an analysis of the associations among the particular elements that build these relationships. Correlation coefficients, mainly Kramer and Pearson's (Churchill and Iacobucci, 2009, Burns and Bush, 2006), were used to analyze the associations among the elements; whereas a Chi square test (Wilson, 2006) was applied to check the independence of the variables. In addition, an exploratory factor analysis (Malhotra, et al., 2008; Zaborski, 2001) was conducted with the use of principal components analysis. It is noteworthy that cross tabulations (Kedzior and Karcz, 2001) were used as a method of statistical analysis since the application of the other methods was limited because of the type of scale used in the questionnaires.

The process-based approach to research into the relationship between patients and medical facilities calls for identification of the dimensions and determination of the strength of these relationships. According to the research assumptions, these relationships are determined and, simultaneously, characterized by four main elements:

- engagement of a healthcare facility with patients (Blythe, 2009),
- engagement of a patient with a medical facility (Karcz and Kedzior, 2001),
- satisfaction of a healthcare services market subject with the relationship (Schiffman and Kanuk, 2010), and
- trust developed by a healthcare services market subject as a result of this relationship (Solomon et al., 2010).

In order to determine the significance of specific **dimensions of relationships** for healthcare services and to identify the **strength of the relationship** with a patient, average assessment of the variables was calculated in the countries representing the various models of healthcare service organizations.

Tab. 5.1: Dimensions and strength of healthcare facility-patient relationships in Europe

Relationship dimension and strength	Activity undertaken by medical facility	Activity undertaken by patient	Satisfaction	Trust	Strength of relationship
	Scale 1–7				Scale 0–1
Germany	4.302	4.443	4.660	4.534	0.410
Great Britain	3.461	3.680	3.870	4.028	0.348
Sweden	5.157	5.236	5.342	5.154	0.507
Belgium	3.628	4.018	4.217	4.436	0.408
Poland	4.027	4.351	4.587	4.544	0.394

It is worth adding that the strength of the relationship between the medical facility and the patient is quite insignificant; and in most of the countries being studied, it is below 0.5 on a 0 to 1 scale. Sweden is the only country where the relationship between the patient and the medical facility is stronger and equals 0.507.

In order to statistically verify the relationships described above, the Spearman's correlation coefficients were calculated with respect to the strength of the relationships and their determinants. The coefficients were tested to determine statistical significance. The results obtained from the calculations are presented in table 5.2.

Tab. 5.2: Spearman correlation coefficients with respect to the strength of the medical facility-patient relationship across Europe

Spearman r	Activity undertaken by medical facility	Activity undertaken by patient	Satisfaction	Trust
Germany	0.365 (0.001)	0.597 (0.000)	0.538 (0.000)	0.372 (0.007)
Greta Britain	0.349 (0.003)	0.416 (0.000)	0.631 (0.004)	0.274 (0.005)
Sweden	0.350 (0.000)	0.504 (0.000)	0.590 (0.000)	0.510 (0.000)
Belgium	0.332 (0.000)	0.307 (0.000)	0.634 (0.000)	0.418 (0.000)
Poland	0.384 (0.000)	0.468 (0.000)	0.698 (0.000)	0.413 (0.000)

The coefficient values reveal a moderate influence for all dimensions, except satisfaction, on the strength of patient and medical facility relationships in Europe. Satisfaction, in turn, constitutes the dimension that strongly affects these relationships in all countries under study. In the group of moderate dimensions, the most influential one with respect to the patient-medical facility relationship is patients' activity and trust placed in a patient. The least influential dimension in this group concerns the activity of the medical facility. Significance levels approaching zero, in the test of the significance of the correlation coefficient in all dimensions, makes it possible to conclude, with high certainty, that all four dimensions have considerable influence over the strength of the relationship with patients.

5.4 Model of the long-term relationship between the medical facility and patients in the European healthcare market

During the process of developing the **model of the medical facility-patient relationship** in the European healthcare services market, it is vital to consider and analyze particularly the determinants that influence the involvement of the medical facilities in the mutual relationship. A great variety of factors taken into account in current relationship models of market subjects, e.g., the EBK (Schiffman and Kanuk, 2010) or Nicosia model (Schiffman and Kanuk, 2010), do not facilitate the analysis and complicate explanation of the mechanisms of relationship development. Hence, there is a need for a relatively simple, measurable, and pragmatic approach to the determinants of medical facility-patient relationships in the European healthcare services market. At this point, some dilemmas arise, namely, what would be a useful (very simple) approach from a practical point of view is not always acceptable from a scientific perspective. On the other hand, too complex a group of determinants, despite methodological correctness, may become pragmatically useless.

In the literature on the subject, many attempts have been made to tackle the problem, mainly by focusing on individual aspects of consumer-company relationships and not taking into account the principle of *ceteris paribus* for variables and interactions (Poiesz and Robben, 1994). Another approach, in turn, recommends finding a criterion followed by market subjects, with a simultaneous rejection of other variables (Stewart, 1989). Such an approach, however, is contrary to the concept of external legitimacy (the influence of the whole environment on the market participants) and the need for a full explanation of the ways and reasons for the interactions between particular market subjects and for the maintenance of those interactions.

Bearing this discussion in mind, a relationship model of health services market subjects can be developed in the virtual environment with the use of the three-factor consumer behavior model, 3F (Smyczek, 2007). Although the model has been designed solely to explain the market behavior of consumers, the universal character of its construction allows it to be applied to medical facilities. The model leaves behind the commonly used practice of the so-called summary of variables, i.e., including variables that are presented only on a general and abstract level. Often identification and explanation of relationships between subjects in various markets leads to limitation (both theoretical and operational) of the number of determinants, which constitute only summary variables in place of a much larger number of more detailed variables.

Nonetheless, by employing a contrary approach (as in the 3F model), i.e., by identifying (determining influence on the relationship of the market subjects) a narrower group of selected general factors, it is possible to learn about their influence and that of other more detailed factors that determine these relationships in practice. Consequently, through more understandable analysis, one can reach a methodologically correct as well as simple and pragmatic level (Antonides and van Raaij, 2003).

Such an approach has already been presented in the literature to describe and explain some selected aspects of customer-company relationships. Consequently, the ELM model (probability of information processing) developed by R.E. Petty and J.T. Cacioppo (1983) utilizes two main factors: motivation and abilities. These determinants affect the whole process of information processing by market subjects. D.J. MacInnes, C. Moorman and B.J. Jaworski (Lambkin et al., 2001), in turn, built a model of three determinants responsible for shaping the attitudes of market subjects and have distinguished motivation, opportunity, and ability (MOA model). The model was further developed into a model of advertising message processing by T.B.C. Poiesz (Lambkin et al., 2001).

All the models have concentrated mainly on explaining the process of information processing by market subjects during the period that they entered into market relationships with another subject. Nonetheless, the models could be more broadly employed, i.e., in a full explanation of the complicated phenomenon of relationships between patients and medical facilities. In order to understand how the relationship model based on motivation, abilities, and opportunities (three-factor relation model of market subjects) can be used to explain the relationship between patients and medical facilities, the following assumptions must be considered.

- Before making 'a decision' about involvement in market relationships, the subjects must define their **motivations** and assess their **abilities** as well as external **opportunities**; it is assumed that the assessment requires minimum intellectual and time engagement on the part of the subject (Hawkins, 2004).
- There are three essential conditions that must be met in order for a relationship to appear between the subjects: motivation to become engaged in a definite relationship, the (perceived) abilities necessary to become engaged, e.g., knowledge, market experience; and (perceived) opportunities favorable for the engagement. Motivation with respect to the patient is connected with, e.g., a need to be healthy or with external stimuli, such as promotional activities or informal information. Motivation with respect to a medical facility relates to, e.g., generating bigger profits. Abilities, in turn, are connected with, e.g., a patient's intellectual predispositions as well as prior knowledge and experience. Abilities of medical facilities correspond to their financial resources or available personnel. Abilities also include elements that are outside the particular market participants; for example, for the patient these include streamlined procedures of medical service delivery, which facilitates involvement in the relationship, and for medical units, an adequate level of patient knowledge. Opportunities are mainly related to the environment (favorable or not) in which the relationships are to develop (market offer, market infrastructure, disturbances, etc.). It is worth emphasizing the fact that the 3F model is based on the assumption that

the determinants are prerequisites for the development of certain market relationships. These conditions are not essential since, for example, lack of one
component can be fully compensated for by an excess of another (Bywalec,
2007).

- In the 3F model, it is assumed that all the factors that affect relationships between market subjects can be reduced to three determinants. This level of generality makes more detailed analysis of various determinants pointless. Consequently, instead of identifying, for example, patients' subjective evaluations of
the credibility and attractiveness of information sources or information quality,
it is sufficient to define a subjective level of patients' motivations. Likewise, instead of asking a representative of a medical facility about the influence of e-
tool knowledge and experience with e-tools on his or her employment in the facility, it is appropriate to ask respondents for an estimation of their ability to get
involved in the use of such instruments. Finally, in the model, opportunities are
not distributed over a great number of possible determinants (time, location, offer); but respondents are asked to point to opportunities that are sufficient for
involvement in definite market relationships. Hence, from the utilitarian (operational) point of view, analysis of these determinants allows for information
about subjective motivation assessments as well as about the level of abilities
and opportunities perceived by patients and medical facility representatives. At
the same time, from a methodological point of view, it is assumed that the observed level (range) of abilities and opportunities does not differ from actual
(objective) abilities and opportunities (Kiezel, 2010).
- It is also assumed that the three main determinants may affect each other, e.g.,
if the level of opportunities perceived by the patient is very low, then high motivation for engagement in a relationship with a given medical facility is also unlikely to be present. If a medical facility, in turn, is insufficiently motivated to
offer definite services for a given segment of patients, then neither a high level
of opportunities perceived by the personnel nor market opportunities are able to
encourage the subject to become involved in the relationship (Schiffman et al.,
2008),
- The combination of determinants, motivation, opportunities and abilities, can
be examined at a high level of generality (whatever the service, brand, etc.) or in
a more detailed manner (depending on the service brand, etc.). If a given medical facility takes into account various determinants, it becomes involved in a relationship in the market (taking into consideration the most suitable variables
included in the 3F model) (Blackwell et al., 2001),
- If there is a need for a more detailed analysis of the determinants that bring
about a relationship between medical facilities and patients then it is possible
to differentiate each variable (Doole et al., 2005).

It should be added that in the 3F model being discussed, each determinant plays a significant role in stimulating and shaping market subject relationships. If any of the factors is not favorable or their combination is rather unattractive for the patients or the medical facility, then (according to the 3F model assumptions) there is a great likelihood that the engagement will not occur, even in a limited scope. The 3F model also focuses on the negative effects of interactions among determinants, such as negative associations with a given medical facility (motivation), misunderstanding of a message conveyed by a medical facility representative (abilities), and wrong choice of a patient segment (opportunities). It is worthy of note that each of the factors is composed of many variables that create 'a bunch', which motivates the subject to become engaged in a relationship. The bunch shows the subject's abilities and creates the conditions for involvement in the relationship.

The attempt to develop a three-factor model of the relationship between patients and medical facilities in the European healthcare services market consisted of a study carried out among representatives of medical facilities. The representatives were asked about their motivation to become involved in relationships with patients, the skills indispensable in order for the relationship to become long lasting, and their assessment of opportunities for creating long-term market relationships with patients.

In order to identify the factors that describe relationships between medical facilities and patients in the European healthcare services market and that, simultaneously, form the basis for the model development, exploratory factor analysis was conducted. The research allowed identification of seventeen variables that may affect these relationships. They were given to representatives of medical facilities, using a Likert scale to determine the level of acceptance of each statement. The list of seventeen statements, one for each of the variables identified follows.

1. Continuous provision of healthcare services through various channels (24/7availability) contributes to the development of long-term relationships with patients.
2. Considerable reduction in service costs at a medical facility is necessary for development of long-lasting relationships with patients.
3. Proper knowledge about relationship-building tools is vital in creating long-term relationships with patients.
4. Investment in long-term relationships with patients is very risky.
5. Rapid development of long-term relationships with patients acts as a protective measure, as rivals also develop such relationships.
6. Higher profits from the relationship and reduced costs of communication with patients may encourage development of long-term relationships with patients.
7. Patients' proper knowledge about healthcare service influences development of long-term relationships with patients.
8. Broad and accessible information about relationship-building tools would encourage their implementation in my medical facility.

9. Introduction of relationship-building tools may help streamline patient service and, consequently, eliminate queues at medical facilities.
10. Trust placed in a patient is necessary for a long-term relationship with the patient.
11. Having knowledgeable personnel in a medical facility is vital for development of a long-term relationship with a patient.
12. Introduction of patient relationship-building tools requires great engagement on the part of a patient.
13. Proper recommendations from representatives of other medical facilities/doctors would persuade me to implement a system of long-term development of relationships with patients.
14. Willingness to broaden what is being offered in the market would make me introduce long-term relationship-building tools,
15. Only a legal obligation would convince me to introduce a system of long-term development of relationships with patients.
16. Willingness to gain new patients would make me implement a system of relationship development with patients.
17. Sound experience in building relationships with patients is necessary for development of these relationships.

After the analysis, the KMO index (McGivern, 2009) for the seventeen variables equaled 0.764. Next, using the MSA_h index, the sample selection adequacy of each individual variable was calculated. Sample adequacy measures showed that the following variables had an MSA_h index too low to be included in the remaining analysis: (1), (4), (6), (9), (13), (14), (16), and (17). The MSA_h index for these variables was below 0.5 and, therefore, they were not included in further analysis. The remaining analysis, therefore, includes nine variables with high KMO coefficients of 0.877. These nine variables are the following: (2), (3), (5), (7), (8), (10), (11), (12), and (15).

Calculation of the eigen value and the percentage of variance explaining subsequent components allowed determination of the final number of factors to be taken into consideration in the remaining analysis. The criterion of the eigen value above single digits demonstrated that the further analysis should retain three factors which explain 62.84% of communality for all variables. Employment of the principal component method with quartimax rotation made it possible to determine the factor loadings for the variables. In table 5.3 significant factor loadings have been marked in bold type, which, after rounding off, are not lower than the absolute value of 0.5.

Tab. 5.3: Factor loadings (obtained by means of the principal component method after quartimax rotation) in the model of relationships between medical facilities and patients

Variable	Component (factor)		
	1	2	3
2.	0.083	**0.731**	− 0.262
3.	**0.561**	0.059	0.179
5.	0.148	0.075	**0.676**
7.	− 0.179	**0.811**	0.041
8.	0.067	− 0.269	**0.755**
10.	− 0.252	**0.577**	0.174
11.	**0.794**	0.281	− 0.016
12.	0.212	**0.597**	0.230
15.	0.259	− 0.053	**0.725**

Thus, three factors describing the tendency of medical facilities for involvement in long-lasting relationships with patients in the European healthcare services market have been obtained.

(1) The first factor is characterized by variables according to which engagement in long-term relationships in the healthcare services market is conditioned by (3) adequate knowledge about relationship-building tools and (11) having knowledgeable personnel in a medical facility. This factor has been referred to as the abilities of medical facilities.

(2) The second factor consists of variables according to which engagement in relationships with patients is encouraged by (2) considerable reduction of service costs at a medical facility, (7) patients' adequate knowledge about healthcare services, (10) great trust placed in a given patient, and (12) considerable engagement on the part of a patient. This factor has been referred to as market opportunities.

(3) The third factor characterizes variables that induce a medical facility to become involved in building relationships with a patient (5) protection against competitors, (8) broad and accessible information about the tools of building relationships with patients, and (15) legal obligation. This factor has been called motivation of a medical facility.

With reference to the findings presented above, a conclusion can be drawn that building long-lasting relationships between medical facilities and patients in the European healthcare services market is based on three factors: the ability of a medical facility to become involved in these relationships, opportunities created by these relationships in the market, and the motivations of medical facilities to get engaged in these relationships.

In the exploratory factor analysis, indexes were assigned to hidden constructs (factors) on factual grounds. In further proceedings, the model based on these constructs was subject to analysis by means of confirmatory factors analysis, CFA, which helped to check the fit of the model to the data (Sztemberg, 2000: 92). Moreover, unlike the exploratory factor analysis, which accepts the correlations of each factor with all indexes, in this model, definite indexes are attributed to a concrete construct. In other words, non-zero regression coefficients between a given construct and its test-assigned indexes are permitted. Thus, CFA tests the quality of a measuring model.

The analysis permitted the existence of correlations between factors because it can be assumed that particular medical facilities engage in relationships with patients when they are motivated to act and have the appropriate abilities to become involved in these relationships. The last indispensable factor that influences the development of a patient-medical facility relationship is a broad availability of relationship-building tools.

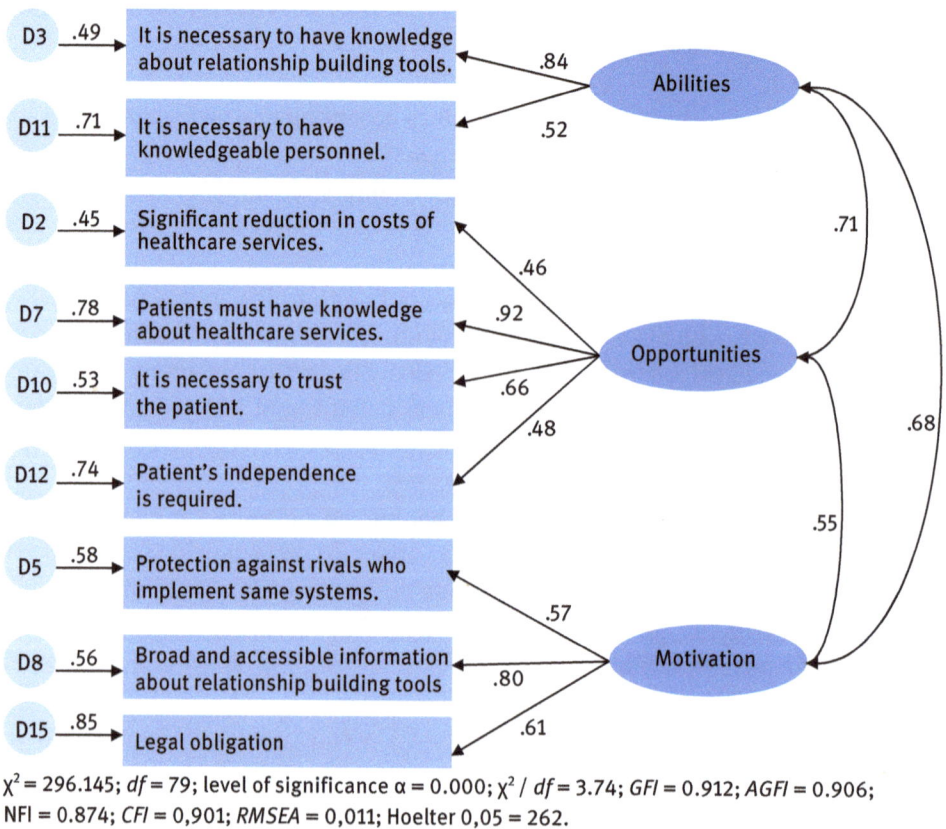

$\chi^2 = 296.145$; $df = 79$; level of significance $\alpha = 0.000$; $\chi^2 / df = 3.74$; $GFI = 0.912$; $AGFI = 0.906$; $NFI = 0.874$; $CFI = 0,901$; $RMSEA = 0,011$; Hoelter $0,05 = 262$.

Fig. 5.1: Structure of dependence in the factor analysis of relationships between medical facilities and patients in the European market of healthcare services (standardized coefficients)

Figure 5.1 shows a path diagram of confirmatory factor analysis in a three-factor model of relationships between medical facilities and patients. The diagrams display standardized regression coefficients between hidden constructs and observable indexes, i.e., factor loadings. They have been placed along one-direction arrows, leading from factors, presented in the ellipses, to indexes, presented in the rectangles. The diagram also shows the coefficient values of correlations between the factors. These values have been located along two-direction arches connecting the factors.

In order to ensure the identification of the model, the variance of the hidden variables (Browne and Mels, 1996) was established at level 1, i.e., these are standardized variables. This solution is currently preferred over establishing the value of one of the factor loadings of each construct at level 1. Both methods have the same standardized value of factors and fit measures. Standardized values were estimated by means of the maximum likelihood method based on the AMOS program. The variables were regarded as interval ones, which usually yields good results with five-point scales (Gorniak, 2000: 133).

The confirmatory factor analysis yielded index values that constitute measures of model fit to the data. Consequently, the χ^2 value with the degrees of freedom summarizing the divergence between the observed covariance matrix and the model-implied matrix is a traditional measure that allows the testing of the hypothesis that there is no divergence between these matrices in the population. The χ2 test leads to rejection of the hypothesis. Nonetheless, its utility, especially in the case of models with more variables, is limited, as it too easily results in the rejection of true models (Hoyle, 1995, Mueller, 1996). Additionally, the popular measure of model fit, χ^2/df, was calculated and the obtained index value equaled 3.7, which is much lower than the upper limit for well-fitted models established at level 5. RMSEA Steiger-Lind is another fit measure gaining positive assessments among experts (Bollen and Long, 1993: 136–162). This measure shows how badly a model is fitted, including the number of parameters that require estimation. Therefore, the more closely its value approaches 0, the better. With respect to the model being analyzed, its value equals 0.011 and lies below the preferred upper limit for well-fitted models, which is 0.05 and well below the limit of 0.1 for well-fitted models. Other measures used to determine the extent of the model fit were the goodness of fit index GFI and the modified adjusted goodness index AGFI by K.G. Joreskog and D. Sorbom. Values of the measures fall within the range of acceptance (> 0.9), although a result of > 0.95 would be more satisfactory. Another measure used for assessment of the model fit was the normed fit index (NFI), which measures a relative decrease in a fit function value caused by a transition from the zero model to the more complex one. This index results in values from 0 to 1 and equals 0.874 for the model being analyzed. This is a satisfactory result because with a good fit, the index approaches 1. It should be emphasized, however, that this index depends on the sample size; therefore, P.M. Bentler came up with another fit index, the so-called normed comparative fit index, CFI (Bentler, 1990: 238). The index for the model being analyzed equals

0.901, which is also satisfactory. Finally, the Hoelter test was applied in order to see whether the model being analyzed would be rejected or not at the conventional level of 0.05 with a sample size of 235 or less. A sample size of 200 is the lower acceptable limit in the case of this measure.

Table 5.4, presents nonstandard regression coefficients and covariance values between factors obtained as a result of evaluation of the model using the maximum likelihood method calculated with the AMOS program. Interpretation of coefficient values is convenient thanks to standardizing the factor variance at 1, whereby covariance between the factors is equal to the correlation coefficients in the figure 5.1. Table 5.4 contains the values of critical quotients for the factors (the relationship of a parameter to its standard error). Thanks to the quotient, it is possible to quickly verify the statistical significance of the indexes by comparison to the common criterion 1.96 (for p = 0.05). In the case of the model being analyzed, all factors are statistically significant.

Tab. 5.4: Confirmatory factor analysis of constructs defining the relationship of medical facilities with patients (nonstandard and critical quotients)

Relationship		Evaluation	Statistical error	Critical quotient	P
P1_3	← abilities	0.753	0.020	34.278	0.000
P1_11	← abilities	1.364	0.037	32.134	0.000
P1_2	← opportunities	1.349	0.028	29.173	0.000
P1_7	← opportunities	1.237	0.043	22.573	0.000
P1_10	← opportunities	0.958	0.019	45.411	0.000
P1_12	← opportunities	2.045	0.026	33.429	0.000
P1_5	← motivation	0.829	0.034	40.728	0.000
P1_8	← motivation	1.216	0.022	39.154	0.000
P1_15	← motivation	1.592	0.029	49.138	0.000
Opportunities	↔ motivation	0.176	0.041	4.610	0.000
Abilities	↔ motivation	0.182	0.027	5.142	0.000
Abilities	↔ opportunities	0.159	0.036	3.554	0.000

On the basis of the findings presented, it can be concluded that the exploratory factor analysis demonstrates that the analyzed relationships of medical facilities in the European healthcare services market is correct. In light of the measures that were presented, except for the χ^2 test, the model is acceptable, although not well-fitted. All the indexes (distinguished through exploratory factor analysis) are significantly related to the constructs.

Conclusions

Bearing in mind the analysis discussed above, it can be stated that relationship marketing activities undertaken by medical facilities in Europe are based on four relationship dimensions: involvement of a medical facility in contacts with patients, a patient's engagement with medical facilities, satisfction gained by a healthcare services market subject from the relationship, and trust of a healthcare services market subject resulting from the relationship.

The research has shown that satisfaction from cooperation with a given patient has the most powerful influence on this relationship. The second most influential factor is the trust placed in a patient by his/her engagement, whereas involvement of a medical facility has the smallest effect on the relationship. It is worth adding that the influence of all the dimensions on the strength of the relationship between medical facilities in Europe and their patients can be described as moderate.

The research results have revealed that relationships between medical facilities and patients are likely to be long-term provided that, with favorable market opportunities, patients are properly motivated and are able to become involved in these relationships. It is worth emphasizing the fact that development of these relationships is considerably dependent on market opportunities, which either foster or prevent their development.

References

Antonides G. & van Raaij, W. F., 2003. *Consumer behavior. European perspective*. New York: John Wiley & Sons, Ltd.

Arnould, E., Price, L., Zinkhan, G., 2004. *Consumers*. Boston: Irwin, McGraw-Hill.

Bentler, P.M. 1990. Comparative fit indexes in structural models. *Psychological Bulletin*, Vol. 107, No. 2, 238–246.

Berry, L.L., Parasuraman, A. 1991. *Marketing services. Competing through quality*. NY: Free Press

Blackwell, R. D., Miniard, P. W. & Engel, J. F., 2001. *Consumer behavior*. Fort Worth: Dryden.

Blythe, J., 2009. *Essentials of marketing*. London: Financial Times Press.

Bollen, K.A. & Long, J.S. (Ed.) 1993. *Testing structural equation models*, Newbury Park: Sage Publications, Inc.

Browne, M.W. and Mels, G. 1996. Path analysis: RAMONA. In: *SYSTAT 6.0 for Windows*, Chicago: Statistics, SPSS Inc.

Burns, A.C., Bush, R.F., 2006. *Marketing Research*, New Jersey: Prentice Hall.

Bywalec, C., 2007. *Konsumpcja w teorii i praktyce gospodarowania*. Warszawa: PWN.

Churchill, G. A. & Iacobucci, D., 2009. *Marketing research: methodological foundations*, South Western: Educational Publishing.

Doole, I., Lancaster, P. & Lowe, R., 2005. *Understanding and managing customers*. New York: Financial Times Press.

Egan, J. 2008. *Relationship marketing. Exploring relational strategies in marketing*. London: Prentice Hall.

Gay, R., Charlesworth, A., Esen, R. 2007. *Online marketing. A customer-led approach*, Oxford: University Press.

Glowik, M., Smyczek, S. 2011. *International Marketing Management. Strategies, Concpets and Cases in Europe.* Munich: Oldenbourga Verlag.

Górniak, J. (2000). *My i nasze pieniądze.*Krakow: Aureus.

Gronrros, Ch., 1994. From marketing mix to relationship marketing, *Asia-Australia Marketing Journal,* Vol. 2, Issue 1., p. 9–29.

Hawkins, D. I. & Best, C. R., 2004. *Consumer behavior: building marketing strategy.* Boston: McGrae-Hill.

Hofstede, G. 2001. *Culture's Consequences: Comparing Values, Behaviors, Institutions and Organizations across Nations.* Thousand Oaks: Sage Publications.

Hoyle, R. (Ed.) 1995. *Structural Equation Modeling. Concept, Issues and Applications,* Thousand Oaks: Sage Publications, Inc.

Karcz, K. & Kędzior, Z., 2001. *Zachowania podmiotów rynkowych w Polsce a proces integracji europejskiej.* Katowice: CBiE AE.

Kedzior, Z. & Karcz, K., 2001. *Badania marketingowe w praktyce.* Warszawa: PWE.

Kiezel, E., 2010. *Konsument i jego zachowania na rynku europejskim.* Warszawa: PWE.

Lambkin, M., Foxall, G., van Raaij, F. & Heilbrunn, B., 2001. *European perspective on consumer behaviour.* London: Prentice Hall Europe.

Malhotra, N., Hall, J., Shaw, M. & Oppenheim, P., 2008. *Essentials of marketing research: an applied orientation.* New York: Prentice Hall.

McGivern, Y., 2009. *The practice of market research: an introduction.* London: Pearson Education.

Mitręga, M. 2005. *Marketing relacji. Teoria i Praktyka.* Waszawa: CeDeWu.

Mueller, R.O. 1996. *Basic Principles of Structural Equation Modeling.* NY: Springer-Verlag.

Petty, R.E, Cacioppo, J.T. 1983. Central and Peripheral Routes to Persuasion: Aplication to Adevertising. In: Petty, R.E., Woodside, W.G., Advertising and Customer Psychology, Cambrige: Lexington.

Poiesz, T., Robben, H. 1994. Individual Reactions To the Advertising: Theoretical and Motodological Development. International Journal of Adevertimg, Vol. 2

Schiffman, L. G., & Kanuk, L. L., 2010. *Consumer behavior: global edition.* London: Pearson Higher Education.

Schiffman, L. G., Bednall, D., O'Cass, A., Paladino, A., D'Alessandro, S. & Kanuk, L. L., 2008. *Consumer behaviour.* New Jersey: Prentice Hall.

Sheth, J.N. and Parvatiyar, A. 2000. The domain and conceptual foundations of relationship marketing. In: Sheth, J.N. and Parvatiyar, A. (Ed.) *Handbook of relationship marketing*: 15–26 Thousand Oaks: Sage Publications, Inc.

Smyczek, S., 2007. *Modele zachowan konsumentow na rynku uslug finansowych.* Katowice: UE.

Solomon, M. R., Bamossy, G., Askegaard, S. & Hogg, M. K., 2010. *Consumer behaviour.* New York: Financial Times Press.

Stewart, D.W., 1989. Meausers, Methods and Models in Adevertising Research. Journal of Adevrtising Research, Vol. 12.

Sztemberg, M. 2000. Konfirmacyjna analiza czynnikowa jako weryfikacja eksploracyjnej analizy czynnikowej. In: Walesiak, M. (Ed.) *Pomiar w badaniach rynkowych i marketingowych.* Wrocław: AE.

Wilson, A., 2006. *Marketing research: an integrated approach.* NY: Financial Times Press.

Żabinski, L. 2001. *Paradygramty współczesnego marketingu.* Katowice: UE.

Żabiński, L., (Ed.). 2000. *Modele strategii marketingowych.* Katowice: UE Publishing House.

Zaborski, A., 2001. *Skalowanie wielowymiarowe w badaniach marketingowych.* Wrocław: AE.

Thuy Nguyen and Mario Glowik

6 Emerging Buying Center Concepts in Healthcare Industries

Abstract The medical cardiology device market in Europe indicates promising growth rates while, simultaneously, medical device unit prices for cardiac implants are decreasing. The introduction of the diagnosis-related group (DRG) system in various European countries, developed for monitoring and controlling reimbursement costs, caused hospitals to be increasingly confronted with business performance issues.

In order to optimize their procurement processes for medical devices, hospitals have started to develop and install buying center structures.

This chapter describes the actors and their roles in a hospital buying center and the corresponding network configurations with external stakeholders, such as group purchasing organizations (GPO) and medical device manufacturers.

Keywords: Medical cardiology devices, Diagnostic related group, Buying center, Group purchasing organization

6.1 Introduction

The following chapter describes developments towards more centralized procurement processes in hospitals for technologically advanced medical devices. Based on the conventional buying center concept developed for industrial products, we depict the recently increasing buying center configurations in hospitals, which represent important institutional units in the healthcare (service) industry. We aim to explain the roles of relevant actors in a hospital's buying center and their bilateral relationships with internal and external stakeholders.

Our empirical study focuses on procurement processes for cardiology medical devices for heart diseases. Based on secondary data analysis in the course of a qualitative research approach (Yin, 2009: 6), the first part of this article is devoted to an analysis of current reimbursement frameworks in German hospitals. The discussion is followed by an overview of European market dynamics for medical cardiology devices, with a particular focus on Germany.

In the course of the field analysis during 2012 to 2013, we conducted, among other things, an interview with a medical director in a large hospital group, which has contributed valuable industry insights verifying our research outcomes.

Finally, as a result of our analysis, we are able to describe modern buying center configurations in hospitals for procurement processes related to advanced cardiology medical devices.

6.2 The reimbursement system as applied in hospitals

Germany represents one of the large member countries of the European Union (EU) with a fine-grained healthcare system. The expenses for healthcare are going up steadily, from 212 billion Euros in 2000 to around 287 billion Euros in 2010 (Berger, 2011: 12). As in other EU member countries, an aging population, advanced health sensitivity of the inhabitants, more sophisticated patient treatments (e.g., medical devices, pharmaceuticals) as well as attractive margins on the supply side (e.g., pharmaceutical firms) compared to other industries, have contributed to an overall increase in healthcare costs.

On the demand (hospitals) side, the introduction of the **diagnosis-related group (DRG)** system, developed for monitoring and controlling reimbursement costs, caused hospitals to be increasingly confronted with business performance issues rather than only healthcare concerns. The DRG system was first introduced in 1983 in the USA to monitor and limit hospital expenditures. The DRG is mainly used to reimburse hospitals for their services and aims to secure transparency and the efficient use of resources in inpatient care. Since the mid-1990s, almost all European countries have introduced DRG systems (Bhattacharjee, 2007: 65; Quentin et al., 2013: 1973), albeit with varying degrees of adoption. Global budgets (set targets for standardized healthcare expenditures) still account for more than 50 percent of funding, for instance in such countries as the Czech Republic, Denmark, Ireland, the Netherlands, and Norway (Paris et al., 2010: 36–37).

By contrast, in the United Kingdom and Sweden, payments per case/DGR already account for more than half of the funding; whereas in Finland, Germany, Italy, Poland, and the Slovak Republic, hospital care is paid exclusively through the DRG system (Paris et al., 2010: 36–37). The DRG-based hospital payment system is adopted for different purposes. While in some countries, for instance in Sweden and Finland, the DRG system is primarily used for performance comparison, budget adjustments, and benchmarking; other countries, such as Germany and France, adopted the system mainly for reimbursement of costs (Geissler et al., 2012: 633–636).

The DRG is based on a patient classification system. First of all, the disease pattern (clinical picture) of a patient is defined. In the second step, expenditures for the patient's treatment are calculated according to 'homogeneous patient cases'. As the process in Figure 6.1 illustrates, the case classification is grounded on pre-defined treatment steps, such as the main diagnosis, procedures, surgical operations, eventual complications, and a secondary diagnosis, as well as the patient's age and weight.

Hospitals apply the DRG calculations through a 'DRG grouper', a software program that has to be licensed by the hospital for its use. Incorrect DRG calculations can arise when necessary information for the patient is not properly recorded (Lauterbach et al., 2009: 167–168). Hospitals receive the reimbursement for their treatment expenditures based on the DRG calculation for each 'homogeneous patient case'. As a consequence, the hospital is unable to recover any extra costs if not defined and classified in the DRG system. The DRG serves as a cost control instrument. On the other hand, physicians and hospital staff are obliged to secure medical and financial-economic success simultaneously. In order to manage this increasingly emerging challenge, hospitals have started to deploy their influence in the medical cardiology devices procurement process because there is potential for cost optimization in this field.

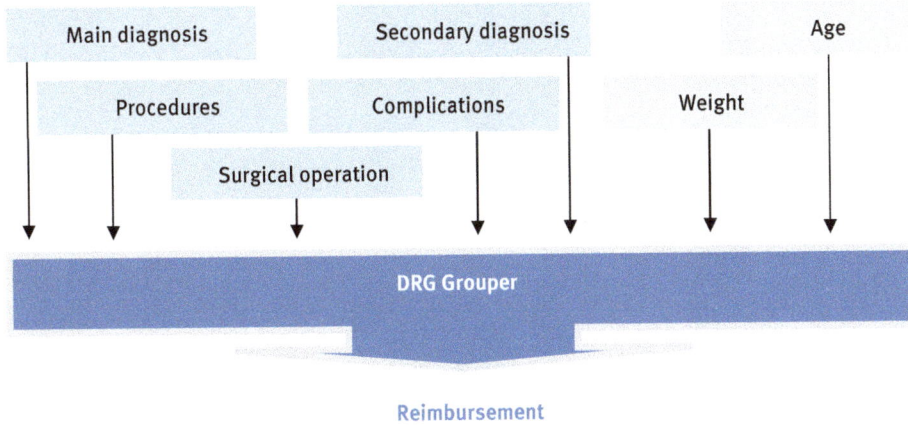

Fig. 6.1: DRG reimbursement system. Adapted from Lauterbach et al. (2009: 168)

6.3 The European market for medical cardiology devices

Diseases of the heart and circulatory system of the human body, described as cardiovascular disease (CVD), are the main cause of death in Europe. According to a 2012 report, published by the European Society of Cardiology, the European Heart Network, and the British Heart Foundation Health Promotion Research Group, each year cardiovascular disease (CVD) causes over 4 million deaths in Europe and 1.9 million deaths in the European Union (EU). In other words, CVD causes 47 percent of all deaths in Europe and 40 percent of all deaths in the EU. Death rates are generally higher in Central and Eastern Europe than in Northern, Southern, and Western Europe (European_Heart_Network, 2012).

An important segment within the cardiology device industry is cardiac rhythm management. Cardiac rhythm management describes the treatment of disorders of the heart's electrical system, which lead to arrhythmias or heart failure. The current lifestyle of a major part of the European population, which is characterized by occupational stress, fast-food, and permanent mobile reachability but often includes fewer sports activities, has increased the risk of cardiac diseases, e.g., arrhythmias and heart failures (York et al., 2004: 465).

As a result, an accelerating number of patients have to be treated within each country's healthcare system. Between 2005 and 2010, market volumes for medical devices such as implantable pulse generators (IPG), implantable cardioverter defibrillators (ICD), and cardiac resynchronization therapy (CRT) have increased significantly. Figure 6.2 illustrates the growth of IPG, ICD, and CRT implantations per million inhabitants in Europe (Eucomed, 2010).

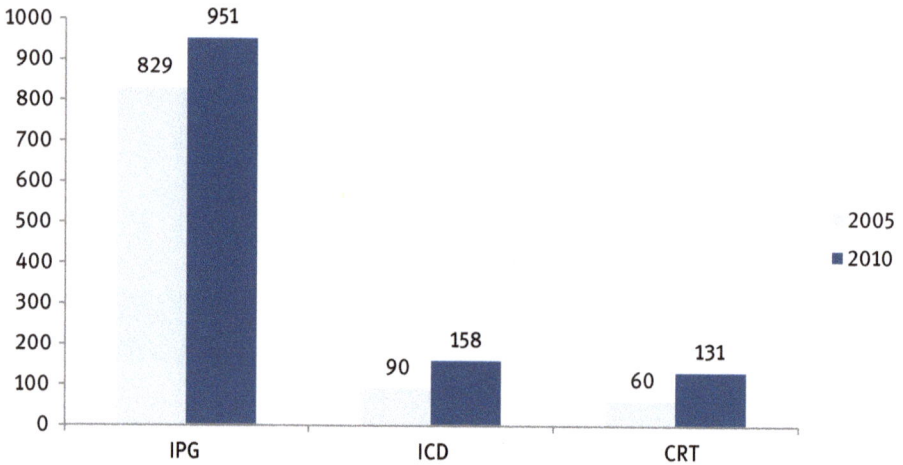

Fig. 6.2: Rate of implantation of IPG, ICD, and CRT devices per million inhabitants in 2005 versus 2010 in Europe
Source: Eucomed (2010)

IPG, ICD, and CRT cardiac devices are briefly introduced in the following description. An IPG is used to stimulate the heart electrically, e.g., when the patient's heartbeat is below 60 beats per minute (normal rate is 60 to 80). In case of an abnormally fast heart rhythm (between 100 and 400 heartbeats per minute), an ICD apparatus interferes by delivering a strong electric shock to restore the normal heart rhythm. Patients with asynchronous heart contradiction suffer from insufficient blood transportation, which leads to less oxygen and lower supplies of nutrients. An implanted CRT device transmits electrical impulses to both heart chambers, which restores the synchronous contradiction of the heart ventricles and, thus, stabilizes the blood pumping performance (Biotronik, 2012).

The market for IPG, ICD, and CRT cardiology devices in Europe is driven by five firms, Medtronic (USA), St. Jude Medical (USA), Boston Scientific (USA), Biotronik (Germany), and the Sorin Group (Italy). These industry-leading firms make use of their advanced cardiology device technology against the background of forty years of research and development assets. Their customers are hospitals with cardiology departments, electrophysiology labs, and private practices (Millennium_Research_Group, 2010). Figure 6.3 illustrates the distribution of the market shares of these firms for cardiology products in 2010 in Europe.

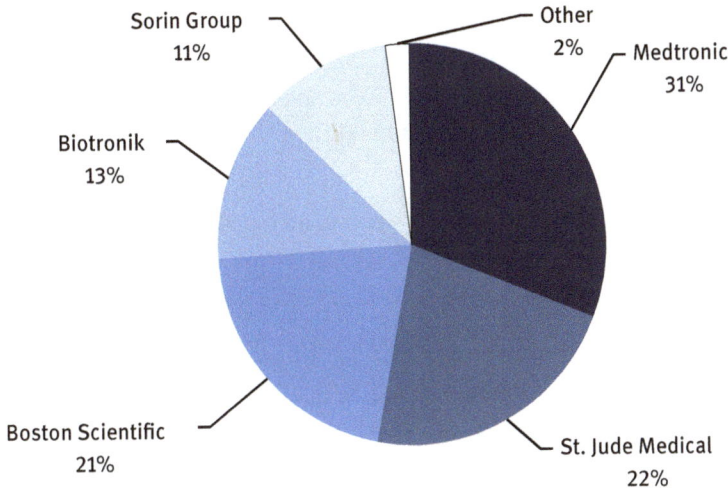

Fig. 6.3: Market share of five leading cardiology medical device companies in the European market in percentage of the total market share (status 2010)
Source: Millennium Research Group (2011)

The market for cardiology medical devices indicates promising growth rates for the future for the following reasons:

- demographic changes, such as an aging population and increasing health sensitivity;
- changing lifestyles causing a tendency towards less physical exercise and increased use of computers and increased communication activities;
- modern work characteristics of the population, e.g., permanent reachability, time pressure, etc.;
- technological innovation (e.g., telemonitoring);
- technologically advanced medical devices for cardiac rhythm management, interventional cardiology, interventional radiology, and neurology, providing the best prerequisites for further product differentiation; and
- oligopolistic market structure (five major firms), preventing intensive competition.

Potential risks for cardiology medical device manufacturers doing business in the European markets are the following:

- reimbursement rates are permanently reviewed by local governments in Europe,
- declining reimbursement rates discourage medical technology suppliers,
- product approval and clinical trial evidence are long-term and cost intensive,
- alternative therapies through basic research (e.g., pharmaceutical, stem cells) may substitute for medical cardiology devices, and
- price pressure increases from intensified competitive market dynamics.

While the market volume for cardiac implants has increased in recent years in Germany, the average selling prices (ASP) for cardiac implants has decreased. For example, in Germany, a CRT device sold for 11,650 Euro in 2006. Beginning in 2013, the same product sold for 6,283 Euro (compare Table 6.1).

Tab. 6.1: ASP development of IPG, ICD, and CRT devices in Germany from 2006 until Q2/2013
Source: Eucomed (2013)

Year	ASP for IPG in Euro	ASP for ICD in Euro	ASP for CRT in Euro
2006	1,453	8,140	11,650
2007	1,320	7,735	10,225
2008	1,230	7,581	9,855
2009	1,107	7,281	9,221
2010	1,027	6,540	8,367
2011	930	5,769	7,611
2012	820	5,019	6,867
Q2/2013	768	4,518	6,283

The major reason for the price decline for medical cardiology devices is the emerging bargaining power of the so-called 'group purchasing organizations', which are explained in the next section in more detail.

6.4 Group purchasing organizations

In the past, medical device suppliers were selected by each hospital based on direct bilateral negotiation (Krütten et al., 2005: 24). The introduction of the DRG provoked a change from the traditional purchasing process of hospitals towards more centralized purchasing systems. In the course of this development, 'group purchasing organizations' (GPO) emerged in the European healthcare market. GPOs are positioned as an interface between the medical device industry (suppliers) and the users (hospitals). GPOs' business models differ regarding their procurement standardization policy (degree of supplier consolidation), their procurement volumes, and their compensation models (Berg and Burdach, 2012: 26).

Larger procurement volumes provide GPOs with considerably greater bargaining power than any single hospital gains when negotiating with medical device manufacturers. Among the leading European GPOs are, for instance, Prospitalia in Germany or HealthTrust Europe in the United Kingdom; and there are a number of smaller group purchasing organizations, such as GPO-Healthcare in the Netherlands, Purch in Sweden, or Proceur in the United Kingdom (Healthcare_Europa, 2013). Some examples of preeminent GPOs in Germany are, Prospitalia, Clinicpartner, and Agkamed (Clinicpartner, 2010; Agkamed, 2014; Prospitalia, 2014). These organizations are growing in importance because hospitals benefit from the cost savings through consolidated and standardized volume procurement processes for medical devices. As a result, an increasing number of hospitals make use of the GPOs bundled bargaining power. As per 2011, 80 percent of the hospitals had already organized around half of their purchasing volumes through GPO organizations in Germany (Berger, 2011; 2012: 43). For a hospital, joining a GPO procurement system becomes an important element since cost efficiency is one of the most crucial criteria related to the question of whether a hospital is able to survive in the future or not.

In general, four major types of GPOs can be identified, depending on the degree, intensity, and legal liabilities related to the medical device procurement processes in the German market. There are so-called **unconsolidated GPOs, non-binding GPOs, binding GPOs,** and **hospital group GPOs** with collective purchasing coordination (Krütten et al., 2005: 16; Berger, 2011: 39). The different missions and organizational structures of these GPOs are explained below.

Unconsolidated GPOs

Unconsolidated GPOs are usually small in size and rather regionally organized and focus their activities on the exchange of product and price information. A centrally organized institution does not exist, and the procurement activities are characterized by unconsolidated volume bundling. In this informal form of cooperation, the purchase decision is up to the individual hospital. Standardization effects are rather marginal due to procurement quantity, which tends to be rather low (Krütten et al., 2005: 16).

Non-binding GPOs

Non-binding GPOs have centralized their activities to manage and implement coordinating tasks. They operate through remote volume bundling with a wide range of products. They mainly negotiate individual price lists with different suppliers for their purchasing cooperation members (e.g., hospitals). However, non-binding GPOs, as the name indicates, do not maintain binding contractual relationships with medical device suppliers. Supplier selection and order placements in the course of the final purchasing decision remain at the hospital (Berger, 2011: 39)

Binding GPOs

Binding GPOs engage in central purchase volume bundling activities. They have a broad range of medical device products in their portfolio. Within the GPO organization, there is a central procurement division that negotiates binding agreements with medical device suppliers. These agreements contain, for example, quantity commitments, price conditions, delivery, and payment terms. Consequently, through bundled procurement volumes, binding GPOs are able to negotiate attractive conditions for their member hospitals. On the other hand, the member hospitals are obliged to select their procurement materials and services from a pre-defined supplier portfolio, which limits their flexibility when making decisions (Berger, 2011: 39)

Hospital groups

Hospital groups represent the highest form of centralized procurement activities, which simultaneously provokes the largest contractual liability for the member hospitals. The purchase is centrally organized and standards are clearly defined for all affiliated hospitals, which are committed to the purchase of goods defined by the hospital group headquarters (Berger, 2011: 39). Hospital groups are the most common centralized procurement model currently applied in Germany (Krütten et al., 2005: 18).

In the following sections of the paper, important GPOs and hospital groups in Germany are introduced (compare Table 6.2). Sana Kliniken AG with an annual purchasing volume of more than 1.1 billion Euros, 400 hospitals, and an additional 400 facilities (e.g., nursing homes, pharmacies, etc.) serves as the largest hospital group in Germany. The largest GPO is Prospitalia GmbH with a procurement volume of 1.1 billion Euros, 690 member clinics, and 800 facilities (Prospitalia, 2014; Sana, 2014).

Tab. 6.2: Procurement volume of leading GPOs in Germany: Prospitalia GmbH (status 2013), Clinicpartner eG (status 2010), and Agkamed GmbH (status 2013); Important hospital groups in Germany: Sana Kliniken (status 2013), Rhön Kliniken AG (status 2013), Helios Kliniken GmbH (status 2012), and Asklepios Kliniken GmbH (status 2012)
Source: Prospitalia (2014), Clinicpartner (2010), Agkamed (2014), Sana (2014), Rhön-Klinikum (2014); Asklepios (2012), Helios Kliniken (2012)

GPO	Procurement volume p.a. (Euro)	Operating units
1. Prospitalia GmbH	1.1 billion	690 clinics/800 facilities*
2. Clinicpartner eG	850 million	112 clinics
3. Agkamed GmbH	580 million	190 clinics
Hospital Group	**Procurement volume p.a. (Euro)**	**Operating units**
1. Sana Kliniken AG	>1 billion	400 clinics/400 facilities*
2. RhönKliniken AG	777 million	90 clinics/54 facilities*
3. Helios Kliniken GmbH	738 million	72 clinics
4. Asklepios Kliniken GmbH	651 million	100 clinics/150 facilities*

* facilities include nursing homes, pharmacies, etc.

Membership in a GPO provides the hospital with the following advantages (Berg and Burdach, 2012: 27):
- reduction of medical device procurement costs through volume bundling and standardization,
- product and supplier selection by the GPO,
- negotiation of contract terms and conditions by the GPO,
- professional development of purchase strategies, and
- increased efficiency through optimization of the product portfolio and supplier pool.

Potential drawbacks for a hospital as a member of GPO come from
- less direct supplier relationships for the hospital;
- limited access to market-related information, which reduces market transparency for the hospital;
- loss of procurement knowledge; and
- increased dependence on a GPO (Berg and Burdach, 2012: 27).

All-in-all, the advantages of becoming a member of a GPO exceed the disadvantages for a hospital. The reason is mainly the cost savings a hospital is able to realize through its GPO network relationships. The rising importance of GPOs in the medical device market and their increasing bargaining power through centralized procurement leads to intensified price competition among medical device manufacturers (suppliers). Purchase process configurations have changed to a considerable extent in hospitals, as described in the next section of this chapter (Berg and Burdach, 2012: 26).

6.5 The centralized procurement process

The **buying center concept**, as first introduced by Webster and Wind (1972: 77) for industrialized manufactured products in the 1970s, describes the internal actors of a firm involved in the procurement process. The more complex the product, the more desirable is the establishment of a buying center, which amplifies the decision role of the procurement department (Bonoma, 1984: 82; Strothmann, 1997: 48). Like other manufacturing industries for technologically advanced products, various hospitals have established **buying center (BC)** configurations that organize the procurement activities for clinical products. The idea behind the BC is that the procurement process for technologically and commercially complex medical devices, e.g., cardiac implants, is shared and managed by BC members with different medical and commercial expertise, perspectives, and objectives. According to our research, verified by an interview in 2012 with a medical director in a large hospital group in Germany, the typical roles and positions of the buying center members in a hospital can be described as below (Nguyen, 2012).

- **User:** a person or group of people who uses the product; in a hospital this role is held by physicians and the medical director. From the user's perspective, the product quality is paramount, while, comparatively, the price has less significance. The products have to adequately meet user expectations, such as performance, safety, and feasibility criteria.
- **Buyer:** the procurement director in a hospital takes control of the budget and formal processing of the purchase.
- **Decider:** usually belongs to the firm's management and makes the final procurement/investment decision. A decider's position in a hospital is typically held by the managing director.
- **Initiator:** creates the idea of procuring a certain product or service. In a hospital the medical director often serves as an initiator.

The GPO, which bundles the procurement volumes of its member hospitals and finalizes the contract negotiation with the medical device supplier amplifies each hospital's buying center through the following roles.

- **Gatekeeper:** the GPO selects, holds, blocks, or transfers information from the external environment (e.g., market surveys, supplier information) to the members of the hospital's buying center.
- **Influencer/Buyer:** affects the medical device procurement decision process through his or her own activities, such as the GPO's negotiations and contract finalization with medical supplier firms.

According to the interview outcomes with the medical director, the procurement for cardiac implants is usually conducted at a hospital every two years by a tender (Nguyen, 2012). Once a tender is open, all relevant medical device suppliers are invited to the hospital group headquarters to present their offerings (pre-negotiating phase). In the next round, the preferred suppliers, based on their first offering, have a chance to present their products and services in more detail and negotiate terms and conditions with the hospital representatives of the buying center.

The participants from the buying center, who have to consider the DRG framework and the corresponding budget constraints, develop a ranking of potential suppliers according to their offers. Once the internal ranking of the preferred medical supplier is set, the users (physicians) get increasingly involved in the process because of their expert opinion. The managing director of the hospital is in charge of making the final procurement decision. The procurement process for medical devices initiated by the hospitals buying center and finalized by the GPO is illustrated in Figure 6.4.

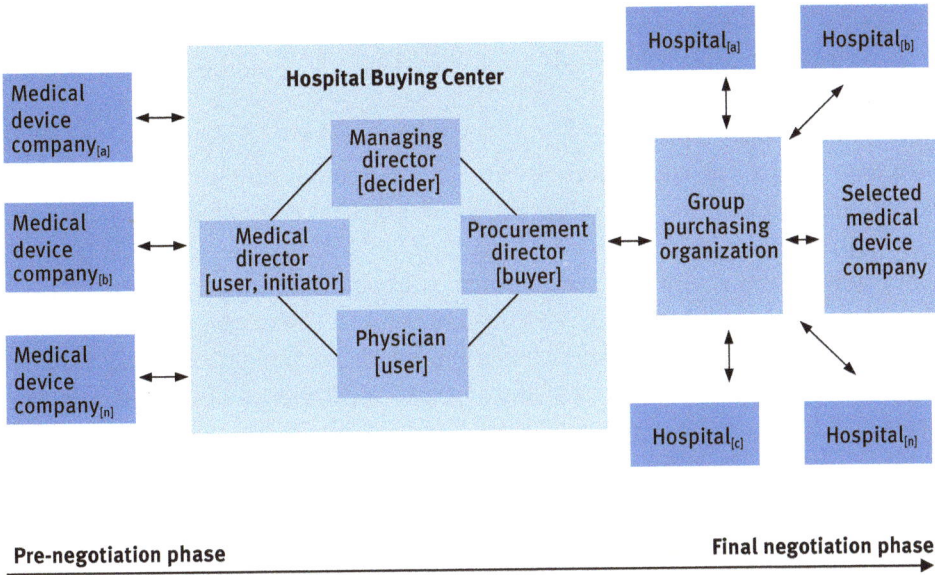

Fig. 6.4: The actors in a hospital's buying center and their positioning in the procurement process for medical devices

Once the medical supplier selection is completed by the members of the hospital's buying center, the procurement process is passed to the GPO (e.g., Prospitalia), which finalizes the contract negotiation directly with the selected medical device supplier (final negotiation). The GPO usually realizes more price benefits than one hospital can because of the bundled purchase volume contributed by various hospitals. The increasing importance of the GPOs leads to continued price competition regarding medical devices on the supplier side.

Conclusions

This chapter describes recent developments in hospitals related to their medical device procurement processes for heart diseases. Research outcomes indicate that buying center concepts, as traditionally known for the procurement of technologically advanced products in manufacturing industries, have been introduced in the healthcare service sector. As result of our field research, we are able to describe actors and their roles in a hospital buying center and network configurations with external stakeholders, such as GPOs and medical device manufacturers.

The medical cardiology device market in Europe indicates promising growth rates for the future, while, simultaneously, medical device unit prices for cardiac implants are decreasing. One of the major reasons is that hospitals make use of their relationships with GPOs. Another reason is that procurement processes, because of the DRG reimbursement systems, have become more professionalized and commercialized in hospitals, which are the most important actors on the demand side for medical device products.

On the supplier side, the qualification profile of the medical device company sales staff necessarily contains profound commercial and product-related medical expertise as well as a fine-grained service mentality (Krütten et al., 2005: 24).

Conventional sales support activities, such as technical services (e.g. maintenance of technical equipment and information about new product releases), are of vital importance for the medical device manufacturer. The customer-specific adaptation of service packages according to a hospital's individual needs and budgets becomes a crucial way to gain competitive advantage for the medical device manufacturer and helps balance the bargaining power of the GPO (Slater, 1997: 164–165; Woodruff, 1997: 139–140).

Medical device suppliers need to understand the hospital's buying center configuration in order to ensure that the product development process is in accordance with the changing demands of their clients (hospitals). Each actor's role in the hospital's buying center needs to be adequately considered by the medical device supplier and effective communication channels have to be installed. Service-based effective communication includes information about product improvements and related training offers to physicians who are experts from the medical point of view but sometimes lack familiarity with the supplier's specific product applications (Yoder et al., 1961: 117–119; Orsenigo et al., 2001: 487).

References

Agkamed, 2014. *Das Unternehmen. Full Service für die Mitgliedseinrichtungen: AGKAMED.* February 08, 2014: http://www.agkamed.de/index.php?id=30.

Asklepios, 2012. *Kennzahlen.* February 08, 2014: http://www.asklepios.com/Kennzahlen.Asklepios?ActiveID=1123.

Berg, M. and Burdach, C. B., 2012. *Strategischer Einkauf im Krankenhaus. Der Einkauf im Spannungsfeld zwischen Klinikleitung und Ärzten. Die Entwicklung vom operativen Abwickler zum strategischen Partner.*

BME-Fachgruppe. Retrieved June 11, 2012 from: http://www.bme.de/fileadmin/bilder/Buchtipps/Leifaeden/Leitfaden_Einkauf_im_Krankenhaus_2012.pdf.

Berger, R., 2011. *Roland Berger Strategy Consultants: Sachkostenentwicklung und Bedeutung von Einkaufsgesellschaften im Krankenhausumfeld.* München: Roland Berger Strategy Consultants.

Berger, R., 2012. *Roland Berger Strategy Consultants: Sachkostenentwicklung im Krankenhausumfeld.* Retrieved February 12, 2014 from: http://www.rolandberger.de/medien/publikationen/2012-05-08-rbsc-pub-Sachkostenentwicklung_im_Krankenhausumfeld.html.

Bhattacharjee, K., 2007. *Diagnostic related groups – Suitable means to an end?* Retrieved May 31, 2012 from: https://www.frost.com/sublib/display-market-insight.do?id=115142822.

Biotronik, 2012. *Patienten. Behandlung & Nachsorge.* May 03, 2012: http://www.biotronik.de/wps/wcm/connect/de_de_web/biotronik/sub_top/patients/Diseases_and_diagnoses_en/#jump.

Bonoma, T. V., 1984. *Managing marketing*. New York: Free Press.

Clinicpartner, 2010. *Zahlen. Daten. Fakten*. February 08, 2014: http://www.clinicpartner-eg.eu/zahlen-daten-fakten.

Eucomed, 2010. *Medical Technology Facts and Figures*. Retrieved May 21, 2012 from: http://www.eucomed.org/uploads/_medical_technology/facts_figure/110518_statistics_for_cardiac_rhythm_management_products_20052010.pdf.

Eucomed, 2013. *Entwicklung der ASP auf dem deutschen Markt*. August 07, 2013: http://www.eucomed.org.

European_Heart_Network, 2012. *European cardiovascular desease statistics*. European Heart Network AISBL. Retrieved January 13, 2014 from: http://www.escardio.org/about/Documents/EU-cardiovascular-disease-statistics-2012.pdf.

Geissler, A., Scheller-Kreinsen, D., Quentin, W. and Busse, R., 2012. DRG-Systeme in Europa: Anreize, Ziele und Unterschiede in zwölf Ländern. *Bundesgesundheitsblatt – Gesundheitsforschung – Gesundheitsschutz*, 55 (5): 633–642.

Healthcare_Europa, 2013. *Procurement in Europe: Part one*. Retrieved March 05, 2014 from: http://www.healthcareeuropa.com/procurement-in-europe-part-one/.

Helios_Kliniken, 2012. *Zahlen und Fakten über Helios*. February 08, 2014: http://www.helios-kliniken.de/ueber-helios/unternehmensportrait/zahlen-und-fakten.html.

Krütten, J. M., Rautenberg, F. and Liefner, M., 2005. *Zukünftige Relevanz und Konsequenzen von Krankenhaus-Kooperationen für Medizintechnologie-Anbieter in Deutschland*. Retrieved June 25, 2012 from: http://www.bvmed.de/stepone/data/downloads/54/a5/00/studie_einkaufskooperationen.pdf.

Lauterbach, K. W., Stock , S. and Brunner, H., 2009. *Gesundheitsökonomie – Lehrbuch für Mediziner und andere Gesundheitsberufe*. Bern: Hans Huber.

Millennium_Research_Group, 2010. *Global Markets for Cardiac Rhythm Management Devices 2011*. Toronto: Millennium Research Group.

Millennium_Research_Group, 2011. *Global Markets for Cardiac Rhythm Management Devices*. Toronto: Millennium Research Group.

Nguyen, T., 2012. Interview with the medical director of SRH hospital.

Orsenigo, L., Pammolli, F. and Riccaboni, M., 2001. Technological change and network dynamics. Lessons from the pharmaceutical industry. *Research Policy*, 30 (3): 485–508.

Paris, V., Devaux, M. and Wei, L., 2010. *Health systems institutional characteristics: A survey of 29 OECD countries*. OECD Publishing. Retrieved March 05, 2014 from: http://www.oecd-ilibrary.org/social-issues-migration-health/health-systems-institutional-characteristics_5kmfxfq9qbnr-en.

Prospitalia, 2014. *Aktuelles aus der Welt der Prospitalia*. February 08, 2014: http://www.prospitalia.de/home/index.php?prospitalia=pecunna4o88268ptbufl9qa0if301im3.

Quentin, W., Rätto, H., Peltola, M., Busse, R. and Häkkinen, U., 2013. Acute myocardial infarction and diagnosis-related groups: Patient classification and hospital reimbursement in 11 European countries. *European Heart Journal*, 34 (26): 1972–1981a.

Rhön-Klinikum, 2014. *Unsere Kliniken*. February 08, 2014: http://www.rhoen-klinikum-ag.com/rka/cms/rka_2/deu/34024.html.

Sana, 2014. *Zahlen und Fakten*. February 08, 2014: http://www.sana-einkauf.de/ueber-uns/zahlen-und-fakten.html.

Slater, S. F., 1997. Developing a customer value-based theory of the firm. *Journal of the Academy of Marketing Science*, 25 (2): 162–167.

Strothmann, K.-H., 1997. *Kompetenztransfer im Investitionsgütermarketing*. Wiesbaden: Deutscher Universitätsverlag.

Webster, F. E. and Wind, Y., 1972. *Organizational buying behavior*. Cliffs, NJ: Englewood.

Woodruff, R. B., 1997. Customer value: The next source for competitive advantage. *Journal of the Academy of Marketing Science*, 25 (2): 139–153.

Yin, R. K., 2009. *Case study research: Design and methods*, 4th ed. Thousand Oaks, California: Sage Publications Ltd.

Yoder, W. O., Cunningham, R. M., Tacy, A. J. and Hankins, F. W., 1961. Industrial marketing. *Business Horizon*, 4 (1): 117–128.

York, D. A., Rössner, S., Caterson, I., Chen, C. M., James, W., Shiriki, K., Martorell, R. and Vorster, H. H., 2004. Prevention conference VII: Obesity, a worldwide epidemic related to heart disease and stroke. Group I: Worldwide demographics of obesity. *Circulation*, 110 (18): 463–470.

Marta Grybś

7 Integrated Marketing Communication in the European Healthcare Market

Abstract Institutions in the healthcare market communicate with patients, who, in the marketing understanding of the process, are the customers of the products and services offered by these institutions. For many years, it has been observed, both in the international and the European arena, that the concept of healthcare marketing communication has been evolving. This chapter consists of analysis, characteristics, examples, and recommendations that consider the integrated marketing communication of healthcare service providers in five countries in Europe, which represent five healthcare systems: Germany, the United Kingdom, Sweden, Belgium, and Poland.

Keywords: Integrated marketing communication (IMC), Healthcare market, Marketing communication, Healthcare marketing

7.1 Introduction

It can be stated that marketing communication plays a crucial and pervasive role in the healthcare marketplace. There are several dimensions of that fact. First of all, marketing efforts of pharmaceutical and medical companies that sell health support devices create demand for branded products and services. There is also a preventive dimension of healthcare marketing, whose aim is to spread awareness of not only treating oneself but also preventing oneself from becoming ill. In addition, more and more hospitals, nursing homes, hospices, physician practices, managed care organizations, rehabilitation centers, and other healthcare organizations have begun to apply marketing communication strategies in their activities in the market. These organizations usually did not focus on marketing until the early 1970s. Nowadays, it can be observed that there is a great deal of marketing taking place in healthcare organizations (Kotler et al., 2008: 16). More and more healthcare organizations have become aware of marketing communication possibilities and have begun to integrate specific tools and channels in order to be more effective.

These are only a few examples that demonstrate the development of one side of marketing communication, namely the use of influential promotion and sales to attract and retain customers. But marketing tasks and tools go beyond developing a stream of persuasive messages, and more and more often turn to true dialog between a company and a consumer – relationship marketing. The aim of this chapter is to characterize the integrated marketing communication concept in the healthcare market with a focus on the European market.

7.2 Integrated marketing communication – notion and characteristics

Integrated marketing communication (IMC) may be understood as a concept in which a company, while communicating a clear and reliable message about the company and its offerings to the environment, has to integrate and coordinate many communication channels (Pickton and Broderick, 2005: 3). On the other hand, according to (Kotler, 2003: 563), integrated marketing communication is based on the idea of looking at the whole marketing process from the viewpoint of the customer. In order to better understand the concept of IMC, the term *marketing communication* will be defined.

Marketing communication is one of the most important spheres of company activity; it determines a company's competitive advantage in the market (Pilarczyk, 2008: 295). It is an important tool of marketing strategy as a result of the fact that it enables an enterprise to meet its practical market aims (Wiktor, 2006: 10). The role of marketing communication is very often underestimated and simplified to refer to advertising or promotion only. The terms *marketing communication* and *promotion* are slightly different. It can be concluded that promotion is one of the components of the wider term of marketing communication (Pabian, 2008: 25). Promotion is a more narrow term because a company possesses a diverse range of tools to communicate with the market and influence the consumers. Throughout the years, the difference between advertising, promotion, and marketing communication has commonly been misunderstood (O'Guinn, 2011: 34). However, it should be emphasized that marketing communication is a much more complex term than advertising or even promotion. Promotion should not be viewed in isolation from other marketing communication tools as it is not the sole communication effort of a company (City, 2005: 12).

For a company, the marketing communication role is crucial, as the nature of the enterprise can be identified through the process of communication with the environment (Wiktor, 2006: 11). Marketing communication consists of all the elements of the marketing mix that consider the communication between the company and the target audience about all issues influencing marketing performance (Smith, 2012: 600). Marketing communication does not consider only the process between the market and company; it involves all stakeholders within and outside the company (Percy, 2008: 23).

The most important aim of marketing communication seems to be reaching the target audience and influencing its behavior. However, among several marketing communication objectives, four main ones can be identified (Rydel, 2001: 28):
- to inform,
- to persuade,
- to educate, and
- to remind.

The informing role of marketing communication is very important because it includes notifying the audience members (present and potential customers) about new products, current offers, or new companies. Very often the message contains information about the price, product parameters, or sale conditions. Creation of brand awareness is made possible through the informing function (Parada and Homan, 2010: 8).

The persuading role of marketing communication is based on influencing and encouraging the customer to act in a specific way, usually to purchase the company's market offering (Bearden, et al., 2001: 369). Customers are meant to change their behavior or their life style in order to purchase the specific goods or services offered by the seller (Keller, 2001: 819–824). Nevertheless, the objective is not always to increase sales. Nonprofit organizations also take advantage of this marketing communication function, for example, by persuading people to quit smoking or eat a healthy diet (Bearden, et al., 2001: 369).

The educating role of marketing communication very often creates positive habits in customers. They learn that the teeth should be brushed, the house should be insured, or fruits and vegetables should be eaten at least five times a day. So this function is usually performed along with the persuasive one (Rydel, 2001: 29).

The reminding function in marketing communication can especially be observed when consumers are already aware of the company and its offer. The aim of reminding is to prevent a situation in which competitors are able to persuade customers to choose a different offer (Blakeman, 2007: 39). Moreover, it reassures customers about the adequacy of their decision. It ensures that customers can remember the brand. Moreover, they become loyal, which they express by choosing the same brand again (Holm, 2006: 23–26).

The market is constantly changing. The arena of competitors is more and more complex, especially in the era of modern technology and globalization. The marketplace is considered in global terms. Every day, there is a growing number of new companies; the Internet is revolutionizing commerce; and, as a result, there is an almost unlimited number of marketing opportunities. Nevertheless, the number of barriers and threats is increasing as well (Madhavaram and Badrinarayanan, 2005: 25).

This situation has led to a changing approach to marketing communication. Companies do not rely on basic methods to reach their customers anymore. In the face of increasingly sophisticated customer demand and a higher complexity of both market conditions and the micro and macro environment of the company, companies have changed their communication strategy (Clow and Baack, 2002: 4). Communication has needed to become more coherent and clear. As a result, the emergence of integrated marketing communication has been observed (Blythe, 2002: 2).

Integrated marketing communication (IMC) is a concept that was defined by the American Association of Advertising Agencies as a method of planning marketing communication that included all the communication possibilities of the company (Szymoniuk, 2005: 31). In other words, it is a program in which all marketing communication tools, sources, and channels are coordinated and integrated in order to maximize the company's influence on consumers and minimize the costs. Such an approach enables clear, coherent, and the most effective communication of messages (Keller, 2001: 819–827).

The IMC concept is constantly developing. As a response to the changing environment, there are an increasing number of tools that can be utilized in the process of communicating with the market. Marketing communication requires the coordination of all marketing communication tools in order to produce a customer-oriented and unified marketing message. Moreover, it is based on inclusion of new media within the context of traditional ones, along with more established and likely to evolve forms of marketing communication (Bearden et. al., 2001: 359). This process demands not only the efforts of marketers but also the involvement of all company departments, especially managerial, during the period of setting objectives. Marketing managers have to set their goals according to the general company objectives. Based on the goals, different marketing communication tools are considered in an integrated communication plan, which is used to reach the target market (Belch et. al., 2008: 50–59). The division of all marketing communication tools and the process of their integration can be understood according to the scheme presented in figure 7.1. The graph displays the six main tools of marketing communication.

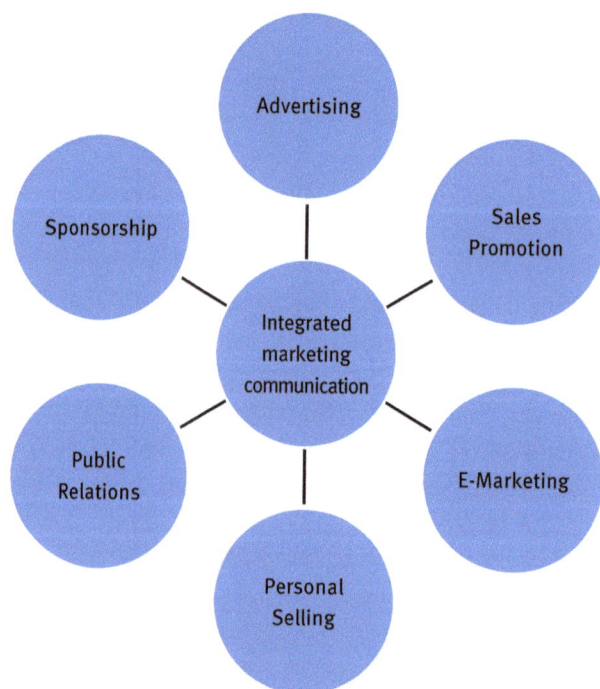

Fig. 7.1: Integrated marketing communication
Source: Author's elaboration adapted from *L. Boone, D. Kurtze:* Contemporary Marketing, *Cengage Education, 2012, p. 489*

The scheme presented in figure 7.1 divides marketing communication tools into six main categories. There is a division between advertising and online marketing because the importance of online advertising is increasing nowadays. The Internet, modern technologies, and social media have influenced the development of marketing communication. Consumer behaviors have changed, and the transparency of consumer needs is greater because of the possibility of following their online behaviors. As a result, the number of online tools that can be engaged in communication with the environment is rising rapidly (Gurau, 2008: 169). Sponsorship, sometimes analyzed as a part of advertising or PR, is classified separately in this chapter because of its ubiquitous character and as a result of the fact that its theory and functions are highly developed (Parada and Homan, 2010: 101–119). The events that are sponsored are gaining in popularity, which leads to the conclusion that sponsorship has to be classified separately from other marketing communication tools. The basis and functions of its personal selling and sales promotion character differ strongly from other marketing communication tools and, as a result, are classified separately (Pelsmacker et. al., 2007: 68–87).

7.3 Healthcare marketing communication

The institutions in the **healthcare market** attempt to communicate with patients, who, in the marketing understanding of the process, are the customers for the products and services offered by these institutions. Throughout the years, it has been observed in the international arena that healthcare marketing has evolved. The term appeared around forty years ago for the first time; and from that moment, the concept of communicating with the market changed dramatically. At the beginning, it was understood mainly as simple usage of advertising or colorful brochures (Weiss, 2011: 8). Numerous debates took place concerning whether or not marketing should be viewed as a profession. Over the years, the importance of dialogue with the community has increased. More and more hospitals, clinics, or community health centers became aware of the marketing communication tools available and engaged in marketing strategies. These strategies involve definition of the target audience, the engagement of employees, creation of a brand, advertisement not only of services offered but also of social issues, and the idea of community engagement (Ziglio, 2000: 143–154). New trends appeared in healthcare marketing that encouraged organizations to be effective in communicating with patients. There are countries where a complex approach toward healthcare marketing has been present for several years, especially Western, more developed countries, while in others, it is at its beginning (Weiss, 2011: 8).

In the marketing communication industry, healthcare is one of the least researched segments. However, despite low investments in research, a huge development of official and unofficial tools of marketing communication has been observed.

Healthcare marketing as a term and as a consciously implemented strategy came into being in the 1980s and 1990s. At the beginning, it focused on advertising, direct mail, and other traditional promotional strategies. The limitations of competition based on product, price, and place have encouraged healthcare providers to differentiate themselves through promotional strategies (Thomas, 2010: 264). In the contemporary healthcare arena, marketing communication strategies involve far more than simply advertising. Healthcare providers, throughout the years, have turned to personal selling and sales promotions to compete more effectively. More and more marketing communication tools have appeared. In order to develop an effective marketing communication strategy, marketers in the area of healthcare had to demonstrate an understanding of the various media available to them and be able to craft a message with appropriate content and tone, as the healthcare market is a sensitive one (Thomas, 2010: 265).

The healthcare market environment is demanding, on the one hand, and sensitive, on the other. As a result, nowadays healthcare marketing is necessary. Moreover, the emergence of the global marketplace can be observed in the case of the healthcare industry. The healthcare market is very dynamic. Marketing communication in that market has to follow demand and utilize new technologies as well as be aware of increasing international competitiveness and consumers who expect a higher and higher quality of services (Berkowitz, 2011: 14). Several examples of healthcare marketing communication tools will be discussed in the next paragraphs.

The majority of consumers have access to the Internet, where lots of time is spent searching for information on preventive medicine, healthcare products and services, support groups, or possible treatments. As a result, the term *marketing 2.0* appeared in connection to the healthcare segment. This is based on the assumption that there is a great opportunity for marketers to reach consumers where they are searching for information, including traditional media like television, but with a major focus on online tools like websites, chat rooms, or social media (Renfrow, 2009: 32–39). A mix of media should be used in communication with consumers; however, the potential of online marketing should be emphasized. It is on the web where patients nowadays begin a dialogue with health experts and where a brand can be formed based on one-to-one communication. Healthcare marketing 2.0 may be defined as a combination of direct response and relationship marketing, usually based on online tools (Renfrow, 2009: 32–39).

Another quickly developing trend in the healthcare market may be described as an integration of IT and information technology into existing marketing communication channels. It is believed that marketing along with IT can revolutionize healthcare information technology to finally position it as one of the most important parts of the mission and strategy of healthcare organizations. Well-developed healthcare information technology can be used as a competitive advantage of a healthcare company because it may demonstrate leadership and differentiate the company in the healthcare market. Implementation of IT into healthcare reduces medical errors, increases support staff productivity, and ensures higher quality and standards of care. But, from the marketing communication point of view, it may be part of a strategic message sent to the consumers – that the healthcare provider is a leader in the market. Moreover, implementation of IT into healthcare extends the amount of possible marketing communication channels to be used in relationships with consumers (Quinn, et.al, 2008: 221–230). There are several major technology tendencies to be observed. The popularity of personal health records, where patients communicate and collaborate with healthcare providers using electronic devices and the Internet, is increasing. This provides a big opportunity for marketers to contact a patient and his family, and it ensures personalized messages. As a response to the growing popularity of mobile devices, the term *mobile marketing* appeared; and it finds an application in the healthcare sector. Mobile applications are one of the fastest growing technologies in healthcare (Garets and Horowitz, 2008: 286–296). Consumers can manage their wellness and chronic health conditions everywhere and all the time as a result it is possible for healthcare providers to gather information about consumers and have personalized communication with them. Furthermore, social media possibilities have also been noticed by healthcare marketers. Social networking is increasing in popularity, and its impact is also growing. Building a community around a brand enables a relationship to begin between consumers and healthcare providers, who can learn a lot about each other. What is more, an interesting trend has appeared called healthy gaming. Consumers are downloading mobile applications or purchasing devices like Wii Fit (part of PlayStation) or software programs and many other interactive programs from healthcare providers in order to manage their health and wellness with a fun element. Interactivity is an important part of the trend, as consumers demand contact with the devices that support them in their health struggles. Applications tell the consumers how to be healthy with healthy eating, running, sleeping and many other things, all in a sort of game that ensures pleasant emotions connected with the healthcare provider that released the device or program (Hollfelder, 2002: 24).

Significant consumer behavior changes have also occurred. Consumers more and more often take care of their healthcare needs on their own by doing research on the Internet or asking for advice from friends. As a result, more and more marketing communication in the healthcare sector is individualized. It is no longer business to business marketing communication, when healthcare products and services were mainly focused on physicians, doctors, and healthcare institutions and, through these 'agents', were communicated to consumers. Nowadays, it is possible to communicate directly with consumers. This is challenging because marketing communication in the healthcare segment has to fulfill several objectives: it needs to educate consumers while at the same time presenting targeted and relevant offers. Another huge dispute that appears in the case of marketing communication in the healthcare market is concerned with emotional, moral, and ethical issues for consumers and other stakeholders with regard to spending money on marketing of services and promotion of drugs instead of proper treatment. Furthermore, healthcare products and services are not the usual products to communicate about as usually it is impossible to touch or feel them. It is a private and sensitive issue especially from a marketing communication point of view. As a result, an assumption was made that for marketing communication to be effective in the case of healthcare, it should be based on trust (Renfrow, 2009: 32–39).

Considering recent consumer behavior changes, it can be concluded that modern marketing communication in the healthcare market is about being integrated and personalized. Integration enables companies to choose the best and the most updated marketing communication tools in order to ensure deep personalization of messages and relevance of information in order to form long-term relationships with consumers (Smith, 2012: 600–602). Each person has a different experience with a disease; as a result, more targeted marketing communication is required to respond to their needs and choices.

To characterize marketing communication in the European healthcare market, a proper analysis of several trends should be done. Direct advertising to consumers in the healthcare market has already been discussed. It can be observed that, especially pharmaceutical industries, have moved from direct-to-physician advertising to direct-to-consumer advertising, called DTCA (L.M. Crawley et. al., 2009: 279). This change occurred because the focus now is placed on the consumer market due to new consumer behavior, the spread of Internet access, and the development of new technologies. DTCA as such is permitted to some extent only in the USA and New Zealand. However, especially pharmaceutical companies influence the countries of the European Union, where a considerable effort has been made to lower the barriers to direct access over the past couple of years. DTCA can now be observed but not in its full potential. The Internet is a powerful tool for direct communication with consumers (World Health Organization, 2009: 644).

It can be observed more and more frequently that companies in the healthcare market utilize ambient media in their marketing communication. Ambient advertising can be defined as unexpected, nontraditional place-based marketing communication. Such a tool has been used by non-healthcare companies for a long time; however, in the healthcare sector it is starting to develop. The strategy is based not only on the consumer but also on the context in which it is placed and in which the consumer will face the message (Reyburn, 2010: 9–11). It is recommended for healthcare providers, especially hospitals, which have tight budgets and should focus their capital on patients' treatment to optimize the marketing communication tools and media performance. As a result, ambient media is recommended as a perfect marketing communication solution. Because of its creativity, it surprises consumers and engages them in a relationship. The cost of advertisement is relatively low, and effectiveness, according to research, is higher (Lega, 2006: 340). Examples of ambient media activities include sponsored goal post pads for a sports medicine practice 'when you break more than a tackle', messages on the floors of hospitals and pharmacies, or posters in buses or trams that promote healthy living like preventing breast cancer (Reyburn, 2010: 9–11).

Branding by healthcare companies is a relatively recent phenomenon. A brand is understood as a name, term, symbol, or design that identifies the goods or services of a seller or group of sellers. Brand identity refers to the visual features that create awareness in the mind of the consumer. These features include things like the brand's name, image, typography, color, package design, and slogans. The aim of the brand image is to distinguish a company's product in the market from the competition in the minds of consumers (Mangini, 2002: 20). Managing a brand was not common among healthcare companies in the past, although some notable exceptions could be observed. An explanation might be the fact that healthcare companies believed that branding is most effective for products that are designed for a mass market, can benefit from advertising, and can be effectively evaluated by consumers. Few healthcare services have these characteristics. Because most healthcare is provided locally, few healthcare organizations need to develop national brand recognition (Gershon, 2003: 12). The lag in managing the brands and application of any brand strategy in healthcare has both a negative and positive influence on healthcare marketing communication. The disadvantage includes a small level of expertise in today's healthcare branding efforts. The advantage, on the other hand, is that the healthcare industry can observe and learn from other industries. The emergence of the new healthcare consumer has provoked an increase in the popularity of branding among healthcare providers (Thomas, 2010: 264).

There are various examples of marketing communication activities, such as hospitals that place ads in newspapers and magazines to promote their facilities and services, run community health programs, have CEOs take part in interviews, or allow a television series to use a hospital image. All of these efforts (advertising, PR, event marketing) go toward building the brand. Many associations turn to social marketing to encourage more people to adopt healthier life styles, like quitting smoking, cutting down on saturated fats in their diet, and increasing exercise (Kotler et al., 2008: 32). In order to really influence the behavior of customers and promote positive health habits, a social marketing relationship with healthcare has developed. Social marketing as a concept can be ideally applied to patient-centered services; however, it demands a deep understanding of the system. Social marketing as connected to healthcare can be understood as promoting healthy behavior changes by first identifying consumers' needs and then using the information gathered to create suitable messages. Social marketing works by eliminating barriers, emphasizing the benefits, and offering incentives to change behavior to healthier ones. Consumers are the main focus of social marketing; as a result, gathering information is crucial. It enables creation of advantageous messages and choosing the most effective marketing communication tools, which can be adjusted to different audience markets (Quinn et. al., 2009: 221–239).

7.4 European healthcare marketing communication

The European healthcare market changed in the 1990s, when the so-called rediscovery of public care took place. Plenty of European countries changed their approach to the health system from a traditional one, which was focused on treating illnesses through use of high-tech hospital services, to community-based healthcare. Countries in Europe started to take measures to integrate health and social care. The challenges faced by the healthcare systems in European countries stimulated the integration strategies (Antunes and Moreira, 2011: 129–135). At the beginning, the concept of healthcare marketing was perceived to be controversial. It can be dated from 1975, when one of the first hospitals formed an official job position as a marketing staff member. This took place in Evanston Hospital in Illinois. Nowadays, more and more institutions present in the healthcare industry, such as rehabilitation centers, doctors, and nonprofit hospitals include marketing in their strategies (Antunes and Moreira, 2011: 129–135).

7.4.1 Healthcare marketing communication in Germany

Germany is one of the largest healthcare markets in the world; it is third largest after the USA and Japan. In Europe, it is the largest healthcare market. The German healthcare market is distinctive because it is composed of health regions with regional and supra-regional cooperation structures aimed at generation of innovations in healthcare (Pfannstiel, 2011: 77–83). This structure creates a health facility that has a bigger impact than within its local borders while ensuring healthcare near the place where people live. It can be assumed that stakeholders saw the need both for a health region with a high level of visibility and pioneering initiative and also an area where stakeholders freely, directly, and actively stand behind it and analyze the course of its development (Lasch, V. et. al., 2010: 15–31). Health regions have become interesting as a brand in Germany, both for private and public institutions, because healthcare offerings, products, and services that cannot be provided on their own power can now be introduced more quickly, less expensively, more reliably, more effectively, and more profitably with the support and cooperation of the regional authorities (Obermann, K. et. al., 2011: online). As a result, a healthcare brand influences a health region and reinforces potential innovation. Moreover, brands applied in innovative healthcare organizational forms are fulfilling the role of symbols for the health region as a whole. Regional healthcare brands are created to increase the general level of healthcare and the health management in a region. The aim of the brand is to support the health region in being a recognized and respected health location in the national health market. It can be stated that innovative organizational forms are unquestionably defined by the stakeholders in a health region. Stakeholders join forces professionally; spread good publicity; and, finally, communicate the healthcare qualities of the initiative to the audience, both on a regional and multiregional level. Stakeholders see the brand as an advantage in terms of high-quality regional healthcare offerings, products, and services (Pfannstiel, 2011: 77–83). The appearance and power of the brand rises and falls with the level of stakeholder and consumer involvement. As a result, it can be concluded that health regions have to create brands in order to be able to emerge and compete effectively. The brand can only be powerful and effective for the health region when both stakeholders and consumers can quickly recall a vibrant brand in their mind. Another condition to be fulfilled is that the healthcare brand is effective when innovative organizational forms are being distinguished by consumers and remembered in a competitive landscape such as healthcare. A brand creates an image and a precisely defined concept of a health region; what is more, it can protect health regions from crises (Schabloski, 2008: 17).

Another important part of healthcare marketing communication in Germany is promotion, which is governed by an authoritative body. The Heilmittelwerbegesetz (HWG) (the Law on Advertising in the Field of Healthcare) governs pharmaceutical promotion, which is only allowed to medical professionals. The communication activities of pharmaceutical companies are also considered advertising under the law, which is challenging for the marketing of prescription drugs (Aspalter, 2012: 25–33). There are also self-imposed restrictions on marketing, with voluntary ethical guidelines outlined by the research and development industry association (Obermann et. al., 2011: online). Communication materials must be issued and fit the tight legal limits. The product cannot be named on promotional materials if patients or public audiences are addressed directly. The press can mention the generic name of the medicine, even though this is also becoming difficult because of changes affecting the media, both financial and in terms of content (Bird and Bird, 2013: online). Campaigns aimed at physicians are allowed in order to promote new products; however, reaching potential customers that are patients is only possible through disease awareness initiatives. Direct-to-consumer advertising is prohibited, so only indications and balanced information about all therapeutic options can be mentioned during health promoting events (International Society for Pharmacoeconomics and Outcomes Research, 2011: online). Another challenge is connected with the need to ensure relationship-based marketing. The marketing communication has to be as tailored as possible, so communication tools and messages must be adjusted to each relevant professional healthcare target group, as there is a huge diversity of specializations and a wide range of professional bodies and associations (Rose, 2001: online).

The Internet as a marketing communication medium is estimated to have a significant role. The 'Cybercitizen Health Europe' study by Manhattan Research indicated that people looking for information about healthcare and pharmaceutical companies, their products, and services are interested in websites but not so keen on becoming fans and getting into relationships on social media communications for that purpose. Germans were the least interested in learning about prescription drugs from pharmaceutical companies. The hypothesized reason for that situation is that they reveal distrust of the industry (Manhattan Research, 2011: online). However, it was found that around 50 percent of doctors use social media, so there are opportunities to connect with medical professionals through social media. Nevertheless, restrictions in promotional tools still apply; and content needs to be maintained and monitored. Growing communities, such as closed networks for doctors, are becoming more important as target audiences. Digital channels usage tends to rise in the case of the healthcare sector (Rose, 2001: online). Digital-based marketing communication is estimated to make up more than 50 percent of all tools used in the healthcare market. In addition, there is a growing emphasis on healthy life education as well as focused activities on the value-added services that have been built up around most major brands (Bird and Bird, 2013: online). The use of smartphones and mobile devices is also spreading in Germany for revealing and accessing medical information online. There are an increasing number of mobile applications available for consumers and doctors, which help with maintaining health diaries used to adjust healthcare services better (Rose, 2001: online).

There are several marketing channels adopted in the healthcare market in order to communicate with the target audience in Germany. Due to the fact that promoting medications to nonprofessionals is legally regulated and in most cases prohibited (Bird and Bird, 2013: online), there are advertisements of the healthcare services provided. Healthcare service providers use both traditional media and ambient ones, like billboards in the subway stations. In the press, an ad might encourage young mothers to go to a doctor to do medical tests. The advertisement is based on an emotional message. The picture presents a mother with a child and says 'I want to protect US when something wrong is happening' and below, is the slogan 'Together it is easier'. The advertisement is meant to show the importance of feeling trustful when going to the doctor. It also indicates that by choosing a particular service provider, the consumer will receive high quality service and care.

Some German healthcare service providers use nontraditional media in marketing communication with consumers; an example is a subway station. In the advertisement, a shocking message is presented. An old woman is shown, dressed in clothes that land a person in a hospital. She has luggage in hand and says 'I want to go home'. The aim of the advertisement is to present the problem of elderly people with memory problems. The advertisement suggests that in a special care center, there are caregivers with more eyes and time to take care of old people with memory problems. The center provides the highest quality of care. On the one hand, there is a shocking image of an old woman without shoes, which is scary; and on the other hand, the image is touching at the same time. The advertisement consists of a promise to take care of relatives when there is not enough time for family members to do so.

It can be concluded that in Germany, plenty of regulations are imposed on healthcare marketing communication. There has been almost no development of marketing communication of medications. The healthcare system, which is very much dependent on the government and with its extraordinary division into regions, results in marketing communication strategies mainly aimed at building relationships with consumers and building the healthcare brand of the region. There are several marketing messages from healthcare service providers; however, they are not well integrated into a coherent message sent through different channels. It is recommended that the healthcare service providers adopt an integrated marketing communication concept because such an approach will support achieving the aim of building a strong brand. Sending a coherent message through traditional channels, like the press and radio; online channels, like e-mails, social media, webpages, and ambient media; or interaction based on new technologies will ensure genuine relationship building and emphasize high quality.

7.4.2 Healthcare marketing communication in the United Kingdom

The United Kingdom healthcare market is governed by an authoritative body called the National Health Service (NHS), which was established on July 5th, 1948. Its mission is to provide healthcare to UK citizens based on need and not the ability to pay (Gray, 2007: 307). In other words, the patients' treatment is free because taxpayers fund the NHS. NHS is constantly developing; and in 2000, it released the NHS Plan, which revolutionized marketing practices in healthcare (Department of Health, 2008: online). Beginning a few years ago, independent health providers could bid for contracts to supply health services on behalf of NHS. Frequently, there is more than just one health provider contracted; so an increase in competition has occurred. As a result, development of integrated marketing communication has been observed in the case of healthcare in the UK.

In general, use of advertising to communicate with consumers is much more popular among private healthcare companies than NHS providers. NHS as a healthcare service provider promotes services to stakeholders instead of directly to consumers. The process usually is more informal, based on the following rule. If there is a primary care practitioner who would like to run a diabetes service in the local town to stop patients from travelling to the main city, such a practitioner goes to the local management body. A discussion is often held on an informal basis. When a contract is concluded, the general practitioner will spread the news to the other general practitioners in the town. Sometimes the general practitioner will inform the local newspaper to spread the news among patients to make them aware that the healthcare service exists locally. This is a combination of personal selling with PR and a kind of advertising in order to communicate with the audience (Gray, 2007: 306–310). Currently, to common practices of marketing communication, online activity is added, with an emphasis on social media. As a result, NHS, along with hospitals, is present on social media sites, especially on Facebook.

Reputation building is also of crucial importance in the case of healthcare marketing communication in the UK. NHS claims that a patient has to trust the quality of treatment; otherwise, the patient will change the healthcare provider. There are ethical standards that rule marketing communication among healthcare providers. What is more, the Department of Health is about to introduce a code for the promotion of NHS services in order to decrease the risk of aggressive marketing. This is a voluntary code that can be applied to service providers under NHS (Bailey, 2007: A35). This change results from the fact that a few years ago, the pharmaceutical industry was accused of being overly generous in giving inappropriate gifts to doctors in order to increase the sale of particular drugs. This led to the situation that in order to save the reputation of healthcare providers, there were numerous ethics codes applied to promote high quality behavior and honest marketing communication. There are authoritative bodies on both the international and national level, which oversee marketing practices. In the UK, that body is the Association of British Pharmaceutical Industries (ABPI). Current codes released by the ABPI have been in place since 2006 and set various regulations on the companies to secure the reputation of healthcare providers by requiring appropriate advertising and communication.

Currently, a change in the environment can be observed, especially in the case of competition in the market. The healthcare market in the UK is more and more fragmented, with a rising number of stakeholders. Competition is increasing as there are healthcare service providers that are alternatives to NHS. These providers observe and identify the errors of the public healthcare system. They provide customers with services of higher quality and communicate this to the audience with greater effectiveness. Alternative healthcare providers indicate the failures of public healthcare to the customers and suggest that private care might be better. To do so, they use marketing communication tools like websites and social media (Norwich Union, 2007: online). It can be concluded that integration of different communication channels and marketing communication tools provides customers with coherent information that matters to the customers. The healthcare market is especially subtle as customers value their health and the reputation of service providers matters a lot (Gray, 2007: 306–310).

In the United Kingdom healthcare market, use of PR marketing communication tools can be seen. A magazine called *Making a Difference* has been seen internationally as a case study of successful use of PR in promoting health itself and also healthcare services. The magazine reaches its audience both online and offline, as it can be downloaded from the website. Moreover, it is useful both for the employees of the healthcare sector and the patients (Gombeski, 2010: 111–114). By examining issues of the magazine, its objectives were identified. First of all, it strengthened the market position of the healthcare service provider that issued the magazine as the 'Advanced Medicine and Patient Care' center. In addition, it enhanced the organizational image and successfully built relationships among UK healthcare employees, patients, referring physicians, and community hospitals (UK Healthy Care, 2013:

online) Another PR tool used by UK healthcare service providers is social media. Social media has enormous potential for contacting consumers any time and every place; and it can ensure interaction between the company and its consumers. There are several profiles of healthcare service providers on social media, and they have a large audience. The United Kingdom is one of the most developed countries in Europe in terms of social media use by hospitals (Van de Belt et. al., 2012: 5).

It can be concluded that in the UK healthcare market, emphasis has been placed on building trust in the quality of services provided and on rescuing the image of healthcare providers. PR as a marketing communication tool is very effective in reaching that goal. Healthcare service providers can observe success stories in the market. Nevertheless, even though some information can be found on the Internet, the potential of the channel is underestimated. The magazines or press releases are not enough to build reliable relationships with the patients. The role of IT and new technology solutions should be appreciated, and professional health advice forums should be created using social media. Special apps, available on mobile phones or laptops, should be utilized in order to ensure constant contact between healthcare service providers and patients. This will ensure effective integration of traditional communication channels, such as the press, with modern ones offered by new technology development. Moreover, PR tools along with online marketing do not seem to be enough. Advertising has been underutilized. This should be changed by adding some advertising in nonprofessional magazines to inform consumers about the necessity of healthcare, even when they do not search for the advice. The UK is the country of origin of several of the most creative and lucrative advertising agencies in the world; as a result, companies very often use unconventional and surprising tools in communicating with consumers. Healthcare service providers should do the same and surprise the consumer by providing original messages using ambient media and guerrilla marketing. Undertaking all the activities advised will ensure full integration of marketing communication and will result in an increase in the loyalty and satisfaction of consumers.

7.4.3 Healthcare marketing communication in Sweden

It can stated that Swedish healthcare marketing communication is, on the one hand, very modern, open minded, and controversial, while, on the other hand, it underlies preventive marketing and emphasizes engaging people in marketing communication. Alcohol prevention occupies a high position in the public health promotion agenda in Sweden. Swedish alcohol policy can be described as a combination of two main barriers to alcohol consumption: first of all, tax-based price controls and second, an alcohol retail monopoly in order to limit the availability and accessibility of alcohol, which is the most controversial policy. Since joining the EU, Sweden has had to change its independent alcohol policy; and alcohol visibility increased. However, it still has one of the most strict policies in Europe, believing this is the most effective health promotion tool. In 2002, there was an innovative plan implemented that was based on cooperation between government and the voluntary sector, whose aim was to promote healthy lifestyles and prevent alcohol consumption. The plan was introduced by the National Board of Health and Welfare. The majority of the projects have had teenagers and children as the target group. Some examples of efforts are symposiums, nationwide conferences, dialogs, consultations, support for voluntary groups to strengthen their competence, and all kinds of promotion events (Eriksson, 2011: 8–14).

Some controversial advertising can be observed. As an example, a description of advertising from the Stockholm South General Hospital in Sweden follows. During the summer of 2012, the hospital decided to launch a campaign to look for nurse employees for emergency departments. The announcement, however, was not a usual one as it contained very humorous and erotic content. The image shown in the TV campaign was a 'hot nurse', looking very attractive and wearing very tight clothes and visible underwear. The aim of the campaign was to generate buzz about the hospital; and, despite the controversial content, the aim was fulfilled successfully. The description of the campaign can be found in international online sources, while nationally it generated enormous buzz both on the Internet and in traditional media like TV and radio. The information about the hospital was spread through multiple channels only because of the original and shocking message. On the website of the hospital, official information could be found that in reality the hospital was looking for a highly qualified nurse, regardless of appearance. Based on that situation, it can be observed that Sweden has tried some experiments with healthcare marketing communication and represents a quite modern approach. As a result, the image of healthcare is fresh and modern (Llorens, 2012).

In Sweden, there are projects that aim to promote a healthy lifestyle. During these projects, the health sector employees are engaged in activities. Coaches are present, whose role is to be local practical ambassadors of the venture, organizing tutorials, contests, and theme-related events. Special books are issued that contain ideas for activities. Several examples of activities are a pedometer competition between different departments, creation of a cookbook with healthy recipes, or production of an educational television show. Healthcare employees play a central role in the show; their aim is health promotion and lifestyle information for stakeholders (patients, society). This kind of project led to the conclusion that healthcare professionals' private lifestyle habits can influence both their attitude and their counseling of patients. Therefore, healthcare marketing communication in Sweden is done using a completely new approach. There are efforts to increase knowledge among healthcare professionals about their own lifestyle and to identify the potential barriers to lifestyle changes for this group, including motivation, as it is the main issue in the attempt to promote healthy behaviors (Jonsdottir, 2011: 448–456). On the other hand, Swedish hospitals use LinkedIn as a channel to connect with potential employees; so, in general, the image of the hospital as an employer is professional (HospitalsEU, 2011: online).

Based on the examples that have been described, it can be stated that healthcare marketing communication in Sweden is very much social based. This means that it engages the community in different types of social events. The healthcare professionals are responsible for providing evidence of how to live a healthy life. When utilizing advertising in marketing communication, the Swedish healthcare sector is not afraid of new, fresh, and controversial images. On the other hand, it cannot be said that the marketing communication is fully integrated. Indeed, online tools like social media combined with direct, personal communication and event-based marketing are used; however, there is little use of traditional advertising on television or radio or in the press, which could increase the awareness of consumers. Nevertheless, marketing communication and its integration in Sweden is judged to be very good; and the choice of healthcare providers seems to be reasonable, based on an understanding of the community.

7.4.4 Healthcare marketing communication in Belgium

The Belgian healthcare market, in terms of healthcare marketing communication, is divided, according to the language of the inhabitants, into two main regions: Flemish and Dutch. Therefore, there are more cultural boundaries than legal ones connected to marketing communication with consumers. The legal situation is somewhat similar to the one in Germany. The system is based on compulsory healthcare insurance, which is managed by insurance funds that might be independent of the government (Lega, 2005: 340). The division into two separate regions is a big marketing communication challenge.

In the Flemish community, the implementation of health promotion and preventive healthcare policies has been decentralized by establishing local health networks called LOGOs. Cooperation of health workers from different sectors facilitates the disbursement of information about healthcare providers and preventive healthcare activities. LOGOs are intended to lead health promotion work at the district level and cover a territory with around 300 000 inhabitants. They are composed of local initiatives and structures already in existence and are meant to include all health and welfare workers, such as general practitioners (GPs), pharmacists, dieticians, representatives of the local hospitals and rest homes, medical school managers, health center representatives, and so on. Each of twenty-six LOGOs is supported and coordinated by a multidisciplinary central team and has to implement evidence-based actions, which aim to reach certain health targets set by the government. Actions are based on relationship marketing and composed of marketing communication tools that engage the community and convey a coherent message about the aims to be fulfilled and about heath care service providers. The main aims are the prevention of infectious diseases, which needs to be significantly improved. In particular, attempts are made to further increase vaccinations for polio, whooping cough, tetanus, diphtheria, measles, mumps, and rubella. Moreover, emphasis is placed on increased efficiency in breast cancer screening: the share of the target group (women between 50 and 69 years old) as a percentage of the total number of screenings should increase to 80%, and the number of women screened from that specific target group should increase to 75% (Corens, 2007: 99–125).

The government of the French community defines its objectives for health promotion in a five-year program. The priorities, which are a pillar for healthcare marketing communication, are prevention of addiction, cancer, infectious diseases, and traumas; and promotion of security, physical activity, dental health, cardiovascular health, well-being, and mental health. In addition, a priority is placed on promotion of children's health. In the French community, healthcare marketing communication is organized mainly by the Local Centers for Health Promotion (CLPS), which aim at coordination of both the local implementation of the five-year program and community plans for health promotion. These centers operate on behalf of all the actors within their territory (Corens, 2007: 99–125).

Belgium's health service is said to have easy accessibility and high-quality treatments. Belgium promotes its healthcare market in the European landscape as one with 4 doctors per 1000 inhabitants. With that statistic, Belgium is well above the OECD 2.9 average. Belgian hospitals are equipped with advanced technology and run by highly qualified staff. The Belgian healthcare system is well developed, with a large number of specialized centers and international approaches. Furthermore, there are several Belgian companies that have become international players in the medical equipment and software sectors. Therefore, the advertisements of healthcare providers are focused on the high quality of the equipment and design. The messages emphasize the modernity and professionalism of the services provided. The marketing communication is based mainly on Internet channels and elegant leaflets.

The Belgian healthcare market can be differentiated from other European markets because it has an international approach in its marketing communication strategies. There is an organization that is aimed at providing foreigners with information about Belgian healthcare. Healthcare Belgium is a nonprofit organization established in 2007 by eleven top Belgian hospital groups. The organization receives substantial support from Agfa Healthcare, Dexia Bank, the Federation of Enterprises in Belgium (VBO-FEB), the Virtual Colonoscopy Teaching Centre (VCTC), and Ion Beam Applications (IBA). Its main goal is to provide information on Belgian medical services to foreign patients and healthcare providers in an ethical and coordinated way. The marketing communication with international customers is based on relationship marketing, in which customer feedback is the most important pillar of communication (Healthcare Belgium, 2011: online).

Despite the statement that the Belgian healthcare market is an international one with multicultural approaches; in reality, the environment is very strict. Even though it is called one of the best healthcare systems in Europe (The Guardian, 2011: online), it is certainly not the best in terms of integrated marketing communication. It is difficult to find any information about the marketing communication that has been adopted. There are several actions undertaken in order to promote a healthy lifestyle and prevention of illnesses or to promote the modernity and quality of highly developed equipment. Several English language websites can be found that provide consumers with full information about the healthcare market in Belgium. All types of updates, from innovative actions undertaken in hospitals to instructions about what to do when sick, can be found on these websites (Health Belgium, 2013: online). Belgium has one of the highest usages of social media (Facebook, LinkedIn, and Youtube) by hospitals in communicating with consumers (van de Belt, 2012: 5). Nevertheless, there are no other straightforward marketing communication tools that have been adopted in order to communicate with patients.

7.4.5 Healthcare marketing communication in Poland

Some legal regulations limit marketing communication in the healthcare market in Poland. It is crucial to emphasize that public healthcare was reformed in order to be ruled by free market regulations so that the quality of the services provided would improve. Rapid reformation of public healthcare turned out to be impossible, but private healthcare is supposed to be competitive, developed, and highly professional. At the same time, there are strict regulations imposed on service providers in terms of marketing communication of healthcare services. In Poland, there were discussions about models of healthcare marketing communication strategies (MedicaPR, 2013: online). According to the first approach, the healthcare sector should not be any different than any other commercial sector; and healthcare services should be treated the same as other services according to free trade rules. The second approach perceives healthcare as an exceptional sector based on rules of the medical profession in which health is the priority. In this approach, healthcare cannot be ruled by free market mechanisms. These discussions led to controversies over marketing communication in the Polish healthcare market. It is hard to differentiate when necessary information is being provided to the market about services and when information provided by doctors should be called promotion, which is prohibited. To regulate the issue, the Naczelna Rada Lekarska got involved. According to that body, several actions can be taken by doctors that are aimed at informing customers but not promoting a doctor's practice (Krzyżowski, 2008: online):

- a limit of two information signs outside the building where the practice is conducted and not more than two signs on the way to the building;
- press releases in the special space devoted to healthcare services;
- information in the yellow pages; and
- electronic information, website special telephone numbers.

This list is all that is allowed, so additional channels providing information about a doctor's practice are not allowed, for example, the postings or flyers.

However, for several years, in spite of the strict regulations, an increasing number of social campaigns organized by public healthcare service providers are occurring. The campaigns are created in order to raise awareness about social and healthcare problems. The dynamic development of programs and plans in the area of public health organized by the World Health Organization influenced the approach of Polish employees in public healthcare institutions, who initiated and got involved in a variety of social marketing campaigns, like prevention programs or campaigns aimed at combating modern social health problems (Kowalski, 2011: 2–5). For example, for several years, there has been an emphasis put on early recognition and, therefore, complete treatment of female diseases. An increasing number of offline and online campaigns encourage women to do necessary medical examinations. As an example, a campaign conducted in Warsaw can be described. The campaign was created in cooperation with the largest lingerie brand: Triumph. After shopping, when leaving the store, women could hear the sound of the anti-stealing gate in the front of the store. Shocked women asked the clerk what was going on because they had not stolen anything. They learned that the clerk had discreetly hidden a special transmitter inside the bag, which made the noise. Along with the transmitter, a leaflet was attached that encouraged them to seek preventive care: 'Don't let yourself be shocked. Go to mammography' (Hatalska, 2011: online). Another example is encouraging women to do a cytology test. Encouragement is based on a simple association with death – 'Don't pack yourself into a coffin; – do cytology'. In addition, there was an integrated online campaign, whose basic idea was to visit a website. On the website, women could find information about cytology tests, cancer, and other sicknesses, along with useful links.

Another example of a campaign encouraging tests is one wholly prepared by a private clinic, which encourages men to have medical tests. The campaign is called 'male things', and its main slogan is 'Tested man – do it once but well'. A picture shows three well-dressed men, who are meant to be perceived as men who think seriously about themselves and about their health too.

Research showed that the private healthcare market (the one in which services are provided for an additional payment) has enormous potential. Public healthcare should focus its marketing activities on building added value for customers because according to customers, it lacks quality in comparison to private care. Use of services that require an additional payment is becoming more and more common. Private clinics, hospitals, and other healthcare service providers operate in an increasingly competitive environment. Private healthcare is not limited to big cities anymore; the range of the private services has spread. The image of private healthcare is that it is trustworthy because of marketing communication based on the promises of professionalism, a friendly atmosphere, or simply availability. This marketing effort seems to have been very effective (Klein and Kubicz, 2007: online).

Research was conducted to analyze whether there is a demand for private healthcare, and a specific customer profile was defined: a customer sensitive to high quality services. Such a profile is used by marketers to develop the most effective approach to marketing communication. It can also be observed that there is increasing competitiveness in the healthcare market. To communicate with an audience that demands high quality and professionalism, careful decisions are made about the marketing communication tools used to communicate the competitive advantage of private healthcare service providers.

The private sector emphasizes the comfort of treatment in its marketing communication. For example, Medicover hospitals use phrases like exceptional comfort; individual, personalized treatment; atmosphere of partnership; and extremely comfortable conditions. Medicover differentiates itself from other private and public clinics by putting an emphasis on relationships, while the other healthcare service providers in Poland focus on modernity. What is more, personalization of services communicates to customers that they will not wait in 'never-ending' queues to see a doctor, which was common in Poland. Medicover does not have a tradition in Poland. It is the first non-public hospital in the country that is so large and that specializes in multiple areas. As a result, in its marketing communication, it sends a coherent message that it is comfortable and personalized, which results in a competitive advantage over its public and private competitors (Nazarko-Ludwiczak, 2012: online). Medicover communicates with patients through multiple marketing channels, which reflects its complex attitude and professional service. There are advertisements in the press and radio that communicate the possibility of doing basic tests in a reasonable amount of time and that indicate that the patient is the focus of care. The message is clearly directed at the feelings of the Polish patient, who for several years did not feel cared about by public healthcare. Medicover makes its campaign available in online channels to emphasize the possibility of staying in touch or registering with doctors through online channels. Medciover advertisements were also placed on buses. It can be observed that Medicover uses IMC concepts in planning its marketing communication strategy.

On the other hand, besides Medicover, there is a competitive healthcare service provider – LuxMed, which uses a different approach in communications with consumers. Its campaigns were based on a concept in which a doctor was compared to an artist. The advertisements were placed on the Internet and in the press. An association with famous arts could be observed, and the slogan said: 'Medicine is an art'.

In general, the price of healthcare services in the private sector are said to be too high. However, if the marketing communication tools are chosen effectively, they decrease the number of negative opinions about the price. The majority of Poles believe, whether they use private or public service providers, that private healthcare providers offer services of better quality. There are two main reasons for this belief. Common criticism of public healthcare together with the colorful advertisements and ubiquitous PR of private healthcare have resulted in private healthcare being perceived as having higher quality. Private clinics use young beautiful people in fresh uniforms, which, even if unbelievable, is highly effective. Advertisements of healthcare services are still perceived as dangerous and unnecessary. However, it can be observed that advertisements stimulate competitiveness in the healthcare market, which is necessary in order to improve the quality of services provided. On the other hand, despite significant levels of legal regulation in connection to medicine, there is an increasing amount of medical advertising. The tendency should be changed because people should be encouraged to have more treatments and medical tests and not encouraged to buy more and more medicine advertised by fake nurses. For the past few months, there have been advertisements of sexual life improvement medicine during every hour of the day. Based on that, it is recommended that legal regulations should focus more on the area of sales of medications and not on advertising from healthcare providers. The attitudes of both society and marketers towards marketing communication of healthcare services are changing, and they should change because of the possible positive consequences of marketing communication on the society. It can be a stimulus to improve the standard of services provided, and the percentage of people cured can be increased because of the greater awareness of different medical tests that need to be done. Moreover, internationally increased use of social media can be observed in communications with the target market of healthcare services. A majority of the population is looking for medical information online (BrandPro, 2013: online); therefore, it is one of the most effective marketing communication channels to think about when planning marketing strategy. It can be stated that the private sector of healthcare services has embraced an integrated marketing communication approach by engaging multiple channels to communicate about its services. Nevertheless, the public sector is not following up at present. It is recommended, therefore, that public healthcare providers activate communication first through Internet channels other than simple websites, which contain contact information only. The approach should be more patient oriented and not patient hostile as it sometimes is at present. Public healthcare providers should send a coherent message about the changes they need to undertake.

Conclusions

Several trends can be observed in the European healthcare market that have a strong influence on marketing communication development and evolution. Almost unlimited access to the Internet, which influences institutions and consumer behavior, can be discussed in several dimensions. First of all, it can be analyzed as a tool in the hands of institutions. It can be used to support creation of a brand and communicate with stakeholders. The web provides the possibility of creating a platform where different types of data can be gathered, exchanged, communicated, and accessed by suppliers, consumers, and buyers. On the other hand, this trend can be viewed as the reason for the greater transparency of information about institutions and their services. Consumers gain access to the information. They have become aware of the ability to form communities on the Internet in order to share the experience they had with an institution and the quality of care provided. The Internet enables more interaction among market members. Healthcare providers turn to relationship marketing in order to build long-term and, as a result, profitable relationships with customers.

The European market is complex. Despite being members of the European Union, the markets differ; and, as a result, the tools utilized in marketing communication differ as well. Nevertheless, it can be observed that there is an increasing awareness of the power of integrated marketing communication in the European healthcare market. More and more frequently, institutions use several marketing communication tools and channels to communicate with customers. What is more, it can be observed that marketing communication practices are more customer-centered. They are focused not only on profits but also on promoting positive health behaviors. There is still a big gap between the integration of marketing communication tools in the majority of other industries and their use in healthcare; however, rapid development can be observed in the health sector. The analysis of five different healthcare markets, illustrated by Germany, the United Kingdom, Sweden, Belgium, and Poland, showed that despite different approaches, building a trustful brand is of crucial importance for healthcare providers. It can be observed that few marketing communication features are common to all the markets. The Internet and PR are one of the most common toosl in the hands of marketers, but many other channels are integrated into marketing communication strategies in order to create a coherent message for building long-term relationships with customers. The culture of the healthcare market is different than a decade ago, and it has the potential to reach genuine excellence. The analysis of integrated marketing communication in the European market was based on secondary sources and contains only a few examples. It is recommended that further research be conducted on the five markets in the future to develop greater insight into the issue.

References

Antunes, V. & Moreira, P. 2011. Approaches to developing integrated care in Europe: a systematic literature review. *Journal of Management & Marketing in Healthcare*, vol.4, no. 2.

Aspalter, C. 2012.*Healthcare systems in Asia and Europe*, New York, Routledge.

Bearden W., Ingram T. & LaForge R. 2001. *Marketing. Principles & Perspectives*, Sydney, McGraw Hill Irwin.

Belch, G. E, Powell, I. & Kerr, G. F. 2008. *Advertising and Promotion. An integrated marketing communication approach.* Sydney, McGraw Hill.

Berkowitz, E. 2011. *Essentials of Healthcare Marketing.* Toronto, Jones&Bartlett Learning.

Biley, J.E. 2007 HealthCARE principles: a model for healthy city collaborative, Prev Chronic Diseases, April.

Bird and Bird, 2013. The evolution of new advertising techniques. Germany, Retrived June 13, 2013 from <http://ec.europa.eu/avpolicy/docs/library/studies/finalised/bird_bird/pub_de.pdf>

Blakeman, R. 2007. *Integrated Marketing Communication. Creative strategy from the idea to implementation.* New York: Rowman and Littlefield Publishers.

Blythe, J. 2002. *Komunikacja marketingowa.* Warszawa: PWE.

BrandPro, 2013. Social media w marketing usług medycznych, Retrieved September 17, 2013 from http://brandpro.pl/social_media_w_marketingu_uslug_medycznych

City, M. 2005. Integrated marketing communications. *Marketing communications management.*

Clow K. & Baack D. 2002. *Integrated Advertising, Promotion & Marketing Communications.* London: Prentice Hall.

Corens, D. 2007. Belgium. Health System Review. *Health systems in Transitions*, vol 9, no.2.

Crawley, L.M., Hisaw, L. & Illes, J. 2009. 'Direct-to-consumer advertising In Black and white. Racial Differences in placement patterns of print advertisements for health products and messages.' *Health Marketing Quarterly*, 26, 4.

Department of Health 2008. The NHS Plan. Retrieved May 02, 2013 from <http://www.dh.gov.uk>.

Eriksson, C, Geidne, S, Larsson, M, & Pettersson, C. 2011. 'A Research Strategy Case Study of Alcohol and Drug Prevention by Non-Governmental Organizations in Sweden 2003–20', *Substance Abuse Treatment, Prevention & Policy*, 6, 1.

Garets, D. & Horowitz, J. 2008. 'Healthcare ICT in Europe. Understanding trends in adoption and governance.' *Journal of Management and Marketing in Healthcare* vol. 1, no.3, p. 286–296

Gershon, H. J. 2003. 'Strategic positioning. Where does your organization stand.' *Journal of Healthcare Management*, iss. 48, vol. 1.

Gombeski: Public Relations in Health services, Making a Difference case study, Health Marketing Quarterly, Haworth Press.

Gray, S.J. 2008. 'Healthcare marketing has five "P"s.' *Journal of Management and Marketing in Healthcare*, vol.1, no.3.

Groom, A.S. 2008. 'Integrated Marketing Communication' Communication Research Center, *Quarterly Review of Communication Research*, vol. 27, no. 4.

Gurau, C. 2008. 'Integrated online communication. Implementation and management. Integrated online marketing communication.' Emerald Group Publishing, vol. 12, no. 3.

Hatalska, N. 2011. Archived article, Retrieved March 27, 2011 from <http://www.hatalska.com>

Health Belgium. 2013. Retrieved June 24, 2013 from <http://www.health.belgium.be>

Healthcare Belgium. 2011. Discover Excellence, Retrieved May 15, 2013 from <http://www.healthcarebelgium.com/fileadmin/user_upload/Healthcare_Belgium/brochure/Brochure_web_new.pdf>

Hollfelder, J. 2002. 'A new era for marketing health services.' *Marketing health services*, iss. 22, vol. 2.

Holm, O. 2006. Integrated marketing communication. From tactic to strategy, *International Journal on Corporate Communication*. Stockholm, vol. 11, iss. 2.

HospitalsEU. 2011. *Use of social Media by Hospitals in Sweden* Retrieved October 2013 from < http://hospitalseu.wordpress.com/2011/01/10/use-of-social-media-by-hospitals-in-sweden-part-2/>

International Society for Pharmoeconomics and Outcomes Research, 2011. Germany. Medical Devices, retrieved June 15, 2013, from <http://www.ispor.org/htaroadmaps/germanymd.asp>

Jonsdottir, I, Börjesson, M. & Ahlborg, J. 2011, 'Healthcare workers' participation in a healthy lifestyle- promotion project in western Sweden', *BMC Public Health*, 11, Suppl 4.

Keller, K.L. 2001. Mastering the Marketing Communications Mix, Journal of Marketing Management, westburn Publisher Limited, Volume: 17 Issue: 7.

Klein, N, & Kubicz, I. 2007. Rynek. Na drodze leczenie – marketing? In: Marketing w praktyce, 4/2007, Retrieved June, 4 2013 from <http://marketing.org.pl/index.php/go=2/act=2/aid=m46012fbb721dc>

Kotler, P, Shalkowitz, J. & Stevens, R.J. 2008. *Strategic Marketing for Healthcare organizations, Building a Customer Driven health System.* San Francisco: Jossey-Bass.

Kotler, P. 2003. *Marketing management-analysis, planning, implementation and control.* New York. Prentice Hall.

Kowalski, P. 2011. *Poradnik Marketing Społeczny dla zdrowia kobiet.* Łódź. Stowarzyszenie Zdrowych Miast Polskich.

Krzyżowski, P. 2008. Marketing w Służbie Zdrowia, Retrieved June, 5 2013, from <http://www.nowoczesna-klinika.pl/pl/artykuly/15/zarzadzanie/1/293/Marketing_w_Sluzbie_Zdrowia>

Lasch, V., Sonntag, U. & Maschewsky-Schneide, U. 2010. *Equity in Access to Health Promotion, Treatment and Care for all European Women,* Kassel. Kassel University Press.

Lega, F. 2006. *Developing a marketing function in public Healthcare systems: A framework for action.* Health Policy 78, Dublin, Elsevier Ireland Ltd.

Llorens, I. 2012. *Swedish Hospital Places Ad Seeking 'Hot" Nurses* Retrieved October 2013 from <http://www.huffingtonpost.com/2012/02/21/swedish-hospital-hot-nurses-ad_n_1291329.html>

Madhavaram, S. & Badrinarayanan, V. 2005. Integrated marketing communication (IMC) and brand identity as critical components of brand equity strategy: A conceptual framework and research propositions, *American Journal of Advertising.*

Mangini, M. K. 2002. Branding 101. *Marketing Health Services* vol. 22 (3), 20–23.

Manhattan Research, 2013. *Cybercitizen Health Europe,* Retrieved May, 20 2013, from <www.manhattanresearch.com>

MedicaPR. 2013. Jak reklamować usługi medyczne bez reklamy. Retrieved September 10, 2013 from <http://medicapr.pl/o-nas/aktualnosci/item/49-jak-reklamowa%C4%87-us%C5%82ugi-medyczne-bez-reklamy>

Nazarko-Ludwiczak, E. 2012. *Atrybuty przypisywane własnej marce – komunikacja marketingowa na witrynach internetowych polskich jednostek ochrony zdrowia.* Retrieved May 29, 2013 from: <http://www.zdrowie.abc.com.pl/ko/czytaj/-/artykul/atrybuty-przypisywane-wlasnej-marce–komunikacja-marketingowa-na-witrynach-internetowych-polskich-jednostek-ochrony-zdrowia>

Norwich Union. 2007. Single-sex scandal hits NHS, retrieved May 20, 2013 from: <www.norwichunion.com>

O'Guinn T., Allen C. & Semenik R. 2011. *Advertising and Integrated Brand Promotion,* Mason. South-Western, Cengage Learning.

Obermann, K, Mueller, P, Mueller, H, Schmidt, B. & Glazinski, B. 2013. Understanding the German Healthcare System, Retrieved June 14, 2013, from <http://miph.umm.uni-heidelberg.de/miph/cms/upload/pdf/GHCS_Kap._7.pdf>

Pabian A. 2008. *Promocja. Nowoczesne środki i formy.* Warszawa: Difin.

Parada H. & Homan M. 2010. Promoting Community Change: Making it happen in a real world. Belmont: Cengage Brain.

Pelsmacker P., Geuens M. & Bergh J. 2007. *Marketing Communications. A European Perspective.* London: Pearson Education.

Percy, L.C. 2008. *Strategic Integrated Marketing Communications.* Oxford. Elsevier Inc.

Pfannstiel, M.A. 2011. 'Positioning and self-presentation of innovative organizational forms on the European healthcare market', *Journal of Marketing and Management in Healthcare,* vol. 4, no.2.

Pickton, D. & Broderick, A. 2005. *Integrated Marketing Communication,* Essex: Prentice Hall.

Pilarczyk, B. 2008. Procesy komunikacji marketingowej a pozycjonowanie marek. In: Sobczyk, G. (Ed) *Współczesny marketing. Trendy. Działania*. Warszawa: PWE.

Quinn, G, Ellery, J., Detman L.A., Jeffers, D., Gorski, P.A, Singer, L.T. & Mahan C.S. 2009. 'Creating patient-centred healthcare practices. Social marketing tools and strategies.' *Journal of Management and Marketing in Healthcare*, vol. 2, no. 3.

Renfrow, J. 2009. Healthcare marketing 2.0, *Response Magazine*, no. 2.

Reyburn, D. 2010. *Ambient Advertising. Healthcare media in new context*, MHS.

Rose, C. 2001. Health Promotion in Primary Healthcare: General Practice. Country Report – Germany, German Society of General Practice, Retrieved May, 14 2013, from <http://www.univie.ac.at>

Rydel, M. 2001. Komunikacja jako element marketingu, In Rydel, M. (Ed.) *Komunikacja marketingowa*. Gdańsk: Ośrodek Doradztwa i Doskonalenia Kadr.

Schabloski, A.J. 2008. Healthcare systems around the world. Insure the unsured Projects, p.17, retrieved June, 15 2013 from: <www.itup.org/Reports/Fresh%20Thinking/Health_Care_Systems_Around_World.pdf.>

Smith, B.G. 2012. 'Communication integration. An analysis of context and conditions.' *Public Relations Review*, vol. 38.

Szymoniuk B. 2005. Komunikacja Marketingowa-istota i proces projektowania. In szymoniuk, B. (Ed) *Komunikacja marketingowa. Instrumenty i metody*. Warszawa PWE.

The Guardian. 2011. How Europeans run national health services, Retrieved June, 24 2013 from: < http://www.theguardian.com/healthcare-network/2011/may/11/european-healthcare-services-belgium-france-germany-sweden>

Thomas, R. K.. 2010. Marketing Health Services, Chicago: Health Administration Press.

UK Healthy Care. 2013. Retrieved September 14, 2013 from: <http://ukhealthcare.uky.edu/pubs/difference/>

Van de Belt, T, Berben, S, Samsom, M, Engelen, L, & Schoonhoven, L. 2012, 'Use of Social Media by Western European Hospitals: Longitudinal Study', *Journal Of Medical Internet Research*, 14, 3.

Weiss, R. 2011. Healthcare marketing today is about more than Sick ads. It's about engaging with communities. *Marketing Health Services*, Fall 2011.

Wiktor J. 2006. *Promocja. System komunikacji przedsiębiorstwa z rynkiem*. Warszawa: Wydawnictwo naukowe PWN.

World Health Organization. 2009. Direct-to-consumer advertising under fire. *Bulletin of WHO*, vol. 87, no. 8.

Ziglio, E., Hagard, S. & Griffiths, J. 2000. Health promotion development in Europe: achievements and challenges, *Health Promotion International*, Oxford. Oxford University Press, vol. 15, no. 2.

Beatrix Dietz and Andreas Zaby

8 Strategic Decisions under the EU Regulatory Framework for Orphan Drugs

Abstract This chapter focuses on the effects of the regulatory framework for orphan drugs in the European Union (EU) on company strategy. We have analyzed all 68 orphan drugs that have received designation and marketing authorization in the EU for the treatment of rare diseases since 2000 and obtain the following key findings: There is supporting evidence that the incentives provided by the EU Regulation No. 141/2000 have a positive effect on small companies' likelihood of developing and receiving designations for orphan drugs. However, of these small companies, only very few are able to take the orphan drugs they developed all the way through to market launch. In order to avoid their strong marketing dependence on big pharmaceutical companies new incentives appear necessary.

Keywords: Biotechnology, Market exclusivity, Marketing authorization, Orphan drug, Rare disease

8.1 Introduction

More than 27 million people suffer from rare and often life-threatening diseases in the European Union (EU) (EU 2009: 7). This market segment has undergone considerable change since the adoption of Regulation (EC) No. 141/2000, which aims at creating incentives for research, development and marketing of **orphan drugs**. In order to shed light on whether the incentives are taking effect and which type of companies are taking advantage of them, a study was conducted at the Berlin School of Economics and Law. The results show that particularly the very small, start-up type, firms participate in the development of orphan drugs. However, these firms rarely turn out to be the holders of the marketing authorization (MAA) for the developed drugs. The incentives, therefore, do not appear to be sufficient to enable sustainable success of such start-ups in terms of independence and profitability.

8.2 Background

8.2.1 Current Situation and the EU Regulatory Framework for Orphan Drugs

The topic of Research & Development (R&D) for and marketing of orphan drugs, i.e., drugs for treating rare diseases, has been receiving increasing attention in the context of health policy in recent years (Zaby 2011: 291–306, Melnikova 2012: 267–268, Franko 2013: 163–172, Drummond and Towse 2014: 1–7). Only about a third of the roughly 7,000 rare diseases can be treated (NIH 2007). The EU uses a prevalence criterion in conjunction with its legislation on orphan medicinal products, i.e., a prevalence of no more than 5 in 10,000 individuals within the EU. In relation to the total population of the EU this results in an absolute prevalence of ~250,000 individuals and a relative prevalence of about 0.05% in the EU. In order to improve the treatment situation of the affected patients the European legislative framework on orphan medicinal products was adopted on 16 December 1999 by way of Regulation (EC) No. 141/2000 of the European Parliament and the Council, and became law upon publication on 22 January 2000. It became applicable as of 27 April 2000, the date of the adoption of the implementing Commission Regulation (EC) No. 847/2000. The purpose of the framework is to lay down a Community procedure for the designation of medicinal orphan products and to provide incentives for R&D and marketing of designated orphan drugs. Similar legislation had already been enacted in the USA, Japan, and Australia in 1983, 1993, and 1998, respectively.

Apart from the centralized MAA procedure, the framework provides for the following incentives:

- **Protocol assistance:** The European Medicines Agency (EMA) is obliged to provide assistance prior to the submission of an application for MAA concerning the conduct of the various tests and trials necessary to demonstrate the quality, safety, and efficacy of a medicinal product. This assistance is referred to as protocol assistance and is free of charge.
- **Market exclusivity:** When an MAA is granted for a designated orphan product, the community and the member states may not, for a period of ten years, accept another application for an MAA, or grant an MAA or accept an application to extend an existing MAA for the same therapeutic indication. This incentive applies without prejudice to intellectual property law and is referred to as the market exclusivity incentive.
- **Other incentives:** Under these incentives, holders of orphan product designations shall be eligible for incentive made available by the Community and member states that support R&D as well as the availability of such products. This type of incentive mainly refers to grants and fee reductions or waivers, particularly for small and medium-size companies.

This relatively small yet complex market segment has become rather dynamic (Moors and Faber 2007: 343–347). Large pharmaceuticals companies are facing severe strategic challenges in their traditional business model to develop so-called blockbuster drugs for indications with very high prevalence. Drug development pipelines are not as full as they have been and R&D productivity seems to be decreasing despite ever increasing levels of R&D expenditures. Many patents for some of the best-selling drugs in the world have recently expired or are about to expire soon like Pfizer's Lipitor. Furthermore, there is considerable downward pressure on drug prices from payers and third-party providers (Kaitin 2010: 356–357). It is against this background that large pharmaceutical and large biotechnology companies appear to become strategically interested in the orphan drug segment. Many of these corporations have created dedicated business units or other forms of focusing on such therapeutics, including global players like AstraZeneca, Eli Lilly, GlaxoSmithKline, Novartis, and Pfizer. Large companies have also been active in forming collaborative alliances or acquiring small biotechnology firms with the goal of gaining access to the target companies' orphan drug pipelines (Phillipidis 2011: 1037–1040; Rzakhanov 2008: 679–681).

Thus, the aim of this study is to determine which type of companies take advantage of the incentives granted by the EU Regulation (EC) No. 141/2000. In a first step, we analyze which type of companies develop orphan drugs and hold an MAA for the developed orphan drug. We also look at which strategic decisions are taken by companies in this field, e.g., acquisitions. Last but not least, we conclude by providing recommendations for changes to the regulatory framework in order to improve the treatment situation of patients afflicted by **rare diseases**.

8.2.2 Analytical Approach

The study includes orphan drugs that have applied for an orphan drug designation between 2000 – when Regulation (EC) No. 141/2000 became effective – and 2011 and have received an MAA. These criteria apply to a total of 68 drugs of which 62 are still registered in the Community register of orphan medicinal products. As MAA withdrawal is assumed to have no effect on the relevance of the incentives all 68 orphan drugs are included in the study. Orphan drugs for which an orphan drug designation application was not submitted prior to MAA are not included as incentives do not apply.

To determine for which companies the incentives are particularly attractive, companies were classified according to their business focus and economic strength.

The business focus is categorized as: Biotech (dependent on a company's core competence in the field of pharmaceutical biotechnology), pharma, generic, service (companies that offer services for selected activities along the pharmaceutical industry's value chain, such as clinical trials or registration), as well as governmental and academic institutions, mainly health research institutes and universities.

Economic strength is categorized according to annual sales for the fiscal year 2010. Prior years were adjusted for inflation. Following the EU's definition of categories, albeit with higher Euro-amount thresholds, companies were classified as micro enterprises (sales < € 20 million), small enterprises (sales < € 100 million), and medium-sized enterprises (< € 500 million) (EU 2003: 39). In addition, the categories large enterprise (sales < € 3 billion) and big pharma (≥ € 3 billion) were formed.

8.3 Market Dynamics and Strategic Decisions in the Orphan Drug Segment

8.3.1 Designation and Holder of Marketing Authorization

To assess for which companies the incentives act as the strongest stimulator, the 68 orphan drugs were analyzed on the basis of which company developed the drug and received the orphan drug designation and which company holds the MAA. The results are summarized in Figure 8.1.

It is notable that neither **generic drug companies** nor governmental and academic institutions are significantly involved in the development of orphan drugs or hold an MAA. However, this is not very surprising given that a high number of orphan drugs are innovative and research intensive medicines for which the required competencies concerning development, marketing and other factors are very different from those in the generics field. The low involvement of governmental and academic institutions was also to be expected. While it cannot be ruled out that such organizations participate in early-stage pharmaceutical R&D they do reach the limitations of their competencies and financial resources when it comes to funding and execution of clinical trials as well as drug marketing. The absence of service providers is, perhaps, more surprising and will be discussed in more detail in section 8.2.3.

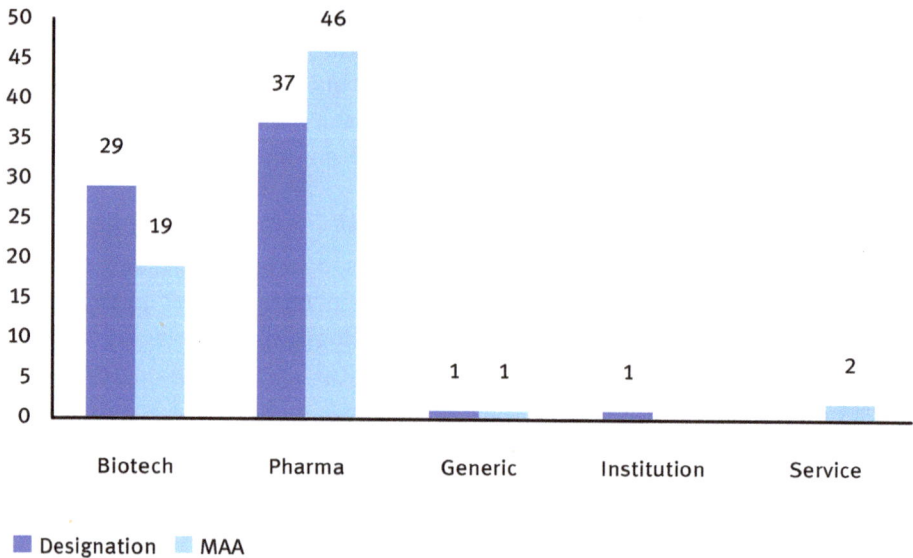

Fig. 8.1: Distribution of developers and MAA-holders according to companies' business focus.

As can be seen in Figure 8.1, **orphan drugs** are being developed almost exclusively by companies from the categories pharma and biotech. Pharmaceutical companies developed and obtained designation for 54 % (37 of 68) of the orphan drugs and biotechs accounted for 43 % (29 of 68).

This distribution changes considerably when it comes to the MAA-holders. Of the 29 biotechs that developed an orphan drug only 19 hold an MAA, representing 28 % of the total. Pharma companies, however, hold 68 % of the MAAs (46 of 68).

Next, the distribution of micro-, small-, medium- and large-sized as well as big pharma companies for the categories biotech and pharma (including generics) deserves further analysis – both, for the development and designation as well as the MAA stage. The results are provided in Table 8.1. It becomes apparent that micro-sized and big pharma companies account for the largest parts of the development and designation of **orphan drugs**. Almost half of the orphan drugs (30) were developed by micro-sized companies, of which 16 belong to the category biotech and 14 to pharma. A total of 18 companies belong to the big pharma group, of which 17 were categorized as pharma and only 1 as biotech (note: some biotech companies are generating such high sales that they qualify to be categorized as big pharma).

Tab. 8.1: Cross-tabulation of developers and MAA-holders according to economic strength and business focus

			Economic Strength				
			Micro	Small	Medium	Large	Big Pharma
Business Focus	Development/ Designation	Total	30	2	8	8	18
		Biotech	16	2	4	6	1
		Big Pharma	14	0	4	2	17
	Marketing Authorization	Total	5	0	9	18	34
		Biotech	2	0	7	7	3
		Big Pharma	3	0	2	11	30
		Generic	0	0	0	0	1

Small, medium and large companies appear to play a rather limited role in the development of orphan drugs. Table 8.1 does not list the two orphan drugs that were developed by a government research institution (Firdapse by Agence Générale des Equipements et Produits de Santé, France) and a private generics company (Peyona by Combino Pharm, Spain) due to the lack of published data. Firdapse was acquired by the US biotech firm BioMarin and Peyona was acquired by the large Italian pharmaceutical company Chiesi Farmaceutici. Concerning MAA-holders two drugs need to be pointed out. Savene, developed by the micro enterprise Topotarget, Denmark, and Photobarr, developed by medium-sized pharmaceutical company Axcan Pharma, Canada, were eventually acquired by service companies (SpePharma, The Netherlands, and Pinnacle Biologics, USA). Furthermore, the generics company TEVA Pharmaceuticals, Israel, which is classified as a large pharma company is the MAA-holder for Trisenox, which had been developed by the micro company PolaRx, USA. TEVA gained access to the drug through acquisition of a company that had acquired the company to which PolaRx had been sold.

The most striking finding, however, is the large difference between the developers and the holders of MAAs in the micro-sized company and big pharma categories. While 45 % (30 of 66) of the focal orphan drugs where attributed to micro-sized companies at the time of their designation, this ratio decreased to about 7 % (5 of 66) concerning the holding of an MAA. In this context it is particularly remarkable that the most significant increase in the number of MAAs is within the categories of large-sized and big pharma companies. While big pharma companies only accounted for the development of 27 % (18 of 66) of the orphan drugs, they however hold the MAA of 52 % (34 of 66) of the orphan drugs. The increase for large firms is also relatively strong from 12 % (8 of 66) to 27 % (18 of 66). This may be seen as a manifestation of the rising interest of renowned pharmaceutical companies in orphan drugs, as referred to earlier. It is also worth emphasizing that biotechs hold only a small part of the MAAs.

On the basis of this data the involvement of micro enterprises appears to be very high. Yet, the analysis has also demonstrated that significant change occurs relating to firms in this size category during the long process from designation to MAA. As a result, micro enterprises only hold a small fraction of the MAAs. It thus appears warranted to assume that the incentives provided by the regulatory framework are not sufficient in assisting companies with relatively low financial strength in bringing their developed orphan drugs to the market on their own. The following sections will analyze this change in detail.

8.3.2 Changes from Designation to Marketing Authorization

Figure 8.2 shows how many companies in each category have retained the rights to the orphan drugs they developed and how many have transferred rights to others, e.g., by means of sale or corporate acquisition. This analysis reveals substantial differences across the categories. While the companies that have been categorized as big pharma pursue 83 % (15 of 18) of their orphan drugs from development to the market, micro enterprises are rarely in a position to obtain an MAA for their developed orphan drugs. In merely 17 % (5 of 30) of the cases do such companies hold the MAAs for the orphan drugs they developed.

A subsequent closer examination of the five micro enterprises and the one small enterprise that actually hold the MAAs for the orphan drugs they developed aims at elucidating the effect of the incentives provided through the EU regulatory framework. The firms, two pharmas (Lipomed and HRA Pharma) and four biotechs (BioMarin, Alexion, Adiennne Pharma & Biotech, and Actelion) were all founded after 1991. They can therefore be considered to be young companies. Actelion and Lipomed each market four drugs and HRA Pharma markets seven drugs. The other companies market only one or two drugs and are likely to have been founded to take the one drug project they developed all the way to the market. All firms for which financial data was accessible were able to increase their sales in the years leading up to 2012. They also reached profitability, with the exception of BioMarin, which, however, did reduce its annual losses. These companies can serve as examples for successful start-ups in the pharmaceutical and biotechnology industries. They demonstrate that it is not impossible to turn such ventures into internationally successful companies. Nevertheless, the data also points to the conclusion that the financial strength a company has before it obtains MAA determines to a large degree its ability to bring the drug to the market. It remains questionable whether the incentives have actually taken effect in the intended manner as these companies were all founded before the EU regulatory framework was enacted. Yet, effects caused by the US Orphan Drug Act, which was passed 17 years before the EU's legislative action, cannot be ruled out.

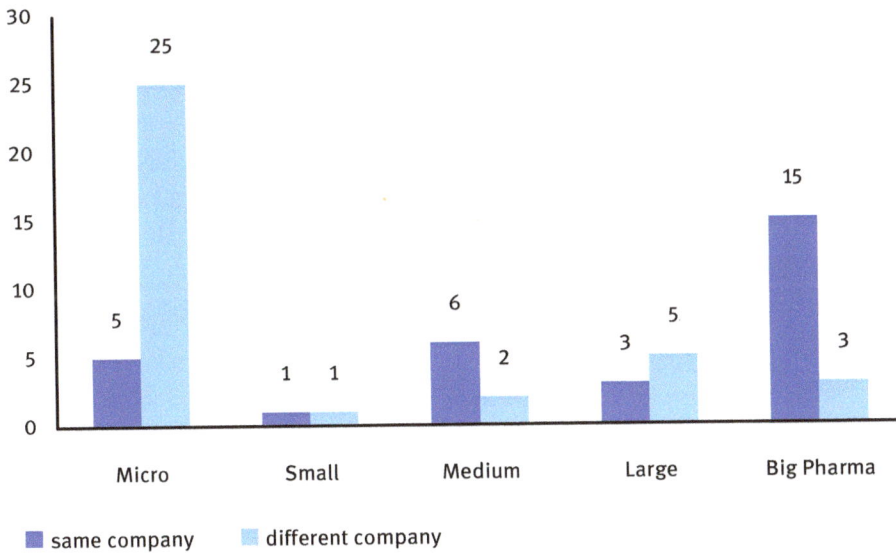

Fig. 8.2: Changes from orphan drug designation to MAA

8.3.3 Role of Service Providers

To gain additional understanding on the impact the incentives are having, the role of **service providers** appears to warrant a closer look.

Service providers were involved in twelve of the studied designation and MAA processes (Cayston, Evoltra, Kuvan, Mozobil, Naglazyme, Revlimid, Soliris, Thelin, Trisenox, Volibris, Vyndaqel, and Xyrem). While large and big pharma companies did not use service providers at all, 83 % of the micro-sized enterprises did use them (10 out of 12). This may be an indication that smaller firms are not capable of following through on designation and MAA processes on their own despite the available incentives. Moreover, the use of a service provider is frequently followed by a licensing or a takeover of the entire company by a big pharma company – a topic that will be addressed in more detail in section 8.4.3.2. Of the twelve drugs with service provider involvement nine were subsequently under the control of big pharma. Interestingly, the three drugs held by micro-sized enterprises showed considerably higher revenues than the other nine drugs. One possible interpretation of this finding might be that the size of the projected revenue potential of a designated orphan drug positively influences the likelihood of filing for an MAA even for a small company.

8.3.4 Strategic Company Decisions

8.3.4.1 Duration from Designation to MAA

Orphan drugs that were held by micro-sized companies at the time of designation received MAAs after an average duration of 46 months, while orphan drugs held by big pharma companies took about half the time. This difference may be due to the experience big pharma companies have with the development and registration processes in general. A different interpretation for the discrepancy is possible if consideration is given to the fact that all regulatory incentives are tied to orphan drug designation. Following this approach, the incentives may very well be offering a strong stimulus for micro-sized enterprises to pursue designation early on in the development process in order to actually benefit from the incentives for as long as possible. This may be of minor importance for big pharmaceutical enterprises for which confidentiality may be more valuable than the incentives – at least during the development phase.

8.3.4.2 Timing and Type of Change of Control over Orphan Drugs

Micro-sized companies participated in the development and designation of a substantial number of orphan drugs (30). However, only a small number of these companies also hold the MAA (5) (see also table 8.1). In this section the 25 drugs that have experienced a change of control are examined more closely in terms of the timing and type (cooperation, licensing, Merger & Acquisition (MA)) of their hand-over.

MAs generally do have a specific execution date, but the pre- and post-transaction process usually takes a long time. In order to address this issue, change of control was split into four categories: continuously, pre-MAA, at MAA, post-MAA. The results are provided in Table 8.2 with the drugs being sorted firstly according to business focus and secondly according to alphabetical order. The analysis reveals that 13 biotechnological micro enterprises and twelve pharmaceutical micro enterprises were unable to bring their orphan drugs to market launch. Ten of the micro enterprises handed over control to big pharma and ten to large pharma companies. This underlines the dynamics in this segment and the strategic importance that micro enterprises hold for larger pharmaceutical companies.

Tab. 8.2: Classification of timing and type of change of control for orphan drugs developed by micro-sized companies

#	Orphan Drug	Development / Designation Company	Business Focus	MAA	Change of Contr.	Holder of Marketing Authorization (MAA) Company	Economic Strength	Business Focus	Type	Timing
1	Arzerra	Genmab	Biotech	Apr 2010	Contin.	Glaxo SmithKline	Big Pharma	Pharma	Cooperation	Contin.
2	Ceplene	Maxim Pharmaceuticals	Biotech	Oct 2008	2006	EpiCept	Micro	Biotech	M&A	Pre-MAA
3	Elaprase	Transkaryotic Therapies	Biotech	Jan 2007	2005	Shire Pharmaceuticals	Large	Pharma	M&A	Pre-MAA
4	Evoltra	Bioenvision	Biotech	May 2006	2007	Sanofi	Big Pharma	Pharma	M&A	Post-MAA
5	Firazyr	Jerini	Biotech	Jul 2008	2008	Shire Pharmaceuticals	Large	Pharma	M&A	At-MAA
6	Increlex	Tercica	Biotech	Aug 2007	2008	Ipsen Pharma	Large	Biotech	M&A	Post-MAA
7	Mepact	IDM Pharma	Biotech	Mar 2009	2009	Takeda Pharmaceuticals	Big Pharma	Pharma	M&A	At-MAA
8	Mozobil	AnorMED	Biotech	Jul 2009	2006	Sanofi	Big Pharma	Pharma	M&A	Pre-MAA
9	Replagal	Transkaryotic Therapies	Biotech	Aug 2001	2005	Shire Pharmaceuticals	Large	Pharma	M&A	Post-MAA
10	Savene	Topotarget	Biotech	Jul 2006	2010	SpePharm	–	Service	License	Post-MAA
11	Siklos	OTL Pharma	Biotech	Jun 2007	2007	Addmedica	Micro	Pharma	License	At-MAA
12	Trisenox	PolaRx	Biotech	Mar 2002	2005	TEVA Pharmaceuticals	Big Pharma	Generic	M&A	Post-MAA
13	Vyndaqel	FoldRX	Biotech	Nov 2011	2010	Pfizer	Big Pharma	Pharma	M&A	Pre-MAA
14	Carbaglu	Orphan Europe	Pharma	Jan 2003	2007	Recordati	Large	Pharma	M&A	Post-MAA
15	Cayston	Corus Pharma	Pharma	Sep 2009	2006	Gilead Sciences	Big Pharma	Biotech	M&A	Pre-MAA
16	Cystadane	Orphan Europe	Pharma	Feb 2007	2007	Recordati	Large	Pharma	M&A	At-MAA
17	Esbrit	Uppsala Med. Information	Pharma	Feb 2011	Contin.	Intermune	Medium	Biotech	Cooperation	Contin.
18	Pedea	Orphan Europe	Pharma	Jul 2004	2007	Recordati	Large	Pharma	M&A	Post-MAA
19	Plenadren	Duocort Pharma	Pharma	Nov 2011	2011	ViroPharm	Medium	Biotech	M&A	At-MAA
20	Thalidomide	Pharmion	Pharma	Apr 2008	2007	Celgene	Large	Biotech	M&A	Pre-MAA
21	Thelin	Encysive	Pharma	Aug 2006	2008	Pfizer	Big Pharma	Pharma	M&A	Post-MAA
22	Vidaza	Pharmion	Pharma	Dec 2008	2007	Celgene	Large	Biotech	M&A	Pre-MAA
23	Volibris	Uppsala Med. Information	Pharma	Apr 2008	2006	Glaxo SmithKline	Big Pharma	Pharma	Cooperation	Contin.
24	Wilzin	Orphan Europe	Pharma	Oct 2004	2007	Recordati	Large	Pharma	M&A	Post-MAA
25	Xyrem	Orphan Medical	Pharma	Oct 2005	2005	UCB Pharma	Big Pharma	Biotech	M&A	At-MAA

Concerning the type of change of control, only three of the 25 drugs originated from a cooperation between the holders of the designation and the holders of the MAA. Only two of the drugs underwent change of control through licensing. The majority was transferred as part of a company takeover (M&A).

As for the timing of the change of control, it becomes apparent that only seven of the 22 drugs (excluding three categorized as continuous) were handed over prior to receiving MAA.

Nine drugs were taken all the way to MAA by the micro enterprises holding the designation, and for the remaining six a participation of the designation holders in the MAA process can at least be assumed. At any rate, it is likely that MAA was imminent at the time of the change of control for the latter group. This signifies that micro enterprises which do not hold on to the drugs they developed after MAA are, indeed, capable of taking the drugs all the way to the MAA or, at least, to a point just prior to the MAA. Thus, it is confirmed that micro enterprises represent attractive takeover targets for big pharma companies.

8.4 Summary and Recommendations

- **Very small enterprises** are highly involved in the development and designation of orphan drugs (30 drugs) which supports the notion that they benefit from the incentives. In particular, biotechnological micro-sized companies take on an important role in developing orphan drugs (16 drugs).
- The duration between designation and MAA is twice as long for **micro-sized enterprises** as it is for big pharma companies, which may also be an indicator that the smaller firms are benefitting from the incentives.
- Of the 30 companies that have developed and received designations for their orphan drugs only 5 hold the MAA. The largest increase in MAA is attributable to big pharma firms.
- Most changes of control were based on **takeovers (M&A)** of the developing firm and less frequently on licensing or cooperation.
- The timing of the change of control occurred most often after MAA was granted or shortly before. Based on the incentives, micro enterprises appear to be able to take the orphan drugs which they have developed and for which designation was received all the way to MAA – however they are not able to launch the orphan drug themselves.
- The ability of a micro-sized company to take the orphan drug all the way to MAA appears to be positively related to the revenue potential of the drug.

Thus we conclude that incentives seem to have a stimulating influence on very small firms regarding development and designation of orphan drugs. Yet, this stimulus does not appear to be sufficient to enable them to actually launch their products after obtaining MAA. To enable micro and small enterprises to gain the ability to market their own products changes to the regulatory framework, e.g. in terms of new incentives are needed.

Proposed future research should be directed at novel financing mechanisms and organizational models. It may be possible to improve the funding of these types of firms through new types of syndication. In addition, local value chains could be optimized within the framework of life-science-clusters. To limit the dependence on big pharma, new modes of marketing assistance for smaller enterprises should be explored. Given the unanimous call for more and better treatment options for patients suffering from rare diseases, progress in the development and commercialization of orphan drugs is necessary.

References

Drummond, M. and Towse, A., 2014. Orphan drugs policies: a suitable case for treatment. *The European Journal of Health Economics*, 3 (1): 1–7.

EU, 2003. Commission recommendation of 6 May 2003 concerning the definition of micro, small and medium-sized enterprises. *Official Journal of the European Union*, 2003/361/EC: 36–41.

EU, 2009. Council recommendation of 8 June 2009 on an action in the field of rare disease. *Official Journal of the European Union*, 2009/C 151/02: 7–10.

Franco, P., 2013. Orphan drugs: the regulatory environment. *Drug Discovery Today*, 18 (3): 163–172.

Kaitin, K., 2010. Deconstructing the drug development process: the new face of innovation. *Clinical Pharmacology & Therapeutics*, 87 (3): 356–361.

Melnikova, I., 2012. Rare diseases and orphan drugs. *Nature Reviews Drug Discovery*, 11 (4): 267–268.

Moors, E. and Faber, J., 2007. Orphan drugs: unmet societal need for non-profitable privately supplied new products. *Research Policy*, 36: 336–354.

NIH, 2007. *Biennial report on the rare diseases research activities at the National Institutes of Health*. Bethesda, Maryland: Office of Rare Diseases.

Philippidis, A., 2011. Orphan drugs, big pharma. *Human Gene Therapy*, 22 (9): 1037–1040.

Rzakhanov, Z., 2008. Regulatory policy, value of knowledge assets and innovation strategy: the case of the Orphan Drug Act. *Research Policy*, 37: 673–689.

Zaby, A., 2011. Orphan drugs: ten years of experience with the EU framework on stimulating innovation for treating rare diseases. *International Journal of Technology, Policy and Management*, 11 (3): 291–306.

Agnieszka Marie

9 Healthcare Business Performance – Control Mechanisms

Abstract Health is the most important asset in human life, and it can be considered to be the basis for all other aspects of existence. For this reason, the healthcare systems play an important role in the modern world, as they maintain the health of the population. The importance of an effective healthcare system can also be considered from an economic point of view, and the effectiveness of healthcare organizations can be ensured through the use of performance business control mechanisms. The objective of this chapter is to provide a clear definition of performance itself and performance measurement in terms of the healthcare sector. Following that, an assessment of performance measurement control mechanisms is provided.

Keywords: Performance measurement, Balanced Scorecard, EFQM Excellence Model, Performance indicator

9.1 Introduction

Health is the most important asset in human life, and it can be considered to be the basis for all other aspects of existence. For this reason, the healthcare systems play an important role in the modern world, as they maintain the health of the population. Access to healthcare is increasing, which has resulted in a longer life expectancy at birth, the average person lives about sixty-six years and, even later, can remain healthy. The importance of an effective healthcare system can be considered also from an economic point of view. With higher retirement ages, people have to be active in the labor market longer than before and pay taxes for a longer period of time, which results in higher public income.

There are several reasons that measuring the level at which objectives are fulfilled in terms of health organizations is important. First of all, there is accountability, which refers to the transparency of resource allocation in the healthcare sector. Due to the specific way of funding, there is a potential risk of inappropriate use of resources, which may have heavy consequences for all relevant stakeholders, especially patients. The performance measurement allows the limitations of the healthcare business to be identified and steps to solve performance problems to be found.

The objective of this chapter is to provide a clear definition of performance itself and performance measurement in terms of the healthcare sector. In addition, an assessment of performance measurement control mechanisms will be provided.

9.2 Business performance control mechanisms

A complex environment, increasing competition, and growing expectations of consumers are forcing modern enterprises to constantly improve their strategies and management systems. Reaching high performance is crucial to gaining a competitive advantage in the market, and effective business performance measurement is indispensable.

Business performance measurement system design should start with clarification of strategies and objectives. Once the priorities are agreed upon, the specific improvement levels can be established. Next a specific measure for each of the objectives should be developed. The measure should indicate how close the company is to the intended target level. Also the frequency of measurement should be clearly stated, and the persons responsible for the measurement should be indicated as well as the sources of data to be used (Fitzroy & Hulbers, 2005: 386–358). An effective business performance measurement should enable the company to develop performance indicators the company will use to measure its performance and business processes. After the key drivers are identified, the company needs to decide how to collect the required data as well as how the data will be presented to the users. In the next step, the performance measurement should be tested; and at the end of the design process, it should be implemented in the company (Andersen & Fagerhaug, 2002).

9.3 Measures of performance in the healthcare system

Performance measurement provides a basis to assess the extent to which an organization has reached its predetermined objectives. It helps to identify areas of strength and weakness and aids in decisions about future projects, with the aim of improving organizational performance (Purbey, 2007: 242). In order to understand the concept of performance measurement in terms of the healthcare system, it is necessary to focus some attention on the term *performance* itself.

There are several perspectives on performance that can be distinguished, as there are many aspects of a healthcare system, such as its efficiency, financial effectiveness, and patient satisfaction. All these elements can be jointly analyzed under the quality of a healthcare system (Purbey, 2007: 242).

The concept of the quality of the healthcare system was developed by A. Donabedian, who identifies three categories of quality: structure, process, and outcome. Structure refers to the attributes of places where healthcare occurs. This includes the features of material resources, like equipment and all necessary facilities; human resources, for example number and qualifications of personnel; and, finally, the organizational structure, such as medical staff organization, methods of reimbursement, or methods of peer review (Donabedian, 1988: 1745). The second category, the process, refers to what exactly is done in giving and receiving care. It refers to the attributes of all the activities that were performed in the course of service provision. These attributes include efficiency of the project organization, degree of service customer involvement, and degree of cooperation during the service provision, as well as other process attributes. The last category of quality in the healthcare system is the outcome, which refers to the degree to which the expected service results were actually achieved, including the level of patient satisfaction with the provided care (Benazic & Dosen, 2012: 53–55).

The term *quality* covers the majority of healthcare system elements; however, it is useful to consider the performance in terms of clinical activities per se, rather than whether the activities were good ones. In a general sense, *efficiency* refers to the relationship between the desired results and the expenditure and efforts expended. In terms of performance measurement, the efficiency measure would, for example, count the number of x-rays within a particular period, while the quality measure would count how many x-rays were provided to people who do not really need such a service (Nerenz & Neil, 2001: 7–8).

In addition, the financial side of the healthcare system needs to be assessed in terms of its effectiveness. Performance in this case relates to the ability of an entity to create revenues. It refers to the relationship between those revenues and expenses (Nerenz & Neil, 2001: 8). Financial performance denotes, then, the general financial condition of the healthcare providers.

The performance measurement of the healthcare system should be considered from the perspective of various stakeholders interested in the sector's condition. There are several stakeholders that can be distinguished (Smith, et. al., 2008: 3):

- government,
- regulators,
- payers,
- provider organizations,
- physicians,
- patients, and
- the public.

The governments need to monitor the health of the nation and set the health policy. As legislative and executive bodies, they have a proprietary role in facilitation, promotion, and extension of health protection (WHO, 2013).

Regulators are those entities that protect patients' safety and welfare. They ensure consumer protection and efficient functioning. Thus they need information on patient safety and welfare as well as information on the efficiency of financial flows (Smith et. al., 2008: 3).

Payers of taxes and members of insurance funds need to be sure the money is spent effectively and in a way that is in line with expectations. For this, they require comparative performance measures and measures of the cost effectiveness of the healthcare system (Smith et al., 2008: 3).

Provider organizations need to monitor and improve the existing services and adjust them to the local needs. For this reason, they require aggregated clinical performance data and information on patient satisfaction, access and equity of care, utilization of service, and waiting times (Smith et. al., 2008: 3).

Another category of stakeholders is the healthcare professional staff. They need to be familiar with current practice and be able to improve performance. They require, therefore, information on current technical standards and available resources (Piligrimiene & Buciuniene, 2008: 105–106). As the physicians, nurses, and other specialists are the employees of healthcare entities, they also need information about the financial position of their employers. They expect to be informed about whether the company is able to continue in business and pay their salary.

Patients should be considered the customers of healthcare services. Consumers need information about possible treatment options, and they need to be able to assess whether the service provided meets accepted safety and quality standards (Australian Government, 2005).

The public are those individuals who are not patients at the moment but who may be in the future. They need to be reassured that specific services will be available when they need them. The public requires information about trends in and comparisons of system performance at the national and local level (Smith et al., 2008: 3).

Healthcare performance measurement must be adjusted for all the stakeholders mentioned above. All of these groups have different information requirements; and, as a result, the indicators used in control mechanisms must deliver the required data.

The **performance indicator** itself refers to the means that allow assessment of whether a particular goal has been reached. Indicators are tied to the goals and objectives and serve as the yardsticks that allow measurement of the level of success in goal achievement. The measures usually take the form of a ratio, rate, or percentage (National Mental Health Benchmarking Project Manual, 2004: 3). The healthcare system has many objectives, such as healthcare acceptability, accessibility, effectiveness, cost effectiveness, public satisfaction, timeliness, safety, responsiveness to individuals' preferences, and others. The fulfilment of these goals cannot always be measured because of their nature (Joumard, 2010: 10).

Taking into consideration all information stakeholders, the indicators in the health sector can generally be used at three levels within the health system. At the policy level, the indicators are used to monitor how effectively and efficiently public resources are being used to satisfy the needs of the community; at the service management level, the indicators deliver feedback on local program strategies; and, at the clinical or service delivery level, the indicators are used to assess the extent to which the services meet the needs of consumers (National Mental Health Benchmarking Project Manual, 2004: 2).

Performance indicators need to be carefully designed to reach specific goals of performance measurement. The development of performance indicators is a cyclical process, called the performance measure life cycle, which consists of planning, developing, testing, evaluating, implementing, modifying, and replacing. The evaluating phase is deciding whether the measure will be accepted and implemented, sent back for readjustments, set aside for some time, or rejected definitely. When the measure reaches a period of declining utilization, it should be replaced; and this constitutes the beginning of new measures (Kazandjian & Lied, 1999: 13–16).

There are three main types of performance measures, which originate from three aspects of healthcare quality (Joint Commissions Resources, 2008: 26):
- structure measures,
- process measures, and
- outcome measures.

Structure measures assess the ability of an organization to provide care – whether it has the necessary resources and arrangements, such as the number, type, and distribution of healthcare equipment and facilities (Joint Commission Resources, 2008: 26). The attractiveness of such measures is based on the availability of data and the lack of complexity. Examples of structure measures are the percentage of intensive care units with a specialty physician available twenty-four hours a day or the number of training sessions for professional staff. The main disadvantage of structure measures is the lack of well-established relationships among the structure, process, and outcomes of healthcare, since it is difficult to prove and assess such associations (Office of Behavioral & Social Sciences Research, 19).

Process measures are supposed to assess the activities carried out by the healthcare services providers. They are often used to assess adherence to the recommended guidelines for medical practice based on scientific evidence. The process measures can to a greater extent than outcome measures identify the areas that require improvement (Pennsylvania Healthcare Quality Alliance, 2013). An important limitation of the effectiveness of such measures is that many care services are provided without evidence of their effectiveness, so the comparison of processes and outcomes is difficult (Office of Behavioral & Social Sciences Research, 15–16).

Finally, there are the outcome measures, which focus on the results of the process. They are the measures of something that is important in its own right, for example, the death rate from a particular disease. By using these measures, the health systems can pay more attention to the needs of the patient (Mant, 2001: 447).

9.4 Balanced scorecard for healthcare organizations

There are several performance measurement systems, among which one of the most popular for the healthcare sector is the **Balanced Scorecard.**

The Balanced Scorecard is a framework that a company can use in order to verify whether it has established both strategic and financial controls to assess its performance (Hitt, Ireland, Hoskisson, 2007: 394). The Balanced Scorecard is based on the assumption that the company needs to balance both financial and nonfinancial measures. An effective scorecard contains a set of strategic and financial objectives tailored to the nature of a particular business (David, 2011: 136).

A balanced scorecard for healthcare organizations should recognize where and how the healthcare adds value. There are three categories of interdependent values affected by healthcare: business value, employee value, and patient value. The healthcare organization itself and its stakeholders receive business value when patients patronize the organization, e.g., return on equity, return on investment. Patients receive value when employees meet their needs. Employees receive work value through employment, benefits and career, and development opportunities that are provided by the healthcare organization and its stakeholders. A balance scorecard should include measures to cover all these value dimensions (Castañeda-Méndez, Mangan, Lavery, 1998: 10).

There are four perspectives creating the balanced scorecard framework (Hitt, Ireland, Hoskisson, 2007: 395):
- financial,
- customer,
- internal business processes, and
- learning and growth.

The four perspectives can be presented in the form of a pyramid, and arranging the levels will be different for not-for-profit organizations and for-profit ones. The basis for both types of organizations is a learning and growth perspective, the foundation for future success. The learning and growth perspective is concentrated in the company's efforts to create a climate that supports growth and innovation (Hitt, Ireland, Hoskisson, 2007: 395). This level includes the proper infrastructure, information systems and organization's people. Long-term success will be ensured by an adequate investment in this area. The next level is the internal business perspective (Voelker, Rakich & French, 2001: 16). The internal business processes are focused on priorities for various processes that create customer and shareholder satisfaction (Hitt, Ireland, Hoskisson, 2007: 395). These must focus on the internal processes that will be necessary to satisfy the organization's customers. Improvement in critical internal processes is an important indicator of future financial and operational success. The differences between the for-profit and not-for-profit organizations appear at the third level of the pyramid. In the for-profit pyramid, anticipating and satisfying customer needs is critical; however, it should be emphasized that the financial perspective is the most important one for these entities (Voelker, Rakich & French, 2001: 16). The financial perspective is connected with growth of profitability and risk from the perspective of shareholders (Hitt, Ireland, Hoskisson, 2007: 395). This perspective measures the financial results that the company provides to its stakeholders. For not-for-profit entities, it is the customer, or rather stakeholder perspective, that is much more important; and the profits are not the ultimate goal. The priority of a healthcare organization is, then, to fulfil the mission and satisfy its stakeholders, while a healthy financial condition ensures a long-term viability (Voelker, Rakich & French, 2001: 16). The customer perspective is concerned with the amount of value customers perceive was created with the company's products (Hitt, Ireland, Hoskisson, 2007: 395).

For each perspective of the balanced scorecard, an organization should establish the objectives, metrics of those objectives, target values, and initiatives that are needed to achieve the goals (Pandrey, 2005: 57).

In order to ensure the successful application of the balanced scorecard, the healthcare provider organization, first of all, should evaluate its ability and readiness to apply this framework. The organization should ensure the hands-on executive leadership has deep content expertise. The organization should focus on patients, their needs, and value propositions. What is more, it should devote a necessary amount of resources, like time, skill set, and information systems, to accelerate the development and implementation processes (Inamdar & Kaplan, 2002: 192–193).

The balanced scorecard may take various forms, and every organization can adjust its structure to particular environmental conditions and circumstances. Some examples will be provided in the analysis below.

9.4.1 Germany – emergency department of the hospital in Friedrichshain

The mission of the emergency department of the hospital in Friedrichshain is to provide care for patients in need, seven days a week and twenty-four hours a day. The vision of the organization is to be considered by its patients and partners to be one of the outstanding emergency departments in Berlin by 2020. The chosen elements of the department's balanced scorecard are presented in the table below.

The balanced scorecard is constructed of four perspectives, which is slightly different from the traditional approach to this performance measurement framework. The mission and vision are consistent with the strategic goals, as set by the organization. The partner perspective focused attention on the satisfaction of the internal partners, mainly the employees. Then the patients and processes perspective is focused on a high quality of care, patient safety, and the patient's overall satisfaction. Next the finance perspective takes into account the resources management and outpatient revenue generation. The last perspective emphasizes the need for improvement of staff qualifications and implementation of innovations.

Tab. 9.1: Emergency department of the hospital in Friedrichshain – Balanced Scorecard
Source: *Adapted from Schachinger* (2009: 28–35)

Partner

Strategic goal	Parameters and units	Operational targets	Initiatives
High level of satisfaction of the internal partner.	Interfaces with satisfactory status.	3-year horizon: ≥ 80%	Case analysis
High rate of medical admissions.	Percentage of emergency admissions per quarter. Decline of emergency admissions per quarter.	3-year horizon: Increase> 5% Maximum −2	Case analysis

Patients and processes

Strategic goal	Parameters and units	Operational targets	Initiatives
High quality of care.	Total number of patients per full-time caregiver per month.	3-year horizon: 120	Negotiations with the Regional Directorate. Definition of tasks and their distribution.
	Number of transfers to ICU within longer than 24h after admission in emergency room. (Number of patients per month in %)	<1%	Case analysis
	Number of patients who come back to hospital within 24h after initial admission (except planned re-appointments). (number of patients per month in%).	<2%	Case analysis
	Total length of stay (administrative recording and treatment). Quantitative analysis of the entries to the treatment reports.	3 year horizon: Inpatients <90 min Outpatients <100 min	Process analysis: qualifications of doctors and personnel assessment.
	Percentage of reanimations in the emergency department in relation to total number of reanimation per quarter with use of a spontaneous cycle < 10 min.	>75%	Case analysis and training
	Percentage of patients without recording despite medical indications (per month).	>1%	Case analysis and feedback

Tab. 9.1: Continued

Patients and processes

Strategic goal	Parameters and units	Operational targets	Initiatives
Patient Safety	Prevention of hospital-acquired infections: use of hand sanitizer (ml) in the areas of the interior medicine, ENT, neurology, (accident) surgery, orthopedics, and gynecology (quantity used per month/ number of patient contacts per month).	Per patient contact >3ml	Training
	Documentation of quality in case of intravenous sedation: number of avoidable sedations with deviations from the documentation requirements (entry of the vital signs, of the applied drugs) per quarter.	<10%	Case analysis and feedback

Finance

Strategic goal	Parameters and units	Operational targets	Initiatives
Optimal occupancy management.	Percentage of patients with discharge against medical advice to all ambulatory patients per month.	3-year horizon: <2%	If necessary, case analysis and consultation with clinic directors, communication, training.
	Specialized admission rate: portion of the specialists taking up patients with indication for the stationary admission per month.	Cumulative interior medicine: > 40% trauma surgery: >20%	Consultation with clinic directors.
Best possible outpatient revenue generation.	Increase of the average proceeds from the private health insurance and statutory health insurance per ambulatory patient/month.	Benchmark: GKV: XXX€/Patient PKV: XXX€/Patient	Personnel and operating cost analysis.
	Billing of all outpatient surgeries as per § 115b SGB V: portion of not seized outpatient surgeries of total number per month.	<10%	Case analysis, consultation with clinic directors.

Potential

Strategic goal	Parameters and units	Operational targets	Initiatives
Staff qualifications.	Number of advanced trainings with a duration of at least 180 min per employee and physician per year.	2	Staff development meeting and individual introduction/expansion of expertise.
Employee satisfaction and innovations.	Number of ideas and suggestions for improvement from the team of the central emergency department per month.	>2	Innovations promotion: incentive and reward system, team meetings etc.
	Percentage of realizations per half-year.	70%	

9.4.2 United Kingdom – Ashford and St. Peter's hospitals

Ashford and St. Peter's Hospitals NHS Trust was formed following the merger of the separate Ashford Hospital and St. Peter's Hospital NHS Trusts (Ashford and St. Peter's Hospitals, 2011). During 2013/2014, the Trust's overarching priorities were to make substantial improvements to both the patient experience (fostering a more open culture and acting on what patients and families are saying) and to staff experience (developing the Trust so that all the staff will be more engaged with decision making and the overall experience of working there). The chosen elements of the Trust's balanced scorecard are presented in Table 9.2 below (Ashford and St. Peter's Hospitals Trust Board, 2013: 1–6).

The balanced scorecard is constructed of four perspectives, which are patient safety and quality, workforce, clinical strategy, and finance and efficiency (stated in Tab. 9.2 as *1–*4). The strategic goals are clearly stated and comply with the hospitals' priorities. There is one strategic goal per perspective and numerous parameters and units for each of them. The workforce perspective focuses, in this case, on the recruitment and development of effectively performing employees. The clinical strategy emphasizes the need to deliver the Trust's clinical strategy of joined-up healthcare. The financial and efficiency perspective measures the financial sustainability of the Trust. All the perspectives seem to be of equal importance.

9.4.3 Sweden – Sahlgrenska University Hospital

Sahlgrenska University Hospital's (SU) mission is to ensure the health and safety of residents and visitors in the region. The hospital is also available to students and tends to develop and implement new knowledge. Sahlgrenska University Hospital's mission is, therefore, to pursue healthcare, research and development, and training (Sahlgrenska Universitetssjukhusets, 2011: 9–65). The chosen elements of the organization's balanced scorecard are presented in the table below.

The balanced scorecard above derives from the organization's mission, and the strategic goals are consistent within the framework. The balanced scorecard in this case is very complex and provides more than one strategic goal per perspective. Moreover the additional description of each strategic goal is provided; and as there are several indicators for each section, they are grouped in a logical way. The perspectives used generally comply with the traditional approach to balanced scorecards, with the exception of customer perspective, which was replaced with patient perspective.

Tab. 9.2: Ashford and St Peter's Hospitals – Balanced Scorecard
Source: *Adapted from Ashford and St. Peter's Hospitals Trust Board* (2013: 1–6).

Patient Safety and Quality

Strategic goal	Parameters and units	Operational targets
To achieve the highest possible quality of care and treatment for our patients.	Summary Hospital-level Mortality Indicator (SHMI)	< 72
	Actual Deaths (Includes Neonatal Intensive Care)	< 945
	MRSA (Hospital only)	0
	C.Diff (Hospital only)	< 13
	VTE (Hospital associated with PE or DVT)	< 24
	Serious Incidents Requiring Investigation (SIRI)	< 75
	Average Bed Occupancy (inc escalation)	< 92%
	Patient Moves (ward changes >=3)	< 7.5%
	Formal Complaints (Total Number)	< 450
	Friends and Family Test Score – Inpatients	70
	Friends and Family Test Score – A&E	70
	Falls (Total Number)	< 700
	Falls – Resulting in Significant Injury (grade 3)	< 15
	Hospital Acquired Pressure Ulcers grade 2 and above	< 139
	Catheter Associated UTI	< 1.2%

Workforce

Strategic goal	Parameters and units	Operational targets
To recruit, retain, and develop a high performing workforce.	Establishment (WTE) *1	3397
	Establishment (£Pay) *1	£ 142m
	Establishment Reduction – CIPs (WTE) *2	55
	Growth (New/Redesigned Roles) *2	88
	Agency Staff Use (WTE)	< 45 WTE
	Agency Staff (£Pay) *3	3.65% of paybill
	Bank Staff Use (WTE)	280 WTE
	Bank Staff (£Pay) *3	6.35% of paybill
	Vacancy Rate (%)	< 10%
	Staff Turnover Rate	< 13%
	Stability	> 85%
	Sickness Absence	< 3.00%
	Staff Appraisals	98%
	Statutory and Mandatory Training	98%
	Staff Engagement Measure *4	3.69

Tab. 9.2: *Continued*

Clinical Strategy

Strategic goal	Parameters and units	Operational targets
To deliver the Trust's clinical strategy of joined-up healthcare.	Trust 4Hr Target (Monitor Compliance)	> 95%
	Emergency Conversion Rate	< 23.8%
	Ambulatory Care Pathways	> 30%
	95% of all LOS < 27 days	< 27 days
	Readmissions within 30 Days – Elective and Emergency	< 6.3%
	Overall Elective Market Share	> 66%
	Overall Elective Market Share (Vascular)	> 50%
	Stroke Patients (90% of stay in Stroke Unit)	> 85%
	% Elective Inpatient Activity Taking Place at Ashford	> 57.53%
	Discharge Rate to Normal Place of Residence (Stroke&FNOF)	> 62.1%
	R&D – Observations and Interventions	797
	Elective Activity (Spells)	> 34,417
	Emergency Activity (Spells)	< 37,644
	Outpatient Activity (New Attendances)	> 110,242

Finance and Efficiency

Strategic goal	Parameters and units	Operational targets
To ensure the financial sustainability of the Trust through business growth and efficiency gains.	Monitor Financial Risk Rating	3
	Total Income Excluding Interest (£000)	£ 232,296
	Total Expenditure (£000)	£ 214,941
	EBITDA (£000)	£ 17,354
	CIP Savings Achieved (£000)	£ 11,839
	CQUINs (£000)	£ 4,950
	Month End Cash Balance (£000)	£ 12,845
	Capital Expenditure Purchased (£000)	£ 17,036
	Emergency Threshold/Readmissions Penalties	£ 3,692
	Average LoS Elective	3.32
	Average LoS Non-Elective	6.99
	Outpatients First to Follow-up Ratio	1:1.5
	Daycase Rate (whole Trust)	> 84%
	Theatre Utilization	>= 75%

Tab: 9.3: Sahlgrenska University Hospital – Balanced Scorecard
Source: *Adapted from Sahlgrenska Universitetssjukhusets* (2011: 9–65).

Patient

Strategic goal	Parameters and units	Operational targets
SU meets the patient's/client's needs and demands, and exceeds patient/client expectations. Activities shall focus on patients' and clients' needs and preferences and on how these should be met. All patients and families are well informed and involved in healthcare. They are treated with dignity, care, and respect for each one's privacy.	(a) Patients who consider themselves as treated in a respectful manner. (b) Patients who believe they have been involved in the planning of their own care. (c) Patients who believe they received individualized information on health status; diagnosis; and methods of examination, care, and treatment.	Measurements of the national patient survey > 90 (weighted value)
	Number of areas/activities that work with patient/relatives/customer dialogue management (or equivalent).	100% of VO
The care at SU is high quality and is conducted in a safe manner.	Proportion of patients with healthcare-associated infections, inpatient somatic care.	≤ 8 %
Each patient should be given the right to safe care and treatment at the right time.	Proportion of patients with healthcare-associated infections, inpatient psychiatric care.	≤ 2 %

Process

Strategic goal	Parameters and units	Operational targets
Introduction of new and rejection of less efficient or obsolete methods is done in an orderly and evidence-based way.	Number of completed HTA analyses.	Higher numbers than 2010, at least 10
The agreed upon care at SU is easily accessible, free of charge, and based on open priorities. SU's operations are characterized by quality, reliability, innovation, and efficiency. Activities work systematically with transfer from inpatient to outpatient care.	(a) Number of patients waiting longer than 90 days for specialized care. (b) Number of patients waiting more than 90 days for operation/action. (c) Number of patients waiting longer than 30 days for visit.	(a) 0 (b) 0 (c) 0
	(a) Proportion of patients who receive an initial healthcare contact within 10 minutes. (b) Percentage of patients visiting doctors within 60 minutes. (c) Proportion of patients that can leave the emergency room within 4 hours.	(a) At least 90% (b) At least 90% (c) At least 90%
Well-defined, standardized, and efficient processes without unwanted variation. Management System is the overall activities, including quality, safety, and the environment.	Number describing overall hospital care processes.	≥ 5

Tab: 9.3: *Continued*

Process

Strategic goal	Parameters and units	Operational targets
The best possible care is ensured through open systematic monitoring. The work is characterized by cooperation, dialogue, and openness.	Proportion of quality parameters that achieves at least the national average in the 'Open comparisons of healthcare quality and efficiency'.	50%

R&D

Strategic goal	Parameters and units	Operational targets
The research and education within the SU are high quality, and daily work involves research to develop new knowledge. Development means to implement new knowledge. Education means to transfer knowledge and develop skills.	Percentage of satisfied students.	Total: 85 %
	Number of scientific publications at SU.	Higher numbers than in 2009 mapping the period 2006–2009.
	Number of operational areas with established strategies and budget for research and development.	Each operational area has written research strategy.
	Number of established educational strategies.	Each operational area has developed the foundations of a written research strategy.

Employee

Strategic goal	Parameters and units	Operational targets
SU is an attractive and competitive employer. SU's employees are highly skilled. Employees of SU should have a sense of security, confidence, participation, and pride in their contribution to the goals' achievment. Executive leadership will be characterized by insight and the ability to exercise the employer's responsibility to achieve the objectives.	Absence from sickness should continue to decrease (% of time worked).	5%
	The number of completed appraisals with individual professional development plan based on business assignments.	90%
	JÄMIX Index	108
	Employees' satisfaction index.	3.8
Employees at SU are characterized by commitment, participation, and responsibility. All employees should feel a personal responsibility for their own performance, development, and environment.	Number of workplaces using a FOCUS model as a method for continuous improvement.	> 50

9.4.4 Belgium – Centre Hospitalier Universitaire de Liège

The mission of the Centre Hospitalier Universitaire de Liège (CHU) is formulated as 'university quality healthcare accessible to all'. The major challenge facing the CHU is, therefore, providing high-quality university hospital care to everyone, whilst safeguarding the long-term financial stability of the institution (Centre Hospitalier Universitaire de Liège, 2005). The characteristics of the CHU's balanced scorecard are presented in the table below.

Tab. 9.4: Centre Hospitalier Universitaire de Liège – Balanced Scorecard
Source: *Adapted from Centre Hospitalier Universitaire de Liège (2005)*

Perspective	Description
Patient	Aims to offer quality care to everyone. It is subdivided into two complementary branches: first, the Medical Plan, where the emphasis is placed mainly on the definition of a clear and coherent multi-site strategy, on the development of centers of excellence (genomics-proteomics, oncology, etc.); and secondly, Patient Care, including the creation of a computerized medical dossier (CMD), improving patient reception, etc.
Finance	Should allow the institution to achieve its mission by rationalizing and planning its revenues, expenditures, and investments. Management control and multi-annual forecasting will be introduced for this purpose. This involves arming the organization with a forecasting system. Theoretically, what will be its situation in one year's time? In three years? In five years?
Internal Processes	Focuses on assessing and improving the organizational procedures: for example, the billing cycle, the IT positioning of the CHU, etc.
Organizational Learning	Aims to improve human resource management: staff training, creation of a mediation service that will attempt to resolve internal conflicts through dialogue and negotiation, etc.

As CHU does not publish a full balanced scorecard, it is not possible to provide a wide analysis of the balanced scorecard's use in this case. The CHU uses four perspectives that do not differ from the traditional approach to the balanced scorecard; moreover, they comply with the organization's mission.

9.4.5 Poland – Specialist Hospital Louis Rydygier in Krakow

The vision of Specialist Hospital Louis Rydygier in Krakow is the achievement of and strengthening of its position as the second largest medical center in the region. The mission of the hospital is to satisfy the most complex health needs of patients with regard to high quality and using highly specialized diagnostic and therapeutic technologies while taking into account high efficiency in the use of resources (Wojewódzki Szpital Specjalistyczny, 2007: 13).

Tab. 9.5: Specialist Hospital Louis Rydygier in Krakow – Balanced Scorecard
Source: *Adapted from Michalak* (2012: 210)

Stakeholders

Strategic goal	Parameters and units
Building satisfaction of patients and their families.	(a) Number of complaints. (b) Percent of patients hospitalized for which individual treatment plans were developed. (c) Patient satisfaction research results.
Improve accessibility to health services.	(a) Number of patients waiting for scarce health benefits. (b) The number of new specialties and medical technology. (c) The occupancy rate of beds. (d) Shorten the waiting time for highly specialized services. (e) The results of patient satisfaction (degree of patient satisfaction).
Strengthen the good reputation of hospital.	(a) Number of publications of the hospital and its workers. (b) The results of patient satisfaction. (c) Number of press releases about the hospital. (d) IDO and CMJ Certification. (e) Place in the national ranking of hospitals. (f) Number of treated patients.
Pursue statutory tasks in terms of financial stability.	(a) The financial results. (b) Level of debt.
Deliver health services of the required quality at a reasonable price.	(a) Percentage fulfilling specific requirements of the payer. (b) Offer of + / í 10% of the average for products from comparable hospitals.
Adjust the range and quantity of health services to the needs of regional communities and payers.	(a) The level of execution of the contract. (b) The degree of shortening waiting lists.

Internal processes

Strategic goal	Parameters and units
Streamlining and simplification of internal regulatory processes.	The percentage of work stations with access to the Intranet.
Create the conditions for the formation and implementation of innovation.	(a) The number of reported/implemented innovations. (b) The number of implemented (3-year cycle) new medical technologies.
Implement quality improvement programs.	(a) Certificates received. (b) Number of implementation of accreditation standards.
Improve and standardize healthcare.	(a) Number of developed standards. (b) Rate of implementation of accreditation standards.
Simplify the process of supply management.	(a) The quantity of contractors. (b) Number of purchased products range.

The balanced scorecard presented above is constructed from only two perspectives, which cannot be enough for measurement of the mission's fulfillment. The stakeholders' perspective focuses on the external stakeholders, like patients and the general public. This section also includes delivering high-quality services, while the internal processes perspective seems to focus on employees and the effectiveness of their work.

The analyzed balanced scorecards show how different the particular entities and their environments are. The healthcare organizations have adjusted the balanced scorecard perspectives and performance indicators to their particular situation. Where an organization prefers to modify the traditional construction of the balanced scorecard, it should be emphasized that a reasonable number of perspectives should be used with a reasonable number of strategic goals, which should derive directly from the organization's mission.

The balanced scorecard is beneficial for organizations that operate in turbulent environments and deal with change, as it allows them to deal with the time delay between decisions, actions, and their consequences (Voelker, Rakich, French, 2001: 20). This model provides a cross-disciplinary and hierarchy-traversing communication process and enables the integration of performance measures for operational objectives at an appropriate level (Striteska & Spickova, 2012: 5).

9.5 EFQM Excellence Model for healthcare organizations

EFQM Excellence Model is a non-prescriptive framework based on nine criteria. Five of them are called 'enablers' and four of them are 'results'. The 'enablers' refer to the things that the company needs to develop and implement for its strategy, while the 'results' cover what the company achieves, in line with its strategic goals (Striteska & Spickova, 2012: 5–6). The framework has nine criteria, which in terms of 'enablers' refer to leadership, policy and strategy, people, partnerships and resources, processes, and products and services. The 'results', which are caused by the 'enablers', cover customer results, people results, society results, and business results (EFQM, 2012).

Each of the enablers and results is well defined and supported by a number of sub-criterion elements. The definition of the criteria and listing of sub-criteria can be found in the table below.

The core of the EFQM model is the RADAR methodology, which is cyclical and continuous. The methodology is based on five steps: determination of required results, planning and developing approaches, deployment of approaches, and assessment and review of achieved results. The model is used as a self-assessment tool, which enables a systematic and regular review of the company's activities and results (Striteska & Spickova, 2012: 4–5).

Tab. 9.6: EFQM criteria and sub-criteria
Source: *Adapted from DTI (2007: 3), EFQM (2012), EFQM(2013)*

Criteria	Definition	Sub-criteria
Leadership	Excellent organizations have leaders who shape the future and make it happen, who act as role models for its values and ethics and inspire trust at all times.	(a) Leaders develop the mission, vision, and values and are role models of a culture of excellence. (b) Leaders are personally involved in ensuring the organization's management system is developed, implemented, and continuously improved. (c) Leaders are involved with customers, partners, and representatives of society. (d) Leaders motivate, support, and recognize the organization's people.
Policy and Strategy	Excellent organizations implement their mission and vision by development of a stakeholder focused strategy. Policies, plans, objectives, and processes are developed and deployed in order to deliver the strategy.	(a) Policy and strategy are based on the present and future needs and expectations of stakeholders. (b) Policy and strategy are based on information from performance measurement, research, learning, and creativity-related activities. (c) Policy and strategy are developed, reviewed, and updated. (d) Policy and strategy are deployed through a framework of key processes. (e) Policy and strategy are communicated and implemented.
People	Excellent organizations value their employees and create a culture that allows the achievement of organizational and personal goals.	(a) People resources are planned, managed, and improved. (b) People's knowledge and competencies are identified, developed, and sustained. (c) People are involved and empowered. (d) People and the organization have a dialogue. (e) People are rewarded, recognized, and cared for.
Partnerships and Resources	Excellent organizations plan and manage external partnerships, suppliers, and internal resources in order to support their strategy, policies, and the effective operation of processes.	(a) External partnerships are managed. (b) Finances are managed. (c) Buildings, equipment, and materials are managed. (d) Technology is managed. (e) Information and knowledge are managed.
Processes, products, and services	Excellent organizations design, manage, and improve processes, products, and services to generate value for customers and other stakeholders.	(a) Processes are systematically designed and managed. (b) Processes are improved, as needed, using innovation in order to fully satisfy and generate increasing value for customers and other stakeholders. (c) Products and services are designed and developed based on customer needs and expectations. (d) Products and services are produced, delivered, and serviced. (e) Customer relationships are managed and enhanced.

Tab. 9.6: *Continued*

Criteria	Definition	Sub-criteria
Customer results	Excellent organizations achieve and sustain outstanding results that meet or exceed the needs of their customers.	(a) Perception measures. (b) Performance indicators.
People results	Excellent organizations achieve and sustain outstanding results that exceed the needs of their employees.	(a) Perception measures. (b) Performance indicators.
Society results	Excellent organizations achieve and sustain outstanding results that exceed the needs of relevant stakeholders within society.	(a) Perception measures. (b) Performance indicators.
Business results	Excellent organizations achieve and sustain outstanding results that exceed the needs and expectations of their business stakeholders.	(a) Key performance outcomes (lag). (b) Key performance indicators (lead).

The EFQM model became the basis for the majority of national and regional quality awards. This framework does not recommend specific performance measures and does not explicitly consider the performance targets. The EFQM model can, therefore, be used by an organization as a tool of self-assessment, as a guide to indicate the areas for improvement, or as a way to benchmark with other organizations (Dror, 2008: 586).

Conclusions

Medical service providers are the main players in the health market; however, the rules governing this specific market should not be the same as those in other industries. Financial performance in terms of healthcare is important; however, the goal of an entity should not solely be considered to be maximizing profit. Health is the basis of human life, and the health business must take this into account.

Performance refers to the level of fulfillment of the goals that were selected by a company. In terms of the healthcare business, performance has many dimensions, like effectiveness, efficiency, consumer satisfaction, and others, which jointly are considered to be quality. The principal objective of these businesses is, therefore, to increase the quality of their services; and for this reason, there is a need to introduce performance control mechanisms.

First of all, the control should begin at the lowest level – with the healthcare service providers. The specific regulations, best practices, and norms should be established at the level of hospitals, medical offices, and all other entities. This is important because the staff directly involved in providing services to consumers can easily assess the quality and identify the limitations of the healthcare business. Also finding solutions for current problems is easier at the local level, and actions taken by the entities themselves would be much more responsive and flexible. The proper management of all healthcare entities is, then, crucial for their further success.

There are several performance measurement frameworks, among which the most useful in terms of the healthcare sector are the Balanced Scorecard and the EFQM model. The choice of the performance measurement framework depends strongly on the nature of the business and should be selected and developed with regard to the particular business objectives and environment in which it operates. The balanced scorecards used as examples in the third part of this chapter show how the entities and their environments differ from each other.

The next level of healthcare system control should be established at the regional level. Benchmarking within the hospitals seems to be an effective solution for quality improvement. The regional authorities are close enough to the healthcare service providers to maintain a constant and consequential control. The audits and surveys should, however, be mandatory; and no exceptions should be made.

The last level of healthcare control mechanisms is the national one, where the government provides legal regulations and national standards. This is the most powerful element of performance control mechanisms; however, its actions and requirements are often outdated and ineffective.

Control mechanisms are a significant element of the healthcare sector. Service providers can use various indicators to assess their current position in the market; however, everything starts with people. It is the medical staff that creates performance; and perhaps by increasing its involvement, high quality becomes the resulting standard.

References

Andersen, B., Fagerhaug, T., 2002. *Eight Steps to a Sew Performance Measurement System.* Retrieved September 25, 2013 from: http://asq.org/quality-progress/2002/02/one-good-idea/eight-steps-to-a-new-performance-measurement-system.html

Ashford and St. Peter's Hospitals, 2011. *About the Trust.* Retrieved December 12, 2013 from: http://www.ashfordstpeters.org.uk/about-us/about-the-trust

Ashford and St. Peter's Hospitals Trust Board, 2013. *Balanced Scorecard*

Australian Government, 2005. *National mental health information priorities.* Retrieved September 12, 2013 from: http://health.gov.au/internet/publications/publishing.nsf/Content/mental-pubs-n-infopri2-toc~mental-pubs-n-infopri2-pt1~mental-pubs-n-infopri2-pt1-9

Benazic, D., Dosen, D., 2012. Service quality concept and measurement in the business consulting market. *Tržište*, 24(1): 47–66.

Castañeda-Méndez, K., Mangan, K., Lavery, A., 1998. The role and application of the balanced scorecard in healthcare quality management. *Journal For Healthcare Quality: Official Publication Of The National Association For Healthcare Quality*, 20, 10–13.

Centre Hospitalier Universitaire de Liège, 2005. *COS Plan and Strategic Contract of the CHU in Liège.* Retrieved September 25, 2013 from: http://www2.chuliege.be/plancos/english.html#history

David, F., 2011. *Strategic Management. Concept and cases.* New Jersey: Pearson Education, Inc.

Donabedian, A., 1988. The Quality of Care: How can it be assessed?. *JAMA*, 260(12): 1743–1748.

Dror, S., 2008. The Balanced Scorecard versus quality award models as strategic frameworks. *Total Quality Management*, 19(6): 583–593.

DTI, 2007. *A Framework of Excellence.* Retrieved December 15, 2013 from: <http://www.businessballs.com/dtiresources/TQM_excellence_model.pdf>

EFQM, 2012. *Results.* Retrieved September 23, 2013 from: http://www.efqm.org/efqm-model/criteria/results

EFQM, 2013. *Enablers* Retrieved September 23, 2013 from: http://www.efqm.org/efqm-model/criteria/enablers

Fitzroy, P., Hulbert, J., 2005. *Strategic management. Creating Value in a Turbulent World*, United States: John Wiley & Sons, Inc.

Hitt, M., Ireland, D., Hoskisson, R., 2007. *Strategic Management. Competitiveness and Globalization: Concepts and Cases.* Retrieved September 10, 2013 from: <http://pro-ex.org/books/archive/files/c51d0336080c1add4c63d31fd5c4c2ed.pdf>

Inamdar, N., and Kaplan, R., 2002. Applying the Balanced Scorecard in Healthcare Provider Organisations. *Journal of Healthcare Management* 47(3): 179–195.

Joint Comission Resources, 2008. *Managing Performance Measurement Data in Healthcare*, Illinois: Joint Commission Resources on Accreditation of Healthcare Organizations.

Joumard, I., André, C., Nicq, C., 2010. Healthcare Systems: Efficiency and Institutions, *ECO/WKP* (2010) 25.

Kazandjian, V., Lied, T., 1999. *Healthcare Performance Measurement: Systems Design and Evaluation.* Milwaukee: ASQ Quality Press.

Mant, J., 2001. Process versus outcome indicators in the assessment of quality of healthcare. *International Journal for Quality in Healthcare,* 13(6): 475–480.

Michalak, J., 2012. Próba oceny korzyści zastosowania zbilansowanej karty wyników w szpitalach. *Acta Universitatis Lodziensis. Folia Oeconomica*, 263: 197–218.

National Mental Health Benchmarking Project Manual, 2004. Retrieved June 21, 2013 from: <http://amhocn.org/static/files/assets/6282c6c7/Benchmarking_Manual_Part_2.pdf>

Nerenz, D., Neil, N., 2001. *Performance Measures for Healthcare Systems.* Retrieved June 20, 2013 from: < www.hret.org/chmr/resources/cp19b.pdf<

Office of Behavioral & Social Sciences Research. *Evaluating the Quality of Healthcare.* Retrieved June 21, 2013 from: <http://www.esourceresearch.org/Portals/0/Uploads/Documents/Public/Cleary_FullChapter.pdf>

Pennsylvania Healthcare Quality Alliance, 2013. *Our Measures.* Retrieved September September 24, 2013 from: http://www.phcqa.org/measures/

Piligrimiene, Z., Buciuniene, I., 2008. Different Perspectives on healthcare Quality: Is the Consensus Possible?. *Economics of Engineering Decisions*, 1(56): 104–111.

Purbey, S., Mukherjee, K., Bhar, C., 2007. Performance measurement system for healthcare processes. *International Journal of Productivity and Performance Management*, 56(3): 241–251.

Sahlgrenska Universitetssjukhusets, 2011. *Sahlgrenska Universitetssjukhusets årsredovisning 2011.* Retrieved September 20, 2013 from:
http://www.sahlgrenska.se/upload/SU/Dokument/arsredovisning/SU%20%C3%85R%202011%20fastst%C3%A4lld%202012-02-03%20rev%200208.pdf?epslanguage=sv

Smith, P., Mossialos, E., Papanicolas, I., 2009. *Performance measurement for health system improvement: experiences, challenges and prospects*. Cambridge, Cambridge University Press.

Striteska, M., Spickova, M., 2012. *Review and Comparison of Performance Measurement Systems*. Journal of Organizational Management Studies Retrieved September 23, 2013 from: <http://www.ibimapublishing.com/journals/JOMS/2012/114900/114900.pdf>

Schachinger, D., 2009. *Mit Kennzahlen steuern Die Balanced Scorecard als strategisches Führungsinstrument einer Rettungsstelle*. Retrieved December 16, 2013 from:
<http://www.dbfk.de/regionalverbaende/no/bildung/Balanced-Scorecard-Schachinger_21112009.pdf>

Voelker, K., Rakich, J., French, R., 2001. The Balanced Scorecard in Healthcare Organizations: A Performance Measurement and Strategic Planning Methodology. *Hospital Topics: Research and Perspectives on Healthcare* 79(3): 13–24.

Wojewódzki Szpital Specjalistyczny, 2009. *Strategia Wojewódzkiego Szpitala Specjalistycznego im. L. Rydygiera w Krakowie na lata 2007 – 2009*. Retrieved December 12, 2013 from:
<http://www.rydygierkrakow.pl/komunikaty/strategia2007_2009_z_aneksami.pdf>

WHO (2013). *Stakeholders*. Retrieved September 24, 2013 from:
http://www.who.int/providingforhealth/topics/stakeholders_p4h/en/

Justyna Matysiewicz

10 E-healthcare Service and Business Strategies in a Virtual Environment

Abstract The importance of the Internet in the health sector in the EU has increased continuously over the last years. Throughout many European national healthcare services, extensive e-health infrastructures and systems are now viewed as central to the future provision of safe, efficient, high-quality, citizen-centered healthcare. Introduction of the concept of e-health also involves high costs and a change in the perception of healthcare services by both physicians and patients. This chapter presents issues concerning the theory of services, the concept of e-services in the healthcare sector, and the main assumptions of e-health strategies currently being implemented in the EU.

Keywords: E-services, E-healthcare, Virtual environment

10.1 Definition of healthcare service and its characteristics

The first task for any manager is to develop an understanding of the product being marketed. Although many healthcare sales involve goods, most deal with services; and the nature of the product depends on who the customer is. The chapter begins with an introduction to the service concept and its characteristics.

A **service** may be described as any activity or benefit that a supplier offers a customer that is usually intangible and does not result in the ownership of anything. The provision of services may or may not be tied to a physical product. Services, according to the International Standard Industrial Classification (ISIC), include the following: wholesale and retail trade; restaurants and hotels; transport, storage, and communications; financial, insurance, real estate, and business services; personal, community, and social services; and government services. The key assets managed by a firm in each of these businesses are a system of people and machines or equipment. These systems are developed by a firm over many years and are the result of investment in human, financial, and physical resources. The unique blend of the assets in a system gives a service firm its differentiated competitive advantage (Hollesen, 2007).

In the literature, two approaches can be identified that capture the essence of services (Lovelock, 2001).

– A service is an act or performance offered by one party to another. Although the process may be tied to a physical product, the performance is essentially intangible and does not normally result in ownership of any product.

- Services are economic activities that create value and provide benefits for consumers at specific times and places as a result of bringing about a desired change in, or on behalf of, the recipient of the service.

More amusingly, services have been described as 'something that may be bought and sold, but which cannot be dropped on your foot'.

Nowadays, it is difficult to think of firms/organizations that are not involved with services in one form or another (Baron and Hariss 2003):
- Some organizations declare the whole business to be a service business, for example, IT, accounting, health, or education.
- Some organizations declare services to be part of their business; many organizations have service providers within their business. For example, multiple retailers rely on administrative services and technical services from within their own organization.
- Some organizations declare services to be an augmentation of manufactured goods, which is seen extensively with sales of traditional manufactured goods. For example, a new car comes with warranties, free delivery, and so on.

An organization must consider **five main service characteristics** when designing marketing programs: intangibility, inseparability, variability, perishability, and lack of ownership. We will look at each of these characteristics in the following sections.
- Intangibility: Pure services, such as a consultancy session with a psychiatrist, cannot be touched, nor can they travel on a train or airplane, although the train and airplane are themselves tangible. You cannot touch the 'atmosphere' on a train or airplane, nor can you touch conversation with fellow passengers. So it can be said that service intangibility means that services cannot be readily displayed, and so cannot be seen, tasted, felt, heard, or smelled before they are bought. The intangibility characteristic of services often increases risk for the purchaser. Some services are perceived to be riskier than others, depending on whether they are high in (Baron and Hariss 2003) these features.
- Search factor: This factor is one about which customers can get prior information as to what they will receive. For example, the suntan store may promise that after five sessions you will look as brown as the person in the photograph.
- Experience factor: A service high in this factor is one that customers must try out (experience) before they can decide whether or not it is a good deal. Paying for a holiday package, for example, is high in the experience factor as it involves so much more than can be conveyed by a holiday brochure.
- Credence factor: A service high in credence factors is one that is difficult to evaluate even after experiencing it. These are services that are often offered by professionals or experts in their field.

Because service offerings lack tangible characteristics that the buyer can evaluate before purchase, uncertainty is increased. To reduce uncertainty, buyers look for signs of service quality. They draw conclusions about quality from the place, people, equipment, communication material, and price that they see. Therefore, the service provider's task is to make the service tangible in one or more ways (Kotler, et al., 1996).

– Inseparability: Inseparability refers to the notion that in many service operations, production and consumption cannot be separated; that is, a service is to a great extent consumed at the same time as it is produced. For example, although a hairdresser may prepare in advance to carry out the service, most of the hairdressing service is produced simultaneously as the customer consumes the service (Baron & Hariss 2003).

Because the customer is also present as the service is produced, provider-client interaction is a special feature of service marketing. Both the provider and the client affect the service outcome. If the audience is composed of ardent fans of the pop group, they are likely to be ecstatic with the service. The teacher who has taught well and is liked by her students will have effectively satisfied her clients. It is important for service staff to be trained to interact well with clients.

A second feature of the inseparability of service is that other customers are also present or involved. The concert audience, students in the class, other passengers on a train, and customers in a restaurant all are present while an individual consumer is consuming the service. Their behavior can determine the satisfaction that the service delivered to the individual customers. For example, an unruly crowd in a restaurant would disenchant other customers dining there and reduce satisfaction. The implication for management is to ensure at all times that customers involved in the service do not interfere with each other's satisfaction (Kotler, et al., 1996).

– Variability: Organizations providing services to consumers know that no two services provisions are exactly the same, whatever the attempts to standardize them. As services involve people in production and consumption, there is considerable potential for variability. Service variability means that the quality of services depends on who provides them, as well as when, where, and how they are provided (Kotler et al., 1996). A concert performed by a group on two nights may differ in slight ways because it is very difficult to standardize every dance move. Generally, systems and procedures are put in place to make sure the service provided is consistent all the time. Training in service organizations is essential for this; however, in saying this, there will always be subtle differences.

– Perishability: This refers to the fact that, unlike physical goods, services cannot be stored for later sale or use. The perishability of services is not a problem when demand is steady. However, public transportation companies have to own much more equipment because of rush-hour demand than they would if demand were even throughout the day (Kotler et al., 1996).

- Lack of ownership: When customers buy physical goods, such as cars and computers, they have personal access to the product for unlimited time. They actually own the product. They can even sell it when they no longer wish to own it. In contrast, service products lack that quality of ownership. The service consumer often has access to the service for a limited time (Kotler et al., 1996). For example, when buying a ticket to the USA, the service lasts maybe ten hours each way; but consumers want and expect excellent service for that time. Because you can measure the duration of the service, consumers become more demanding of it.

Healthcare services are an example of professional services. Additional characteristics describe professional services as distinguished from non-professional, more routinized services (Løwendahl, 2007). The most important healthcare characteristics are those listed below.

- Asymmetric information: The healthcare practitioner who provides healthcare typically has more knowledge of the service being provided than does the patient who is the consumer. The patient's lack of expertise means he or she is ill-equipped to judge the quality of healthcare. To make matters worse, the quality of healthcare is notoriously difficult to measure and opinions amongst healthcare practitioners themselves may vary about what the best quality healthcare is. When customers buy physical goods, such as cars and computers, they can easier and much better judge of product quality.
- Personnel qualification and knowledge: This is one of the most important characteristics of healthcare services. Healthcare services are highly knowledge intensive, delivered by people with higher education, and frequently closely linked to scientific knowledge development within the healthcare area of expertise.
- Involves a high degree of customization: Customization deals with the efficient adaptation of healthcare services to customer needs and the active co-designing of the customer. Customization is an interactive process between the patient and the provider.
- Involves a high degree of discretionary effort and personal judgment
- Delivered within the constraints of professional norms of conduct: The delivery of healthcare services includes setting patient needs higher than profits and respecting the limits of professional expertise.

Many healthcare organizations offer a variety of services and products to their customers. An organization's product mix refers to the combination of goods, services, and even ideas it offers. Certainly, a hospital is an example of an organization that offers a wide range of goods and services. Indeed, a major hospital will offer hundreds, if not thousands, of different procedures. In addition, hospitals offer a variety of goods (in the form of drug doses, supplies, and equipment) that are charged to the customer (Thomas, 2004).

10.2 Planning healthcare service offerings: the customer value hierarchy

The patient purchasing a specific healthcare service focuses on the values and benefits that come from the service or good. In planning its market offerings, the healthcare organization needs to address **five levels in order to fulfill patient expectations** (Kotler, Shalowiz, Stevens, 2008). The fundamental level is the core benefit that the customer is really seeking. A patient visiting a hospital to deliver a baby wants a safe, healthy birth. The purchaser of aspirin is buying headache relief. Marketers, therefore, must see themselves as benefit providers.

At the second level, the marketer has to turn the core benefit into a basic product. Thus a patient hospital room in a maternity department includes a bed that also serves as a delivery table, a scale, and a recliner; and it provides high-intensity lights and an ultrasound machine.

At the third level, the marketer prepares an expected product: a set of attributes and conditions buyers normally expect when they purchase this product. Expectant mothers can expect a clean gown, fresh bedding, working lamps, acceptable food, and a relative degree of quiet.

At the fourth level, the marketer may offer an augmented product that exceeds customer expectations. For hospitals in developed countries, these augmented products often include the following features: access to care, coordination of care, information and education, physical comfort, continuity and transition to home, emotional support, involvement of family and friends, and respect for patient preferences. This augmented offering arises from the intense competition for patients in these markets. In developing countries and emerging markets, competition occurs mostly at the expected product level.

Differentiation takes place mainly at the level of product augmentation and leads the marketer to look at the user's total consumption system: the way the user performs the tasks of getting and using products and related services.

At the fifth level is the potential product, which encompasses all the possible augmentations and transformations the product or offering might undergo in the future. This is where companies search for new ways to delight customers and distinguish their offerings (Kotler, Shalowiz, Stevens, 2008).

In the process of planning market offerings in healthcare, how the **concept of product** is approached is also important. We can identify a traditional approach, based on the idea described previously, but also a systemic one. Systemic products are products that most often concomitantly satisfy the needs attributed to more than one level of needs. The consumers/purchasers recognize them as sets (clusters) of needs that appear simultaneously in some period of human life, for example, those related to the set of needs linked to healthcare. According to classical expressions of consumption economy, sets of needs defined in this way are satisfied by so-called strategic goods (services); but their consumption, to be satisfactory and sometimes possible at all, additionally requires a separate purchase and consumption of complementary products/services. In case of systemic products, there is usually no such necessity because these products are offered simultaneously (Zabinski, 2008).

Therefore, the distinctive feature of a systemic product is the fact that it contains, in itself, but also in a physical and spatial meaning, not only one, but a few (or even several) products. Healthcare services are an example of a systemic product. Technological advancement, and also a growing level of expectations for the quality and efficiency of this type of service, results in the formation of medical multi-products. Healthcare organizations established nowadays are institutions that offer medical services that are highly advanced with respect to technology, science, and quality, the so-called multi-values, for which such a product is both purchased by the patient and also designed and individualized with his/her participation.

Healthcare systemic products (medical service packages) do not need to demonstrate always the highest technological level what is reflecting the dominant human role (doctor) in the provision of that kind of services. Another characteristic feature of healthcare systemic products is the fact that they are network products. As a rule, they appear in the networks of cooperating medical, ambulatory, and pharmaceutical units and companies that offer technical equipment and financial services established under the patronage of a coordinating unit, the promoter of the systemic product. All the elements mentioned above are offered together in the form of a product (complex offer). This product is formed and modified according to the patient's needs (Matysiewicz, Smyczek, 2012).

10.3 E-health: a new approach in healthcare

With escalating costs in healthcare, increasing turbulence in the Internet commerce environment, and growing uncertainties, traditional healthcare providers are under enormous pressure to provide new ideas and innovative ways of delivering healthcare products and services. Healthcare planners, administrators, and managers today are challenged to rethink, redesign, and reshape the current healthcare system (Tan, 2005).

The appearance of the category of systemic products is one of the symptoms of changes that have taken place in the healthcare sector. The major actions that have impact on development of healthcare systemic products include the rise and diffusion of modern information, communication, and production technologies. The concept of **e-health** is the expression of the application of new technologies in medicine. It facilitates rapid access to information for all stakeholders involved in e-healthcare processes – for example, e-patients, e-physicians, e-care providers, e-vendors, and e-insurers or e-payers.

E-health is defined as the transfer of health resources and healthcare by electronic means (WHO, 2013). It encompasses three main areas:

- delivering health information for health professionals and health consumers through the Internet and telecommunications;
- using the power of IT and e-commerce to improve public health services, e.g., through the education and training of health workers; and
- using e-commerce and e-business practices in health systems management.

The vision of e-health can develop because of the fact that more and more people notice the benefits of the application of mobile technologies, and because of the rapid growth in the capability of mobile devices and the speed and reliability of wireless connections. Owing to wireless technologies and mobile devices, access to the patient's data and the medical information system is possible in the place where medical care is provided, which ensures that the medical staff obtains the complete information that is necessary to specify an efficient therapy. What is crucial is the fact that these technologies also ensure the security of access to the patient's data. The expectations of healthcare specialists towards the e-health system include among others:

- reducing the number of paper documents and the amount of information stored up in various places and providing faster access to information,
- ensuring the ability to react rapidly to patients' needs, and
- supporting better management of therapy plans through remote access to all necessary information.

In addition, the following are included in the potential benefits from e-health (American College of Physicians 2008):

- increased patient access to high-quality healthcare through established relationships with a physician and his or her clinical team by making healthcare guidance and specific preventive, acute, and chronic care available without requiring a face-to-face visit;
- support for modern diagnostic methods, including evidence-based diagnosis;
- better ability to trace medical procedures;
- improved patient-physician communication by broadening communication beyond office visits and telephone care to include other effective and convenient strategies using technology;
- improved patient satisfaction by enhancing access to high-quality healthcare from his or her physicians and their healthcare team;
- improved efficiency of healthcare for patients, physicians, and employers through more appropriate use of resources and lowering the cost for payers;
- facilitating patient participation in healthcare decision making and self-management;
- enabling virtual teams to contribute to enhanced patient care processes; and
- increased possibility of remote delivery of information to medical staff and better coordination of the staff's work.

It is expected that the application of mobile technologies will increase the business value of healthcare because it will become more convenient and efficient in the following four spheres: search for information, information analysis (medications, alternative therapies, check-ups), problem solving, and assistance in decision making. Therefore, e-health can significantly complement existing healthcare and increase the benefits it offers to the patients while providing the grounds for the formation of healthcare products.

10.4 E-healthcare services: characteristics and classification

In the literature, it is possible to identify different e-service definitions. **E-services** has been defined as *those services that can be delivered electronically* (Javalgi, Martin, and Todd, 2004) and as *provision of services over electronic networks* (Rust and Kannan, 2003). Another definition describes it as *interactive services that are delivered on the Internet using advanced telecommunications, information, and multimedia technologies* (Boyer, Hallowell and Roth, 2002). The main point of these definitions is the fact that delivery is electronic or a concern with the infrastructure necessary to deliver an e-service (Hofacker et al., 2007).

Development of the concept of e-health caused a growing interest in the specificity of e-services in healthcare. According to Car et al. (2008), *e-Health is a relatively new and rapidly evolving field and so many of the concepts, terms, and applications are still in a state of flux*. This is the reason there is no clear definition of e-healthcare service. Hadwich et al. (2010) suggest that to better understand the complexity of e-health services it is useful to distinguish four different areas of e-health, the four Cs: commerce, content, care, and connectivity (Meyers et al., 2002).

- E-health commerce: This refers to products and services that are researched and paid for online. One example would be e-pharmacies offering medications online. Other services could include links to health publications or, more progressively, health insurance products (Meyers et al., 2002; Hadwich et al., 2010).
- E-health content: This refers to offerings of health information via an electronic exchange. Patients are able to inform themselves on health portals, including online patient educational documents and video presentations. The information is mostly standardized as it addresses the need of the general population. Other examples may include administrative linkages to appointment systems, lab results, and claims management (Hadwich et al., 2010).
- E-healthcare: Healthcare is evolving through the development of 'virtual services and information-rich bedside services' (Meyers et al., 2002). Internet capabilities will be useful for providers to extend existing clinical treatment capabilities. For example, providers can make virtual house calls using medical devices that report information through in-home monitors linked to the Internet (Meyers et al., 2002). Other options include interactive home monitoring sys-

tems that continuously monitor patients' vital functions at home, transmitting real-time information and retrospective patient data via wireless point-of-service communication to health professionals located outside the home (Meyers et al., 2002).

– E-health connectivity: This refers to Internet-based services that link the various participants in the healthcare marketplace (Meyers et al., 2002). Examples include virtual customer service, online access of claim history and payment, transmission of electronic patient data among members of the healthcare system, e.g., among physicians and insurance companies (Hadwich et al., 2010).

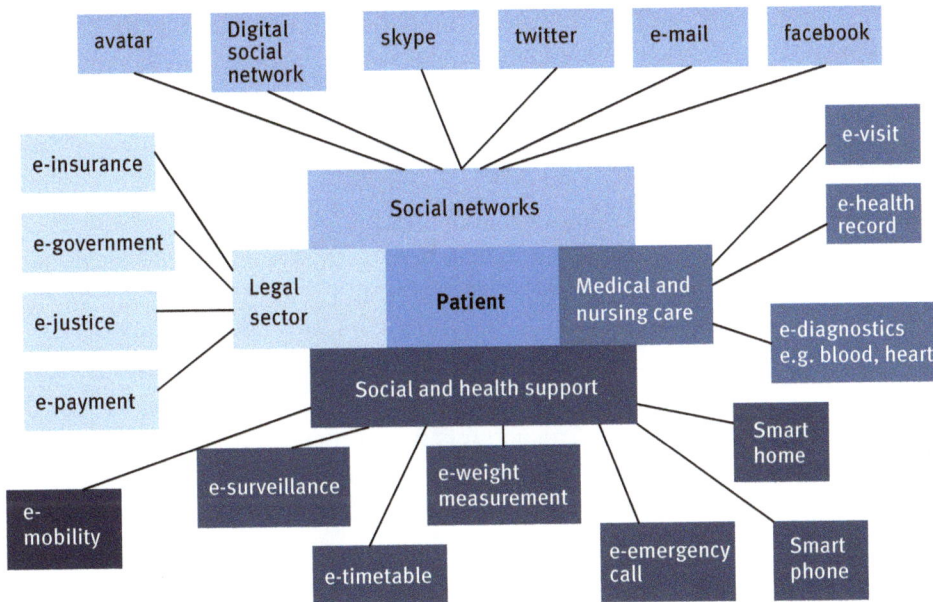

Fig. 10.1: Combination or composition of service parts of the ICT solution for patients
Source: adapted from Kriegel J., S. Schmitt-Rüth, B. Güntert, P. Mallory: New service development in German and Austrian healthcare – bringing e-health services into the market, International Journal of Healthcare Management 2013, Vol. 6, No. 2, p. 81

An additional element can be communities (Kirchgeorg and Lorbeer, 2002). **Virtual communities** are places on the Web where people can find and then electronically 'talk' to others with similar interests e.g., diabetes, depression, and other topics of interest. All the elements differ with regard to the degree of individualization as well as the degree of provider-patient interaction.

Particularly with regard to patient-focused services, e-health solutions can be part of a number of different, larger modules. Depending on the needs and priorities of the individual patient, the several services can be used continuously or temporarily (Figure 3.1.), (Kriegel, 2013).

These patient-related services are not the only traditional e-health options in the context of medical and nursing care (Bitterman, 2011). Based on the environment of the patient or his interaction sphere, other options include support from the sectors of social-health support, social networks, and legal administrative areas (Chan et al., 2008).

It is reasonable to assume that implementation of e-health services becomes more difficult as the degree of individualization and interaction of service delivery increases (Hadwich et al., 2010). Furthermore, legal regulations and privacy concerns regarding online health-related patient data may restrain the implementation of services in the areas of care and connectivity (Lerer and Rowell, 2000).

10.5 E-health business structures

E-business means 'doing business electronically'. It comprises 'Internet-based business', 'e-commerce', and 'e-markets'. It considers business that is conducted exclusively over the Internet (e.g., Priceline.com) to be business that exploits the potentiality of the Internet as a complement to a firm's traditional operations, such as click-and-mortar-based businesses (Zott et al., 2010).

Health e-commerce enterprises, built within the last fifteen years, populate all the main e-business models. Among them the following can be found (Parente, 2000).

– Health e-commerce portals. The portal is the most common face of the Internet for the consumer, providing a launch point for various online activities. Health e-commerce portals are the face of the medical Internet for both consumers and providers seeking medical guidance and information on new innovations. As with other portals, healthcare portals are financed primarily through advertising revenue. An example is *OnHealth*. This site provides consumer-oriented health information through standard medical references as well as original content from the site's writers and editors.

– Health e-commerce connectivity. One of the unique developments of e-commerce is businesses that link information systems seamlessly. Health e-commerce connectivity initiatives include Internet accessible EMRs (*Electronic Medical Records*), assessment of provider quality based on clinical outcomes, and use of quality data in physician selection. Internet connectivity is similar to infrastructure projects in the brick-and-mortar economy in that the enormous initial costs are usually taken for granted once the structure is built. Emdeon is an example. It is a leading provider of revenue and payment cycle management and clinical information exchange solutions, connecting payers, providers, and patients in the US healthcare system.

– Business-to-business e-commerce. Business-to-business e-commerce represents the sale of goods and services directly to other firms and government agencies.

Health e-commerce models are extensions of general business e-commerce, which includes examples such as biotechnology Web sales directly to providers and the sale of refurbished medical equipment through online auctions. Manufactured products are often sold in this way; but services, such as consulting or benefits management, are beginning to be sold as well. *Neoforma*, as an example, provides online solutions that enable buyers to reduce product-procurement costs and suppliers to access a highly efficient direct marketing channel.

– Business-to-consumer e-commerce. Business-to-consumer e-commerce involves manufacturers and retailers selling goods directly to consumers. A model allows consumers to purchase health products ranging from vitamins to health insurance. *PlanetRx* is an example of an online pharmacy.

Strictly focusing on healthcare organizations (HCOs) according to the character of their activity, all those offering e-services through the Internet can be divided into (Chmielarz, 1999) the following groups.

– Internet HCOs with traditional outlets: They use the Internet as an alternative distribution channel; patients have access to services in traditional branches through the Internet and other electronic channels (Model I).
– HCOs operating only by means of the Internet: These are virtual HCOs without traditional branches; patients have access to services only through the Internet or other electronic channels (Model II).
– Internet HCOs created by traditional HCOs but operating separately: There is no relationship between services offered through the Internet and traditional branches (Model III).

Nowadays, HCOs that offer services in traditional branches and support their activities with the Internet (Model I) are the most popular in the European market. They have competitive advantages in the market compared to other HCOs because they have already been operating with a large number of patients. Model II has a complementary role in the market; whereas Model III is less popular form of Internet organization (Matysiewicz, Smyczek, 2011). In table 3.1, a simplified categorization of e-health business structures is shown.

Tab. 10.1: E-health business structure
Source: adapted from J. Tan: E-Healthcare Information System. An Introduction for Student and Professionals, *Jossey-Bass, San Francisco 2005, p. 371*

	Click-and-Mortar E-Health Models (Model I)	Virtual E-Health Models and Services (Model II)
Definition and Characteristics	Uses the Internet as a supplement to traditional marketing, delivering additional benefits to customers and building relationships with them.	Uses the Internet to construct an independent, profitable venture that exists mainly on the Internet.
Competitive Strategies	– Builds brand awareness and improves image. – Uses the Web as a cost-effective way to augment core products with related information and service functions. – Obtains cost savings from automating routine customer services.	– Provides convenience to customers that competitors cannot match. – Provides extra information in a form that competitors cannot imitate. – Uses the Internet to produce superior economic benefits for customers that competitors cannot imitate.
Merits	– Provides large quantities of information to customers. – Gives a company an instant global presence and attracts people who are not the company's current customers but potentially will be. – Opens a new communication channel, allowing a company to develop further relationships with customers, all at a reasonable cost.	– Provides a larger or more specialized selection of products than competitors can offer. – Offers higher-quality information, more economic benefits, and more convenience than competitors can offer. – Provides a sense of community for customers.

10.6 E-health: strategic approach

The healthcare industry is diverse but the Internet appears capable of supporting some common strategic interests. It could, for example, help organizations to do the following (National Research Council, 2000):

– improve the efficiency and effectiveness of processes that customers use to judge organizational performance (e.g., scheduling an appointment) or processes that form the core of the organization's business (e.g., medical management);

– develop partnerships with related organizations in an effort to leverage respective strengths (e.g., MCOs partnering with pharmaceutical companies to develop

disease management programs or regional alliances of providers partnering to form a continuum of care);
- reach consumers directly to solidify brand names and eliminate intermediaries (disintermediation);
- improve, differentiate, and deliver new services to key customers; and
- improve organizational decision making.

Using the Internet can really create multiple benefits for healthcare organizations; but, on the other hand, there are some threats, like losing the confidentiality and security of patient data. To deal with these implications, it must be realized that Internet technology is nothing else but a complementary tool, which has to be integrated into an overall strategy. Indeed, IT does not guarantee profitability unless its adoption is related to the company's strategy (Powell and Dent-Micallef, 1997).

So to make the most of the Internet, both traditional and e-health providers need to look beyond the short-term challenges of cost cutting and staff reductions to embrace a long-term vision and commitment to the opportunities offered by e-health initiatives. A successful **e-health strategy** needs to emphasize the primary benefits that e-health offers to the business goals of the organization. Customer acquisition and retention, customer satisfaction, relationship building, and provision of better-quality healthcare are but a few of the many benefits that await e-providers with the proper vision (Tan, 2005).

The cornerstone of a healthcare strategy is the physician-patient relationship. Doctors make up the front line of healthcare and are the key gatekeepers to health service delivery systems for patients. Effective doctor-patient communication is shown to be highly correlated with patient satisfaction with healthcare services. An increasing number of e-consumers are planning to change health plans and physicians in order to fulfill their desire to receive healthcare services online (Tan, 2005). Therefore, it is important to draw attention to defined standards that build good relationships with patients.

Standards for professional interactions should be consistent across all forms of communication between the patient and physician, whether in person or online. Encounters between patients and physicians should only occur within the bounds of an established patient–physician relationship, which entails rights and obligations for both parties. Table 3.2 presents the implications of online activities for patients, physicians, the profession, and society and contains recommendations that address online communication with patients, the use of social media sites to gather and share information about patients, physician-produced blogs, physician posting of personal information that patients can access, and communications among colleagues about patient care (Farnan et al, 2013).

Tab. 10.2: Online physician activities: benefits, pitfalls, and recommended safeguards
Source: adapted from J. Farnna et al : Online Medical Professionalism: Patient and Public Relationships: Policy Statement From the American College of Physicians and the Federation of State Medical Boards, Annals of Internal Medicine 2013;158, p. 621

Activity	Potential Benefits	Potential Pitfalls	Recommended Safeguards
Communications with patients using e-mail, text, and instant messaging.	Greater accessibility. Immediate answers to noncurrent issues.	Confidentiality concerns. Replacement of face-to-face or telephone. Interaction ambiguity or misinterpretation of digital interactions.	Establish guidelines for types of issues appropriate for digital communication. Reserve digital communication only for patients who maintain face-to-face follow-up.
Use of social media sites to gather information about patient.	Observe and counsel patients on risk-taking or health-averse behaviors. Intervene in an emergency.	Sensitivity to source of information. Threaten trust in patient–physician relationship.	Consider intent of search and application of findings. Consider implications for ongoing care.
Use of online educational resources and related information with patients.	Encourage patient empowerment through self-education. Suplement resource-poor environment.	Non-peer-reviewed materials may provide inaccurate information. Scam 'patient' sites that misrepresent therapies and outcomes.	Vet information to ensure accuracy of content. Refer patients only to reputable sites and sources.
Physician-produced blogs, microblogs, and physician posting of comments by others.	Advocacy and public health enhancement. Introduction of physician 'voice' into such conversations.	Negative online content, such as 'venting' or ranting that disparages patients and colleagues.	'Pause before posting'. Consider the content and the message it sends about a physician as an individual and the profession.
Physician posting of physician personal information on public social media sites.	Networking and communications.	Blurring of professional and personal boundaries. Impact on representation of the individual and the profession.	Maintain separate personas, personal and professional, for online social behavior. Scrutinize material available for public consumption.
Physician use of digital venues (e.g., text and Web) for communicating with colleagues about patient care.	Ease of communication with colleagues.	Confidentiality concerns. Unsecured networks and accessibility of protected health information.	Implement health information technology solutions for securemessaging and information sharing. Follow institutional practice and policy for remote and mobile access of protected health information.

As J. Farna et al. stress, online technologies present both opportunities and challenges to professionalism. They offer innovative ways for HCOs and physicians to interact with patients and positively affect the health of communities, but the tenets of professionalism and of the patient–physician relationship should govern these interactions. Institutions should have policies in place on the uses of digital media. Education about the ethical and professional use of these tools is critical to maintaining a respectful and safe environment for patients, the public, and physicians. As patients continue to turn to the Web for healthcare advice, physicians should maintain a professional presence and direct patients to reputable sources of information.

References

American College of Physicians. E-Health and Its Impact on Medical Practice. Philadelphia: American College of Physicians; 2008: Position Paper. (Available from American College of Physicians, 190 N. Independence Mall West, Philadelphia, PA 19106.)

Baron S. & Harrism K., 2003. *Service marketing*. Texts and cases, Palgrave.

Bitterman N., 2011.*Design of medical devices: a home perspective*. The European Journal of Internal Medicine, Vol.22, 39–42.

Boyer, K. K., Hallowell R., & Roth A.V., 2002. E-Services: Operating Strategy – a Case Study and a Method for Analyzing Operational Benefits, Journal of Operations Management, 20 (2), 175–188.

Car, J., Black, A., Anandan, C., Cresswell, K., Pagliari, C., McKinstry, B., Procter, R., Majeed, A. & Sheikh, A., 2008. *The impact of e-health on the quality and safety of healthcare: a systemic overview and synthesis of the literature*, Report for the NHS Connecting for Health Evaluation Programme, Imperial College, London, March, Retrieved February 06, 2010 from www1.ic.ac.uk/resources/1636368E-DDEE-42A0-85AC-BDE9EC3B9EA1/.

Chan M., Estève D., Escriba C. & Campo, 2008. *A review of smart homes: present state and future challenges*, Comput Methods Programs Biomed, Vol. 91(1), 55–81.

Chmielarz, W., 1999. *System y elektronicznej bankowości i cyfrowej płatności*, Warszawa: PWE.

Farnan J., et al : *Online Medical Professionalism: Patient and Public Relationships: Policy Statement From the American College of Physicians and the Federation of State Medical Boards*, Annals of Internal Medicine 2013;158, p. 621

Hofacker F., Goldsmith R.E., Bridges E. & Swilley E., 2007.*E-Services: A Synthesis and Research Agenda Charles*, This manuscript is currently in press in the Journal of Value Chain Management, Retrieved February 20, 2010 from http://www.researchgate.net.

Hollesen S., 2007. *Global Marketing*, Prentice Hall, p. 228.

Javalgi D., Rajshekhar G., Ch.L. Martin, & Todd P.R., 2004. *The Export of E-Services in the Age of Technology Transformation: Challenges and Implications for International Service Providers*, Journal of Services Marketing, 18 (7), 560–573.

Hadwich K., Georgi D., Tuzovic S., Büttner J. & Bruhn M, 2010. Perceived quality of e-health services: A conceptual scale development of e-health service quality based on the C-OAR-SE approach, International Journal of Pharmaceutical and Healthcare Marketing, Vol. 4 Iss: 2,112–136

Kirchgeorg M., Lorbeer A., 2002. *Kundenbindungsstrategien von e-health-services anbietern*, in Bruhn, M. (Ed.), Electronic Services. Dienstleistungsmanagement Jahrbuch 2002, Gabler-Verlag, Wiesbaden.

Kriegel J., Schmitt-Rüth S., Güntert B., & Mallory P., 2013. *New service development in German and Austrian healthcare – bringing e-health services into the market*, International Journal of Healthcare Management, Vol. 6, No. 2, p. 81

Kotler, P., Armstrong, G., Saunders, J.,Wong, V. 1996. *Principles of Marketing*, The European Edition, Prentice-Hall, Hemel Hempstead,

Kotler Ph., Shalowitz J., & Stevens R.J., 2008. *Strategic Marketing For Healthcare Organizations*: *Building A Customer-Driven Health System*, John Wiley & Sons.

Lerer, L. & Rowell, N., 2000. *The e-Health Consumer*, INSEAD Healthcare Management Initiative, The Healthcare 2020 Platform, Paris.

Lovelock Ch., 2001. *Services marketing. People, Technology, Strategy*, Prentice Hall, p. 5.

Løwendahl B., 2007. *Strategic Management of ProfessionalService Firms,*3rd edn, Copenhagen Business School Press, Copenhagen, p. 22

Matysiewicz J., Smyczek S., 2011. *Building Consumer Loyalty – Challenge for Global E-healthcare Organizations* [in:] *Technology, Internationalization and Customer Experiences*, ed. V. Jauhari, G. Sanjeev, M. Rishi, Viva Books Private Limited, New Dehli.

Matysiewicz J., Smyczek S. 2012. *Modele relacji jednostek medycznych z pacjentami w otoczeniu wirtualnym*, Placet Warszawa.

Meyers, J., van Brunt, D., Patick, K. & Greene, A., 2002. *Personalizing medicine on the web: e-health offers hospitals several strategies for success*, Health Forum Journal, Vol. 45 No. 1, 22–6

National Research Council, 2000. *Networking Health: Prescriptions for the Internet*. Washington, DC: The National Academies Press.

Parente S.T. , 2000. *Beyond the hype: a taxonomy of e-health business models*, Health Affairs, Vol.19, no.6, 89–102

Powell T, Dent-Micallef A., 1997. *Information technology as competitive advantage: the role of human, business, and technology resources*. Strategic Management Journal, 18 (5), p. 375

Rust R.T. & Lemon K.N., 2001. *E-Service and the Consumer*, International Journal of Electronic Commerce

Tan J.(2005): *E-Healthcare Information System. An Introduction for Student and Professionals*, Jossey-Bass, San Francisco 2005, p. 371.

WHO: *E-Health Report*: Retrieved February 20, 2014 from http://www.who.int/trade/glossary/story021/en/,

Zott Ch., Amot R. & Massa L., 2010. The business model: Theoretical roots, recent developments, and future research, Working paper IESE Business School, University of Navarra, 1–45 Retrieved February 20, 2014 from http://www.iese.edu/research/pdfs/di-0862-e.pdf.

Żabiński L., 2008. *Marketing produktów systemowych. Nowa domena współczesnego marketingu* in: Współczesny marketing. Trendy. Działania, ed. G. Sobczyk, PWE, Warszawa

Marcin Młodożeniec

11 Social Media Implementation in the European Healthcare Sector

Abstract Social media have become an immanent part of social life all around the globe. Users look there for new contacts, entertainment, and information. Organizations use them more and more frequently for marketing communication. The significance of social networking services has also been growing in the healthcare sector. Patients look there for, among other things, information concerning disease prevention, healthy lifestyles, and opinions about healthcare centers and doctors. At the same time, entities operating in healthcare search, via social media, for new forms of communication with their clients. This chapter presents the results of research regarding the activity of selected hospitals operating in five European markets that are using the most popular social media, with particular attention paid to Facebook.com.

Keywords: Healthcare, Social media, Implementation, Facebook

11.1 Introduction

The twenty-first century is witnessing an explosion in Internet-based messages transmitted through **social media**. These messages have become a major factor influencing various aspects of consumer behavior, including awareness, information acquisition, opinions, attitudes, purchase behavior, and post-purchase communication and evaluation (Mangold and Faulds, 2009: 358).

There are many definitions of social media. One of the most popular ones, developed by A. M. Haenlein, says that social media is a group of Internet-based applications that build on the ideological and technological foundations of Web 2.0 and that allow creation and exchange of user-generated content (Kaplan and Haenlein, 2010: 61).

Applications of this type allow Internet users to implement at least three activities: participation, sharing, and cooperation (Kaplan and Haenlein, 2010: 65). Social media encompasses a wide range of online sites, blogs, and word-of-mouth forums, including company-sponsored discussion boards and chat rooms, consumer-to-consumer e-mail, consumer product or service rating websites and forums, Internet discussion boards and forums, moblogs (sites containing digital audio, images, movies, or photographs), and **social networking sites**, to name a few (Mangold and Faulds, 2009: 358).

From the point of view of establishing contacts and building relationships among consumers, the most popular forms of social media are the so-called social network sites (SNS) on the Internet. They allow users and organizations to reflect, in virtual space, a network of contacts and relationships that they have in the real world. Owing to their functions, social network sites increase opportunities with regard to acquisition of new relationships and maintaining (developing) existing relationships with already established contacts ('Friends').

The number of people using social network sites is constantly growing. In 2013, the number of users of social media reached 1.74 billion and is expected to keep growing until by 2017, the number will be up to 2.55 billion (Emarketer, 2013).

Globally, the most popular social network site is **Facebook**, which, in May 2013, announced that the site is used by 1.11 billion users a month (News.Yahoo, 2013). The most popular social media also include Youtube – more than a billion unique users (YouTube, 2013), Google Plus – more than 500 million (The Faster Times, 2013), Twitter – 500 million recipients (The Telegraph, 2013), LinkedIn – 200 million (LinkedIn, 2013), and Pinterest – 70 million users (Search Engine Watch, 2013).

The number of users of social media also continues to increase in Europe. In 2011, social network sites were used by 34.5 percent of its population; and it is estimated that this ratio will increase by 2017 to 49.4 percent. The largest percentage of social network site users in Western Europe is observed in the Netherlands (69.6 percent), while in Sweden, it is 64.5 percent; in the UK, 50.2 percent; in Germany, 39.9 percent; and in Italy, 32.6 percent (New Media Trend Watch, 2013). The most popular social network site in this part of the world is Facebook: UK, 29.9 million; Germany, 22.1 million; France, 22.0 million; Spain, 18.3 million; Italy, 18.0 million; Netherlands, 10.8 million; Sweden, 5.4 million; Poland, 10.3 million (Wirtualnemedia, 2013); and in Belgium, ca 5 million users (Internet World Stats, 2013).

11.2 Social media in the economy

The high popularity of social media is taken advantage of by organizations for various marketing purposes. Eighty-seven percent of Fortune 100 companies have a presence on at least one social media site (The Social Skinny, 2013). The site of Coca-Cola is liked on Facebook by more than 73 million people, the site of Red Bull by more than 40 million, and the site of McDonald's by nearly 30 million users. The Vine brand (an application for an edition of videos) on Twitter is followed by more than 4.8 million users, Starbucks by 4.3 million, and Chanel by 2.7 million people (Social Bakers, 2013).

According to the 2012 social media marketing industry report, How Marketers Are Using Social Media to Grow Their Businesses, more than 80 percent of marketers believe that social media are important for their organization (Social Media Examiner, 2013).

For marketing purposes, top global brands use these social media the most: Facebook (99.6 percent), Twitter (95.5 percent), and Youtube (95.1 percent) (International Business Times, 2013).

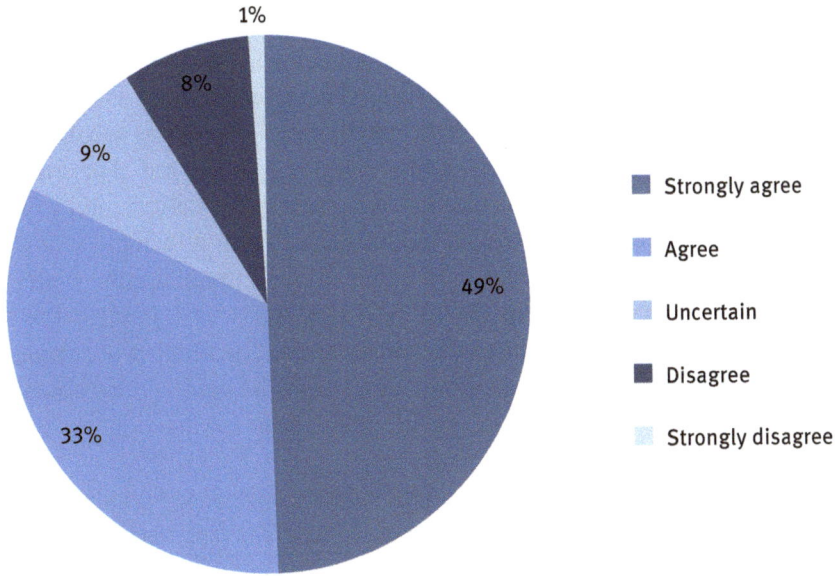

Fig. 11.1: Social media importance for organizations
Source: Adapted from Socialmediaexaminer.com, 2013. Homepage – Reports – 2013 Social Media Marketing Industry Report. Retrieved September 21, 2013 from:
http://www.socialmediaexaminer.com/SocialMediaMarketingIndustryReport2013.pdf

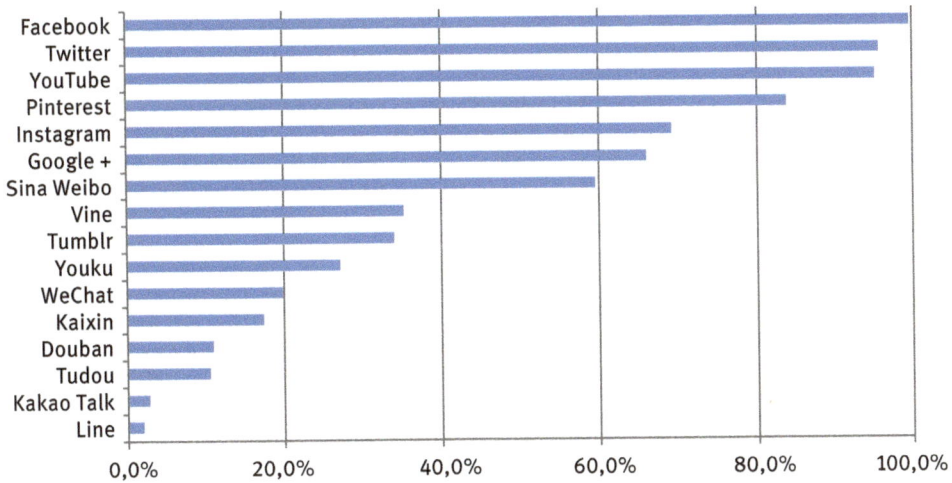

Fig. 11.2: Social platforms, ordered by how many top brands use them
Source: Adapted from Ibtimes.com, 2013. Homepage – Tech/Sci – Social media – Social Media Marketing: How Do Top Brands Use Social Platforms. Retrieved September 21, 2013 from:
http://www.ibtimes.com/social-media-marketing-how-do-top-brands-use-social-platforms-charts-1379457.

The most popular SNS used by companies is Facebook. Brands build and develop communities here thanks to the opportunities for advertising (Facebook Ads) as well as create and publish their own content (the so-called posts) in the form of publication of status (in the form of a text message), publication of pictures (posting a graphic file with the possibility of adding a text message), organization of an event (announcing information about the event, e.g., a conference, seminar, or picnic with a possibility to invite the participants), and asking a question (using a special application that enables asking a question to the fans in the form of a quiz) (Tutaj, 2013: 248). Additionally, organizations themselves can create and publish their applications on Facebook (e.g., for organization of contests). The number of posts is the main indicator that demonstrates the level of activity of the brand on Facebook. The most valuable global brands add, on average, more than twenty-eight posts a month (Młodożeniec and Tutaj, 2012).

The multitude of social media and their specific character enable various applications in marketing. Distinguished by the type of applications used, Cristina Castronovo and Lei Huang provide examples of applications of selected social media (2012: 123).

Tab. 11.1: Social media tools and their objectives
Source: Adapted from Castronovo C., Huang L., 2012. Social Media in an Alternative Marketing Communication Model. Journal of Marketing Development and Competitiveness, 6(1), 123.

Tools	Objectives
Chat Rooms	– improve coustomer service – create a sense of community – garner customer feedback
Blogs	– drive WOM recommendations – build meaningful relationships – increase loyality
YouTube	– harness power of video to increase embedding of content in other sites
Facebook	– advertising – develop a community – target specific audiences
LinkedIn	– connect with professional communities
Twitter	– customer engagement – conversation propagation
Google Wave	– increase collaboration and engagement – crowdsourcing
Four Square	– increase local and mobile connectivity – increase network engagement

Research shows that the most involving posts, i.e., those providing the most interaction on the part of Facebook users in the form of comments, clicks on the 'Like' button, and sharing, are generated by adding posts with photographs. The level of interaction is a significant indicator showing the willingness of fans to take part in the 'brand life'.

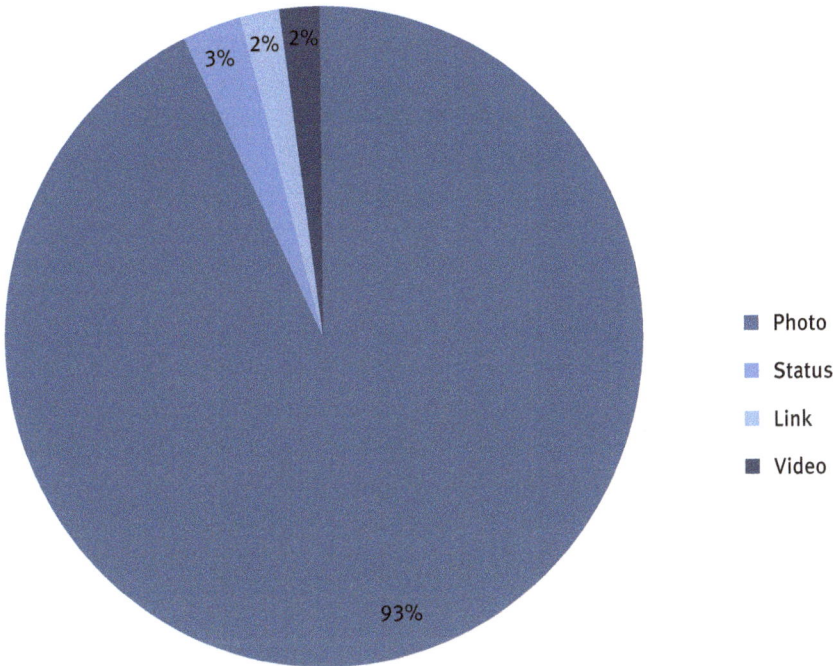

Fig. 11.3: The most engaging post types on Facebook
Source: Adapted from Socialbeakers.com, 2013. Homepage – Facebook statistics – Photos Make Up 93% of The Most Engaging Posts on Facebook! Retrieved September 21, 2013 from: http://www.socialbakers.com/blog/1749-photos-make-up-93-of-the-most-engaging-posts-on-facebook.

The scale and the dynamics of the development of social media as well as their effect on consumer behavior have thus a significant impact on the marketing activity of the organization. This applies to most sectors of the economy worldwide. The same phenomena are visible in the healthcare industry, both in the United States and in Europe.

11.3 Healthcare and social media

Development of Internet use has significantly influenced the healthcare sector. The most popular websites associated with health are visited by 7 to more than 20 million users a month. The most popular site according to ebizmba.com is Yahoo!Health and is visited each month by 2,150,000 users (Ebizma, 2013). The National Institute of Health website enjoys popularity with 20,000,000 visits and WebMed, with 19,500,000 visits. Along with the popularity of websites related to health, there is an increase in patients using SNS as a tool supporting 'management' of their health. According to the report *Social Media 'Likes' Healthcare: From Marketing to Social Business*, published by PWC, 42 percent of consumers in the American market have used social media to access health-related consumer reviews (e.g., of treatments or physicians). Nearly 30 percent have supported a health cause, 25 percent have posted about their health experience, and 20 percent have joined a health forum or community (PWC, 2013). Development of Internet users and the Web 2.0 philosophy has even led to creation of a constantly evolving term of Health 2.0/Medicine 2.0. Health 2.0 refers to technology, patients, professionals, social networking, health information/content, collaboration, and change of healthcare (Van De Belt et al., 2010: 18). Thus we are dealing with developing activities utilizing Web 2.0 technology that connect patients, doctors, and entities of the healthcare industry via social media.

As a result, healthcare entities more and more often include activity in social network sites in their marketing processes. Business strategies that include social media can help health industry companies take a more active, engaged role in managing individuals' health. Social marketing can evolve into social business with the right leadership and investment of resources. Insights from social media also offer instant feedback on products or services, along with new ideas for innovation. Organizations that can incorporate this information into their operations will be better positioned to meet the needs of today's consumers (PWC, 2013).

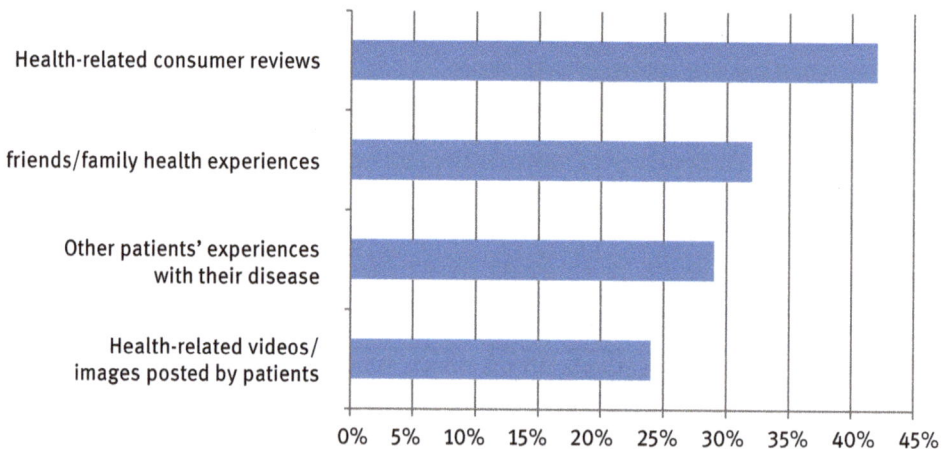

Fig. 11.4: Percentage of consumers viewing health information through social media
Source: Adapted from Pwc.com, 2013. Homepage – Industries – Health industries – Our perspective – Thought Leadership – Social media likes healthcare: From marketing to social business. Retrieved September 21, 2013 from: http://www.pwc.com/us/en/health-industries/publications/ health-care-social-media.jhtml.

The experience of early adopters demonstrates that social media can be used to accomplish healthcare goals in four broad areas (Computer Sciences Corporation, 2013):

- communications,
- information sharing,
- clinical outcomes, and
- speed of innovation.

11.4 Use of social media in healthcare entities in the examined markets

Considering the popularity of social media and their growing importance in the market of medical services, analysis was conducted to determine the presence and the activity of selected entities operating in the field of health protection. For the purpose of this study, research first examined the actions of institutions involved in management of health protection systems in five countries: UK, Belgium, Germany, Poland, and Sweden. Then the activity of the most popular social media of selected European hospitals, also operating in the above markets, was verified.

In the first part, account was taken of actions in social networking sites by eleven entities responsible for the organization and implementation of health protection services. In the case of the UK, research covered the activities of the National Health Service (NHS); in Belgium, L'Institut national d'assurance maladie-invalidité (INAMI); in Germany, seven organizations: Der Verband der Ersatzkassen e. V. (vdek), Der EBL-Bundesverband, Der BKK Bundesverband, Dem IKK/e.V., Die Knappschaft, Der LandwirtschaftlichenSozialversicherung (LSV-SPV), and Der GKV-Spitzenverband; in Poland, the National Health Fund (NFZ); and in Sweden, the Swedish National Institute of Public Health.

Table 11.2 implies that the greatest number of social media is used by the British National Health Service. This organization is present on the social networking sites Facebook and Google+ and on Twitter microblog. It also publishes video materials on YouTube.

The Swedish organization, the Swedish National Institute of Public Health, uses, from the range of social media, only the blog by the CEO of the Institute. Additionally, it is available only in Swedish (Public Health Agency in Sweden, 2013).

On the other hand, four organizations from Germany: Der Verband der Ersatzkassen e. V., Der AOK-Bundesverband, Der BKK Bundesverband, and Der GKV-Spitzenverband use the so-called social plugs (these are special applications installed on the website that enable sharing content directly from the website in the selected social media). The organizations do not have their sites or profiles in the social media themselves; but thanks to social plugs, they make it possible for users to share their content.

Tab. 11.2: Use of social media by entities responsible for health protection in five selected countries of Europe (May 2013)

State	No.	Organization name and website	Presence in social media				
			Facebook	Twitter	Google+	YouTube	Other
Germany	1.	Der Verband der Ersatzkassen e. V. www.vdek.com	No	No	No	No	Social Plug-ins
	2.	Der AOK-Bundesverband www.aok-bv.de	No	No	No	No	Social Plug-ins
	3.	Der BKK Bundesverband www.bkk.de	No	No	No	No	Social Plug-ins
	4.	Dem IKK e.V. www.ikkev.de	No	No	No	No	No
	5.	Die Knappschaft www.knappschaft.de	No	No	No	No	No
	6.	Der Landwirtschaftlichen Sozialversicherung www.lsv.de	No	No	No	No	No
	7.	Der GKV-Spitzenverband www.gkv-spitzenverband.de	No	No	No	No	Social Plug-ins
Great Britain	8.	National Health Service www.nhs.uk	Yes	Yes	Yes	Yes	No
Belgium	9.	L'Institut national d'assurance maladie-invalidité www.inami.fgov.be	No	No	No	No	No
Sweden	10.	Swedish National Institute of Public Health www.fhi.se	No	No	No	No	Blog
Poland	11.	The National Health Fund www.nfz.gov.pl	No	No	No	No	No

The popularity of social media among Internet users and companies does not go hand in hand with the activity of entities involved in the management of health systems in the surveyed countries. This confirms the thesis that healthcare organizations have been slower to adopt social media than other business organizations (Computer Sciences Corporation, 2013).

However, this does not apply to organizations operating in the field of health protection. Hospitals, as a group, have higher adoption rates than other sectors of the healthcare economy. As a cohort, hospitals in Europe are leading in their adoption of social media. In particular, more hospitals in the Netherlands and the United Kingdom use social media than hospitals elsewhere in Europe, the United States, or Australia (Computer Sciences Corporation, 2013).

Table 11.3: Social media use among hospitals internationally (2009 to 2011)
Source: Adapted from CSC.com, 2012. Homepage – Healthcare – Health Services Insights – Should Healthcare Organizations Use Social Media?: A Global Update. Retrieved September 21, 2013 from: http://assets1.csc.com/health_services/downloads/CSC_Should_Healthcare_Organizations_Use_S ocial_Media_A_Global_Update.pdf.

Social media use	Country
High adopters	Netherlands, United Kingdom, Norway, Sweden
Mid-rangeadopters	United States, Austria
Low adopters	Australia, Switzerland, Germany

Hospitals examined in Western Europe, in terms of basic activity on the most popular social media, are increasingly active. In the years from 2009 to 2011, the percentage of hospitals having an account on YouTube increased from 2 up to 20 percent; on Twitter, from 1 percent to 18 percent; on LinkedIn, from 20 to 32 percent; and on Facebook, from 10 to as much as 67 percent (Van De Belt et al., 2012: 18).

The most popular social network site on the Internet used by hospitals in the surveyed countries is Facebook. Facebook accounts were found in all countries, ranging from 15 percent (n = 13) in the Netherlands to 93.1 percent (n = 163) in the United Kingdom.

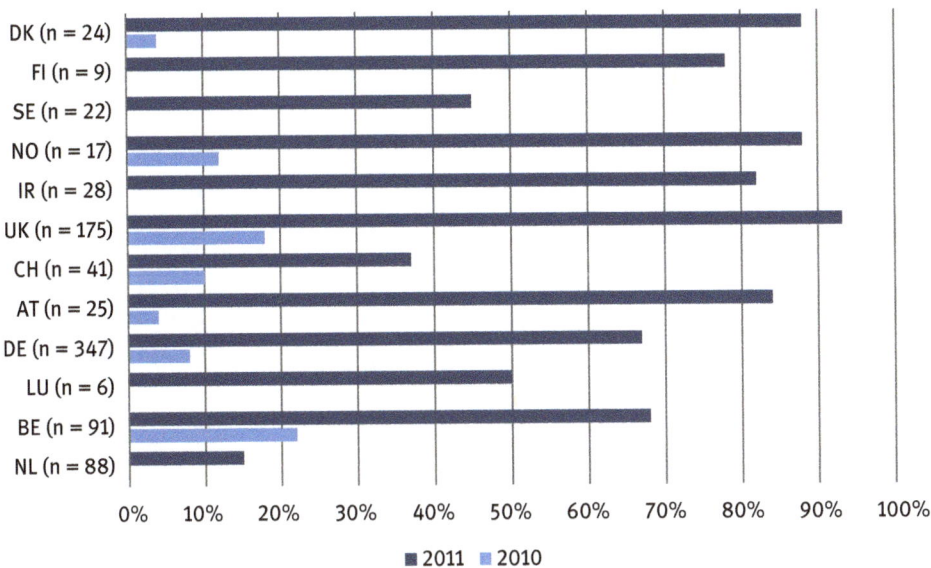

Fig. 11.5: Percentage of European hospitals using Facebook. NL = the Netherlands, BE = Belgium, LU = Luxembourg, DE = Germany, AT = Austria, CH = Switzerland, UK = United Kingdom, IR = Ireland, NO = Norway, SE = Sweden, FI = Finland, DK = Denmark
Source: Adopted from Van De Belt T.H., Engelen L. J., Berben S. A. A., Schoonhoven L., 2012. Use of Social Media by Western European Hospitals: Longitudinal Study. Journal of Medical Internet Research, 14(3)

The analysis of the available literature and the results of the research show, among other things, that the efforts conducted so far are of a general nature. It is difficult to analyze implementation of specific activities in social media on their basis. There is a need for more thorough analysis of the actions of entities in the healthcare industry on social media in order to identify trends and good practices, which are the object of analysis in this chapter.

To attempt to identify promising trends and practices, research was conducted as to the activity on social media implemented by selected hospitals operating in significant markets (Swedish, German, Polish, British, and Belgian). The purpose of the study was to identify the social media that are most popular among the hospitals and to analyze the methods and forms of activity implemented by them on the social network sites used most often.

11.5 Test method

The subject of the research was the hospitals operating in UK, Belgium, Poland, Germany, and Sweden. Because of the level of detail needed for this chapter, it was not possible to analyze all hospitals operating in the markets being studied. An important factor was thus selecting the research sample because statements, rankings, and other information that can be used as the key to selecting the institutions to be surveyed were not available.

To select the research sample, the decision was made to use the hospitals assessed as the best in terms of their activity on the Internet. This information is available at http://hospitals.webometrics.info/en/Europe. The web page shows the ranking of hospitals in terms of the level of their activity online. For the scoring, account is taken, first of all, of visibility (number of links on other websites leading to the site of a given hospital) and size of the site (the amount of information published online). It has been assumed that hospitals assessed well in terms of online activity are also worth examining in terms of activities on social media as they are institutions that are aware of the importance of online activity in marketing communication.

Tab. 11.4: List of selected hospitals

No	Country	Name of hospital
1	Germany	University Clinic Heidelberg Universitätsklinikum Heidelberg
2		HELIOS Kliniken Gruppe
3		Asklepios Klinikum Bad Abbach
4		Universitätsklinikum Jena Klinikum der Friedrich Schiller Universität
5		Klinikum und Fachbereich Medizin der Johann Wolfgang Goethe-Universität Frankfurt am Main
6	UK	Institute of Cancer Research Royal Cancer Hospital
7		Guy's and St Thomas' Hospital NHS
8		Bury Road Surgery
9		King's College Hospital NHS Foundation Trust
10		NHS Greater Glasgow and Clyde
11	Belgium	Universitair Ziekenhuis Leuven
12		International Centre for Reproductive Health
13		Universitair Ziekenhuis Brussel
14		Hôpital a Bruxelles Cliniques Universitaires Saint Luc Universite Catholique de Louvain
15		Centre Hospitalier Universitaire de Brugmann
16	Sweden	Landstinget I Östergötland
17		Landstinget I Uppsala Lan
18		Karolinska Institute & University Hospital
19		Jamtlands Lands Landsting
20		Norrbottens Lans Landsting
21	Poland	Instytut Psychiatrii i Neurologii
22		Slaskie Centrum Chorób Serca W Zabrzu
23		Centrum Zdrowia Dziecka
24		Wielkopolskie Centrum Onkologii
25		LuxMed

From the rankings, the five best hospitals in each country were selected. These hospitals were the subjects of the research. To begin, the research examined the presence of these institutions on the five social media most popular in the world.

Tab 11.5: Presence of hospitals in selected social media (May 2013)

		Fb	Tw	YT	LI	G+
GER	University Clinic Heidelberg Universitätsklinikum Heidelberg*	1	0	0	0	0
	HELIOS Kliniken Gruppe	1	1	1	0	0
	Asklepios Klinikum Bad Abbach	1	1	1	0	1
	Universitätsklinikum Jena Klinikum der Friedrich Schiller Universität	1	0	0	0	0
	Klinikum und Fachbereich Medizin der Johann Wolfgang Goethe-Universität Frankfurt am Main	0	0	0	0	0
UK	Institute of Cancer Research Royal Cancer Hospital	1	1	0	0	0
	Guy's and St Thomas' Hospital NHS*	1	1	0	1	0
	Bury Road Surgery	0	1	0	0	0
	King's College Hospital NHS Foundation Trust	1	1	0	0	1
	NHS Greater Glasgow and Clyde*	1	0	0	1	0
BEL	Universitair Ziekenhuis Leuven	0	0	0	0	0
	International Centre for Reproductive Health	1	0	0	0	0
	Universitair Ziekenhuis Brussel	1	1	1	1	1
	Hôpital a Bruxelles Cliniques Universitaires Saint Luc Universite Catholique de Louvain*	1	0	1	0	0
	Centre Hospitalier Universitaire de Brugmann	0	0	1	0	0
SW	Landstinget I Östergötland	1	1	1	0	0
	Landstinget I Uppsala Lan	1	1	1	1	0
	Karolinska Institute & University Hospital*	1	0	1	0	0
	Jamtlands Lands Landsting	1	1	1	0	0
	Norrbottens Lans Landsting	1	1	0	1	0
PL	Instytut Psychiatrii i Neurologii	0	0	0	0	0
	Slaskie Centrum Chorób Serca W Zabrzu	1	0	0	0	0
	Centrum Zdrowia Dziecka	1	0	0	0	0
	Wielkopolskie Centrum Onkologii	1	1	1	0	1
	LuxMed	1	0	1	0	0
		20	12	11	5	4

* sozial site, not fan page

It seems from the analysis that the hospitals selected for the research use Facebook most frequently. Because use of Facebook was the most popular tool (presence on Fb for 20 out of 25 hospitals) compared with others (Twitter, 12 out of 25; YouTube, 11 out of 25; LinkedIn, 5 out of 25; and Google+4 out of 25), the activity of hospitals in this social network site has been examined in more detail. Looking at the hospitals in each country, currently all of the hospitals in Sweden are using Facebook

(5/5, with the additional detail that one does not have its own fanpage, but has a social site). In Germany, Poland, and the UK, four out of five of the hospitals in the study are using Facebook (in Germany and UK, one hospital has a social site instead of a fanpage); and in Belgium, three out of five use Facebook (including one social site).

Next the hospitals were analyzed in terms of the intensity of their activity on Facebook and the most popular forms of this activity.

Tab. 11.6: Activities of hospitals on Facebook (May 2013)

			Posts	Statuses	Links	Photos	Videos	Questions	Events	Apps	Fans
1	GER	University Clinic Heidelberg Universitätsklinikum Heidelberg	29	0	15	2	0	0	12	0	2010
2		HELIOS Kliniken Gruppe*	0	0	0	0	0	0	0	0	0
3		Asklepios Klinikum Bad Abbach	3	0	0	1	0	0	2	0	300
4		Universitätsklinikum Jena Klinikum der Friedrich Schiller Universität	0	0	0	0	0	0	0	0	99
5		Klinikum und Fachbereich Medizin der Johann Wolfgang Goethe-Universität Frankfurt am Main	0	0	0	0	0	0	0	0	0
		Sum	**32**	**0**	**15**	**3**	**0**	**0**	**14**	**0**	**2409**
6	UK	Institute of Cancer Research Royal Cancer Hospital	0	0	0	0	0	0	0	0	35
7		Guy's and St Thomas' Hospital NHS*	0	0	0	0	0	0	0	0	0
8		Bury Road Surgery	0	0	0	0	0	0	0	0	0
9		King's College Hospital NHS Foundation Trust	20	0	20	0	0	0	0	0	4994
10		NHS Greater Glasgow and Clyde	0	0	0	0	0	0	0	0	0
		Sum	**20**	**0**	**20**	**0**	**0**	**0**	**0**	**0**	**5029**

Tab. 11.6: *Continued*

			Posts	Statuses	Links	Photos	Videos	Questions	Events	Apps	Fans
11	BEL	Universitair Ziekenhuis Leuven	0	0	0	0	0	0	0	0	0
12		International Centre for Reproductive Health	1	0	1	0	0	0	0	0	139
13		Universitair Ziekenhuis Brussel	18	8	10	0	0	0	0	0	703
14		Hôpital a Bruxelles Cliniques Universitaires Saint Luc Universite Catholique de Louvain*	0	0	0	0	0	0	0	0	0
15		Centre Hospitalier Universitaire de Brugmann	0	0	0	0	0	0	0	0	0
		Sum	**19**	**8**	**11**	**0**	**0**	**0**	**0**	**0**	**842**
16	SW	Landstinget I Östergötland	10	5	2	2	1	0	0	0	244
17		Landstinget I Uppsala Lan	7	0	4	3	0	0	0	0	93
18		Karolinska Institute & University Hospital*	0	0	0	0	0	0	0	0	0
19		Jamtlands Lands Landsting	15	0	5	10	0	0	0	0	123
20		Norrbottens Lans Landsting	11	2	5	4	0	0	0	0	214
		Sum	**43**	**7**	**16**	**19**	**1**	**0**	**0**	**0**	**674**
21	PL	Instytut Psychiatrii i Neurologii	0	0	0	0	0	0	0	0	0
22		Slaskie Centrum Chorób Serca W Zabrzu	0	0	0	0	0	0	0	0	981
23		Centrum Zdrowia Dziecka	12	6	2	4	0	0	0	0	6893
24		Wielkopolskie Centrum Onkologii	20	0	14	3	3	0	0	0	483
25		LuxMed	64	0	0	63	1	0	0	0	23732
		Sum	**96**	**6**	**16**	**70**	**4**	**0**	**0**	**0**	**32089**
			210	21	78	92	5	0	14	0	41043

* sozial site, not fan page

In the course of the analysis, it was discovered that the most active fanpage, belonging to the Luxmed brand, is kept not for a single hospital, but for the whole Luxmed Group, the hospital being just a part thereof. At the same time, Luxmed, as opposed to other entities being studied, is a commercial company, focused on gainful activities. Owing to this special character of the Luxmed brand, for the purpose of most comparisons, the activity of this brand was omitted (quantitative indicators for the Luxmed brand are specified in parenthesis); and its actions were subjected to a separate analysis.

In the audited period, all the hospitals added 146 (210) various posts, of which 78 (78) were links to other websites, 29 (92) contained information with photographs, 21 (21) were statuses containing text only, 14 (14) were events, and 5 (4) were published videos. None of the institutions asked questions or used any dedicated application on their fanpage. The hospitals gathered communities with a total number of fans amounting to 17,311 (41,043). The largest total number of fans was observed in Polish hospitals: 8,357 (32,089) fans; followed by British, 5,029; German, 2,409; Belgian, 842; and Swedish, 674 fans.

The kinds of activities are thus dominated by adding links and images. The first activity (adding links) is the most popular in all countries, except for Sweden (more images than links). Adding links is the simplest form of activity, not requiring creativity (like, e.g., when creating the status itself) or involvement (like, e.g., when creating and publishing images or video material). To post a reference (the so-called hyperlink) to the content published on the Internet, it is enough for the fanpage to display a fragment of the text and a link to the promoted content. On the other hand, the least popular activities turned out to be forms requiring the most involvement and creativity, which are creation of one's own applications for Facebook, preparing and asking questions, and preparation and publication of video materials.

The activity of the hospitals on Facebook is hardly diverse. The most posts in the study period were added by hospitals in Sweden – 43 posts; in Poland, 32 (96); in Germany, also 32; in the UK, 20; and in Belgium, 19.

Taking into account the aggregated data covering the number of added posts, it is possible to observe similar indicators illustrating the number of posts added monthly in hospitals in relation to the number of active fanpages in a given country. On average, hospitals having their own profiles on Facebook add the following number of posts:

- hospitals in Sweden: 10.75 posts/month [43 posts, 4 fanpages],
- hospitals in UK: 10 posts/month [20 posts, 2 fanpages],
- hospitals in Germany: 10.7 posts/month [32 posts, 3 fanpages],
- hospitals in Poland: 10.7 (24) posts/month [32 posts, 3 fanpages; 96 posts, 4 fanpages including Luxmed], and
- hospitals in Belgium: 9.5 posts/month [19 posts, 2 fanpages].

Therefore, if we exclude the aforementioned Luxmed, the average number of posts added by hospitals varies between 9.5. and 10.75, which is an average difference of only 2 posts a month between the most and the least active hospitals with break-down into countries.

The most numerous community was created by the Polish hospital, the Silesian Heart Diseases Centre in Zabrze, with 6,893 fans, and the least numerous by the British Institute of Cancer Research Royal Cancer Hospital, with 35 fans. It should be added, however, that the latter institution, apart from joining Facebook, does not conduct active operations there. (It does not add posts.)

A definitely outstanding entity turned out to be the Polish Luxmed. This brand covers a group of enterprises operating nationwide in the healthcare industry. They include, among others, a commercial hospital, a network of clinics, and a residential home. The profile on Facebook is kept for all activities of this brand, including the hospital. In the study period, the brand definitely added the greatest number of posts on Facebook – 64, while the average of posts added by other hospitals amounted to 10.43 posts. Luxmed also had the most numerous community – 23,732 fans, which is more than half the number of all the other institutions that were analyzed combined. Posts published by the brand were dominated by images, the most involving type according to research. Luxmed turned out to be, therefore, the most active entity on Facebook, and proved to have the most professional approach to marketing commu-nication on social media from among all of the entities being studied.

Moreover, the content published by LuxMed on its fanpage was examined. The posts were divided according to their subjects into the following categories: lifestyle (e.g., for mothers –'Where do you mostly buy clothes for your babies?'), health (e.g., 'Do you know what impact phones have on your health?'), events (workshop on overcoming fear of flying), and an offer (e.g., 'We recommend our special offer to all those who dream about a fresh smile'.).The results are presented in figure 11.6.

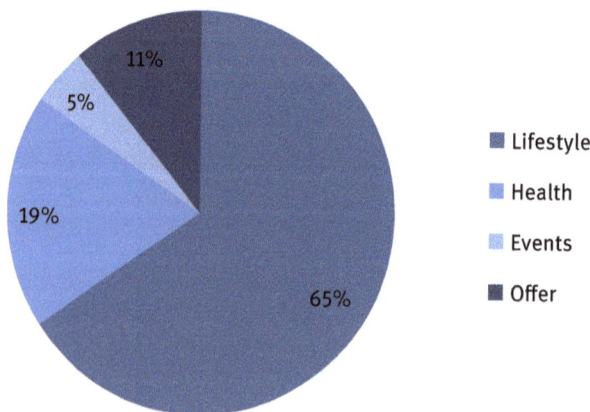

Fig. 11.6: Types of posts published on Luxmed fanpage (May 2013)

The analysis shows that a little less than two-thirds of the posts refer, in their content, to the lifestyle of patients. Luxmed usually addresses the fans with questions related to, among other things, a long May weekend, Mother's Day, the coming Child's Day, shopping, and so on. Information related to health is included in less than one-fifth of the posts. The information most often concerns health education (e.g.,'Hiccups as the result of strong cramps of the diaphragm, which are defensive reflexes of an organism', 'Do you know how many kcal are burnt during one round of golf'?'). Eleven percent of posts draw attention to the medical offer of LuxMed (e.g.,'May is the last chance to lose extra kilograms before you go on holiday. How to do it? With the LUX MED Group programme: Lose weight in a healthy way'). Then, five posts concern events organized by the brand or in which the brand participated (e.g.,'Already on the 23rd of May at 3.00 p.m. you shall have a unique chance to chat with Doctor Barbara Jerschina, a specialist in aesthetic and anti-aging medicine'.).

It seems that the LuxMed brand may be used as a source of good practices for other medical centers in terms of the quantity of published content, its kind as well as types. In addition, the number of brand fans and the numerous interactions (replies of the fans in comments to published posts) demonstrate the effectiveness of LuxMed activity on Facebook.

Conclusions

The research conducted shows that in the entities being studied, social media are used. In the entities coordinating the activities of health service, this use is minute. Only one of eleven of the institutions being analyzed has and actively manages content on social network sites. A more visible activity is typical of hospitals in all five of the surveyed countries, although it differs significantly from the market standards defined by the commercial brands (e.g., the most valuable global brand, Luxmed) both when it comes to the percentage of entities using social media and the intensity of the activities (measured, e.g., by number of posts added each month on Facebook).

On the basis of the analysis, it is difficult to find a connection between the implemented activities on social media and the tax-financial system valid in a given market.

Definitely the most common social network site used by the entities is Facebook, which is used by the entities most often as a tool for sharing other content published online (posts with links) and communication with patients. The more involvement is necessary to prepare a post (publication of video material, adding a question/quiz, posting one's own application), the lower its popularity is in the activity of the institutions being studied.

The activity of European healthcare entities on social media is also not strictly correlated either with the popularity of social media among the inhabitants of the country in which these entities operate or with the size of the country.

The current analysis shows that the degree of activity of healthcare entities may be most strongly linked to the form of an entity's organization. The more an entity is focused on commercial operations and the more its results depend on the number of customers/patients, the greater the activity of entities will likely be within social media regardless of the country and the tax system there. To confirm this thesis, it will be necessary, however, to conduct further research and analysis that looks at the activity of public entities as compared to non-public ones.

The public healthcare institutions that were studied should gain inspiration from activities conducted by commercial entities and the most popular global brands. Effective actions will be, first and foremost, the following improvements related to implementation of activities in social media.

– Presence in a greater number of social media: The institutions should, to a greater extent, use Facebook, Twitter, and YouTube because they are the social network sites most popular among the users-patients.
– Intensity: Activities on Facebook should be implemented with greater frequency as measured by the number of posts. A suggested good practice is publication of on average of one post a day.
– Involvement: Healthcare entities should, to a greater extent, focus on posts offering the greatest opportunities for interactions on the part of the fans of an institution. The simplest form, in the light of the available reports, seems to be posting proportionally more posts containing images, rather than posts with links.
– Lifestyle: In the content of posts, it is worthwhile to refer to the patients' life-style and to disease prevention. Then it is easier to get interaction with fans. Lifestyle is also a rich source of various content that helps to generate a larger number of posts.

References

Castronovo, C. & Huang, L., 2012. Social Media in an Alternative Marketing Communication Model. *Journal of Marketing Development and Competitiveness*, 6(1), 123.

CSC.com, 2012. *Should Healthcare Organizations Use Social Media?: A Global Update*. Retrieved September 21, 2013 from:
http://assets1.csc.com/health_services/downloads/CSC_Should_Healthcare_Organizations_Use_Social_Media_A_Global_Update.pdf.

Ebizma.com, 2013. *What are the top health websites*. Retrieved September 20, 2013, from http://www.ebizmba.com/articles/health-websites.

Emarketer.com, 2013. *Social Networking Reaches Nearly One in Four Around the World*. Retrieved October 02, 2013 from: http://www.emarketer.com/Article/Social-Networking-Reaches-Nearly-One-Four-Around-World/1009976.

Fhi.se, 2013. Homepage – Aktuellt – GD Sarah – Wamalas – blog. Retrieved September 25, 2013 from: http://www.fhi.se/Aktuellt/GD-Sarah-Wamalas-blogg/.

Ibtimes.com, 2013. *Social Media Marketing: How Do Top Brands Use Social Platforms*. Retrieved September 21, 2013 from: http://www.ibtimes.com/social-media-marketing-how-do-top-brands-use-social-platforms-charts-1379457.

Internetworldstats.com, 2013. Homepage – EU Stats. Retrieved September 2, 2013 from: http://www.internetworldstats.com/europa.htm.

Kaplan, A.M. & Haenlein, M., 2010. Users of the world, unite! The challenges and opportunities of social media. *Business Horizons*, 53(1), 61.

Kaplan, A.M. & Haenlein, M., 2010. Users of the world, unite! The challenges and opportunities of social media. *Business Horizons*, 53(1), 65.

LinkedIn.com, 2013. Homepage – Blog. Retrieved September 2, 2013 from: http://blog.linkedin.com/2013/01/09/linkedin-200-million/.

Mangold, W. G. & Faulds, D. J., 2009. The new hybrid element of the promotion mix. *Business Horizons*, 52(4), 358.

Młodożeniec, M. & Tutaj, M., 2012. *Aktywność marek w serwisie Facebook.com jako sposób na budowanie relacji z interesariuszami*, PR Forum Conference, Wisla.

Newmediatrednwatch.com, 2013. *Regional Overview. Europe*. Available from World Wide Web http://www.newmediatrendwatch.com/regional-overview/103-europe?start=5.

News.Yahoo.com, 2013. *Number of active users at Facebook over the years*. Retrieved September 2, 2013 from: http://news.yahoo.com/number-active-users-facebook-over-230449748.html.

Pwc.com, 2013. *Social media likes healthcare: From marketing to social business*. Retrieved September 21, 2013 from: http://www.pwc.com/us/en/health-industries/publications/health-care-social-media.jhtml.

Searchenginewatch.com, 2013. *Pinterest Tops 70 Million Users; 30% Pinned, Repinned, or Liked in June*. Retrieved September 2, 2013 from: http://searchenginewatch.com/article/2282835/Pinterest-Tops-70-Million-Users-30-Pinned-Repinned-or-Liked-in-June-Study.

Socialbeakers.com, 2013. *Facebook Pages Statistics & Number of Fans*. Retrieved September 21, 2013 from: http://www.socialbakers.com/facebook-pages/brands/.

Socialbeakers.com, 2013. *Photos Make Up 93% of The Most Engaging Posts on Facebook!* Retrieved September 21, 2013 from: http://www.socialbakers.com/blog/1749-photos-make-up-93-of-the-most-engaging-posts-on-facebook.

Socialmediaexaminer.com, 2013. *2013 Social Media Marketing Industry Report*. Retrieved September 21, 2013 from: http://www.socialmediaexaminer.com/SocialMediaMarketingIndustryReport2013.pdf

Telegraph.co.uk, 2013. *Twitter in numbers*. Retrieved September 2, 2013 from: http://www.telegraph.co.uk/technology/twitter/9945505/Twitter-in-numbers.html.

Thefastertimes.com, 2013. *Google Forces 500 Millionth User to Join Google Plus*. Retrieved September 2, 2013, from: http://www.thefastertimes.com/tech/2013/06/03/google-forces-500-millionth-user-to-join-google-plus/.

Thesocialskinny.com, 2013. *216 Social media and Internet Statistics*. Retrieved September 2, 2013 from http://thesocialskinny.com/216-social-media-and-internet-statistics-september-2012/.

Tutaj, M., 2013. Activity of NGOs in Facebook social network and mechanisms of interaction with users. In: Smyczek, S. (Ed.) *Technology-Driven Promotion for NGOs. Experiences against social exclusions*: 248–265. Katowice: Wydawnictwo UE w Katowicach.

Van De Belt, T.H., Engelen, L.J., Berben, S.A.A. & Schoonhoven, L., 2010. Definition of Health 2.0 and Medicine 2.0: A Systematic Review. *Journal of Medical Internet Research*, 12(2).

Van De Belt, T.H., Engelen, L.J., Berben, S.A.A. & Schoonhoven, L., 2012. Use of Social Media by Western European Hospitals: Longitudinal Study. *Journal of Medical Internet Research*, 14(3).

Wirtualnemedia.pl, 2013. *10,3 mln Polaków korzysta z Facebooka. Serce i Rozum liderem*. Retrieved September 2, 2013 from: http://www.wirtualnemedia.pl/artykul/10-3-mln-polakow-korzysta-z-facebooka-serce-i-rozum-liderem.

YouTube.com, 2013. Homepage – Press – Statistics. Retrieved September 2, 2013 from: http://www.youtube.com/yt/press/statistics.html.

Sławomir Smyczek

12 Customer Values and Attitudes towards e-Healthcare Services

Abstract Customer attitudes and customer value are essential components of behavior in the market. They develop through the process of thinking and feeling based on one's individual knowledge and life experiences as well as other people's opinions. However, attitudes are difficult to define and directly identify in the market. Described as relatively regular, they can be subject to alterations. Development of definite attitudes concerning e-medical services depends, to a large extent, on value for customers – patients that benefit from services provided in the virtual environment. Nonetheless, the final assessment of the gained value will depend on the value expected by patients. At the very initial stage of virtualization of medical services in Europe, it is possible to identify only the value that is expected by the consumer. This chapter describes, with respect to evaluation of customer attitudes, the value that customers/patients expect from medical facilities and from the services offered by them in the virtual environment in Europe and presents a model showing these attitudes.

Keywords: Customer attitudes, Customer value, Virtualization, Healthcare market

12.1 Introduction

The following chapter describes the nature and scope of customer attitudes and customer value in the market, especially the types of those phenomena and the methodological aspects of identifying both categories. Our empirical study focuses on the value expected by customers in the European e-healthcare market and presents a model showing customers' attitudes toward e-healthcare services. The chapter shows the results of surveys with customers–patients of different types of medical facilitates. Field research was conducted in 2013 in five European countries, which represent the different models of the healthcare system in Europe.

12.2 Consumer attitudes and value as objects of research in the healthcare market

12.2.1 Consumer attitudes

Attitudes are an essential component of human behavior. They develop through the process of thinking and feeling based on one's individual knowledge and life experiences as well as other people's opinions. They reveal themselves through expressions of individual convictions, subjective assessments, and prejudices. Thus, attitudes act as a driving force of human behavior since they affect people's decision making. Some research has demonstrated that certain attitudes lead to relatively consistent behaviors towards similar events or problems. This results from automatizing human reactions in the mental process with respect to thinking, feeling, self-expression, and acting. In general, these processes are harmonious and consistent (Swiatowy, 2005: 254).

In the literature on the subject, many attempts have been made at defining the term *attitude*. They mostly depend on a theoretical concept employed for a definition of attitude or on some targeted aspect of attitude. In general, one can distinguish three major definitions of **customer attitudes**.

(1) Definitions related to the behaviorist tradition or to the psychology of learning, where focus is placed on the behavior of an individual and his/her reactions to surrounding objects, including the social ones. This group comprises, among others, definitions formulated by W. M. Fuson, W. A. Scott, and D. Drob (Fuson, 1943). Generally, a great majority of authors who refer to the behaviorist concept define attitudes as certain inclinations to demonstrate certain behavior.

(2) Definitions that have their sources in a sociological concept, where special attention is given to an attitude assumed by an individual towards the object of the attitude. The sociological concept became a starting point for definitions developed by L. L. Thurston, H. A. Murray, C. D. Morgan, and J. Reykowski (Murray and Morgan, 1945). According to these authors, attitude is a definite, relatively consistent emotional or evaluative approach towards a certain object, or an inclination to assume such an approach, expressed in positive, neutral, or negative categories.

(3) Definitions referring to cognitive theories in psychology. Here, scientists point out that attitude comprises not only some definite behavior or evaluative and emotional approach towards an object, but also all cognitive elements relating to the object. This view has been shared by S. E. Asch, M. J. Rosenberg, M. B. Smith, S. Nowak, and T. Mądrzycki (Madrzycki, 1970: 24).

The definitions presented in the third group are more widely accepted and are employed by a growing number of economists. A similar approach towards attitude is represented by S. Mika, according to whom, an attitude is a relatively regular structure (or an inclination for development of such a structure) of cognitive and emotional processes as well as tendencies to assume behavior that reveals a definite attitude towards a certain object (Mika, 1982: 116). Attitude is not only determined by the three groups of factors but also by their mutual relationships as well as human tendencies to assume a certain type of attitude. Attitude always has some definite direction (positive or negative) and range. Thus, it can be concluded that behavior (including consumer market behavior) is 'the end-product' of an attitude.

Bearing this in mind, it can be stated that attitudes have a significant effect on consumer behavior and vice versa. In the long run, consumer behavior modifies consumer attitudes (through perception and through the process of learning) or gives rise to the development of new attitudes.

In most cases, customer behavior is consistent with customer attitude; however, in some circumstances, they may be contradictory, which is determined by many factors including the following:
– personal factors, and
– situational factors (Rudnicki, 1996: 47).

The first group of factors consists of the following:
– other attitudes contradictory to a definite attitude whose relationship to some behavior is interesting from the individual's point of view,
– motives contradictory to a definite attitude,
– verbal abilities that are vital when a given individual is unable to voice his/her real attitudes, and
– social skills that pertain to knowledge about behavior in a given social situation.

Situational factors include these:
– the presence of other people,
– rules on roles: each person plays many social roles governed by some relevant rules of proper behavior,
– the existence of alternative behavior,
– changes in the level of generalization of an attitude subject,
– predictions of sequences of events, and
– the occurrence of unpredictable external events that may display the existing attitude (Mika, 1998).

When analyzing the structure of attitudes, it is worth emphasizing its correspondence with consumer external stimuli (other people, situations, symbols, marketing activities of companies, etc.), which affect consumer attitudes, and its relation with consumer verbal reactions: verbal expressions of consumer beliefs, opinions, assessments, and buying intentions. In most cases, these verbal reactions present a body of empirical material and constitute a set of indexes of attitudes that are the subject of scientific research.

Getting to the actual core of consumer attitudes is possible only through indirect media, through looking into various consumer reactions to presented stimuli (situations, concepts, products, advertising messages, etc.). The role of attitude as an agent between external stimuli and consumer reactions has a special impact on marketing, as an attitude is often of an instrumental character with respect to a value system of individuals and to their consumption needs (Mika, 1998).

Bearing in mind the considerations discussed above, it can be concluded that attitudes are difficult to define and directly identify in the market. Described as relatively regular, they can be subject to alterations. Moreover, they cannot be analyzed in isolation, but should be considered in a more complex perspective alongside other factors determining individual behavior. It should be remembered that attitudes refer to all objects within the vicinity of an individual. Hence, it is possible to distinguish consumption attitudes (connected with, e.g., online buying of specific medical services) and attitudes towards medical facilities or virtual healthcare services. Consequently, these approaches to attitudes are useful in situations where behavior is analyzed with respect to the consumer regarded as a buyer of virtual healthcare services or a user of medical services as a whole.

12.2.2 Customer value

With regard to the third group of definitions of an attitude, it should be emphasized that they refer more to cognitive elements rather than to definite consumer behavior or a consumer emotional attitude towards a given object. Hence, development of definite attitudes towards cognitive elements concerning e-medical services depends, to large extent, on the value for customers-patients who benefit from services provided in the virtual environment. Nonetheless, the final assessment of the gained value will depend on the value expected by patients. At the very initial stage of virtualization of medical services in Europe, it is possible to identify only the value expected by the consumer. Moreover, the category of value frequently appears in social sciences, including economics. Despite this, scientists find the category difficult to define and often avoid precise definitions thereof, which results in ambiguities hindering the process of researching value for patients. Due to the subjective and situational character of value, a decision was made to refer in the research to the concept of **customer value** as a basis for development of a research tool and for further analysis, both in terms of value for patients and value to be delivered by medical facilities.

The term *customer value* was first introduced in marketing theory in 1954 by P. Drucker when the concept of marketing corporate management was presented (Drucker, 1954). Towards the end of the 1960s, this category appeared in the theory of consumer behavior and referred to the concept of utility (benefit) and satisfaction, part of the theory of consumer choice (Howard and Sheth, 1969, Kotler and Levy, 1969). Later, the use of its original sense was dropped, and the concept of 'value' appeared only in studies into consumer behavior, where it was considered to be declared and respected value, or value preferred by buyers (customer value). The notion of **value for money** recurred in its broader use in economic sciences at the end of the 1980s, thanks to M. Porter's research into corporate competitive advantage and his development of a chain model of added-value (Porter, 1985).

M. Porter's views on customer value (he called it value for buyer) were based on his abundant scientific work on consumers, including the results of research into consumer satisfaction carried out in 1980. Thanks to M. Porter's study, the term customer value has been widely adopted in contemporary concepts, including Total Quality Management, Business Process Reengineering, Supply Chain Management, Value Based Management, and Customer Relationship Management (Szymura-Tyc, 2003).

Also in the 1990s, customer value reappeared as a subject of scientific interest in the theory of marketing supported by the theory of consumer choice, consumer behavior, and consumer psychology. The term *customer value* was used alongside such notions as utility, benefits, needs, and satisfaction.

The reasons for the development of research into customer value were diverse. First, the concept of utility, a basic category of consumer choice theory, did not place enough emphasis on the costs borne by the consumer in the process of buying and using some definite goods. In consumer choice theory, utility was regarded as tantamount to consumer satisfaction with the benefits from using a product (Kamerschen et al., 1991: 446). Research into consumer satisfaction demonstrated, however, that satisfaction experienced by the consumer depends not only on the benefits that the consumer gains from buying and using a product (utility) but also from the relevant costs that he/she must bear – Theory of Exchange Fairness (Jachnis and Terelak, 1998: 172). This necessitated development of a category that could reconcile both the benefits gained and the costs borne by the consumer. Second, research into consumer satisfaction showed that satisfaction appeared only when the results from buying and using a product exceeded the customer's expectations of a product at the very moment of product selection – Model of Expected Discrepancy (Furtak, 2003: 146). Considering product utility and satisfaction to be equal did not allow for identification of this relationship. Thus, it was necessary to find a category that would enable researchers to study the relationship between consumer satisfaction, his/her expectations with respect to products, and the results of purchase and consumption of products, with full consideration of both the benefits to be gained and the costs to be borne by the buyer.

All the research into the consumer and marketing has resulted in the development of the notion of customer value. The definition of the category was based not only on classical marketing theories but also on modern theories of behavior and consumer psychology. Development of the notion was also supported by achievements in service marketing and conclusions drawn from a contemporary concept of relationship marketing. Researchers have also referred to M. Porter's chain model of added-value, which combines value for the customer with added-value for the buyer and the company. Many attempts have been made to define the concept of value for the customer as well as to determine attributes of the category and ways of measuring it.

V. Zeithaml defines customer value by exploiting the concept of product utility. Here, value is an aggregate consumer evaluation of product utility based on the consumer's perception of what is gained against what is given (Zeithaml, 1988: 14).

V. Zeithaml emphasizes that customer value is a subjective and differently perceived category; whereas price constitutes a significant criterion, but its influence on consumers may vary. The author also observes that a clear and legible instruction manual or an assembly manual may be an important factor in a consumer's perception of product value. Moreover, value may be looked upon differently, depending on the circumstances of its consumption.

K. Monroe, in turn, claims that the value perceived by buyers comes from the relationship between the quality or benefits that the buyer recognizes in a product and the perceived sacrifices (loss) he/she makes by paying a given price. K. Monroe claims that perceived benefits are composed of the physical attributes of a product, attributes connected with accompanying services and technical support during product utility, as well as the price and other quality indexes. Perceived costs, in turn, comprise costs borne by the buyer during the purchase, such as the product price and the costs of purchase related to, for example, transfer of title deeds, costs of assembly, costs of exploitation, maintenance (repair) costs, failure risk, or product malfunction risk costs. By assuming that most buyers operate within financial constraints (in the theory of consumer choice, K. Monroe maintained that buyers were more susceptible to borne costs – sacrifices and losses – than to potential benefits), K. Monroe proposed that customer value be measured by the ratio of benefits to costs, and not by the difference existing between them. It is worth adding that the proposed concept did not elicit a big response in the marketing literature. However, the majority of researchers are inclined to define value as a difference (excess) between the perceived benefits and the costs. This seems justified inasmuch as the concept of the perceived costs signifies the cost that is subjectively perceived by the customer. Nonetheless, it should be borne in mind that different customers have different reactions to particular cost components (price, effort, time, etc.). With financial constraints related to their income, buyers may be more or less susceptible to price and other components of perceived costs (Szymura-Tyc, 2005: 69).

A considerable contribution to the definition of customer value was made by A. Ravald and Ch. Gronroos, researchers studying the concept of relationship marketing, who extended the definition of value proposed by K. Monroe. They pointed out that apart from the value of the product itself (the company's offer), there exists a distinct value, which is the result of the relationship between the transaction parties. In their opinion, there are many situations where, despite consumer dissatisfaction with one of the transactions, some prior positive experience that contributed to development of the relationship between the customer and the company encourages him/her to seek compromise. With regard to this, A. Ravald and Ch. Gronroos proposed to take into account the costs and benefits ensuing from the relationship between the buyer and the seller, along with the unpredicted "accidental" costs and benefits connected with a given transaction because they jointly influence the value perceived by the customer. Thus, they referred to concepts elaborated by consumer psychology, known as transaction and accumulated satisfaction, and to the Affective Model of consumer satisfaction. According to the authors, the so-called aggregate unpredicted accidental value is represented by the ratio of accidental benefits and benefits resulting from the relationship to accidental costs and costs resulting from the relationship (Ravald and Gronroos, 1996).

The concepts of transaction satisfaction, accumulated satisfaction, and the so-called attributive satisfaction were used at great length by R. Woodruff in his approach to customer value, which he defined as a composition of preferences experienced and evaluated by the customer. These preferences refer to attributes of the product itself; of its functioning; and, finally, of product consumption effects, thanks to which the customer can (cannot) achieve his/her goals and intentions in the process of product consumption (Woodruff, 1997: 142). This definition represents a hierarchical system of customer value, which implies a need for its assessment at the level of the attributes of a product and product consumption as well as customer goals and intentions. Moreover, this system reveals not only the process of value development but also best represents the relationship between customer value and satisfaction. Thus, it can be treated as a basis for measuring the satisfaction derived from the assessment of value delivered to the customer (Woodruff, 1997: 143). In his approach to the value definition, R. Woodruff demonstrates the dynamic character of customer value, which means that it may change with time. The need for a dynamic approach to customer value is also emphasized by A. Parasuraman, who points out that customers who make a purchase for the first time tend to concentrate on product attributes, whereas those who do it repeatedly pay more attention to the effects of product consumption and the possibilities of achieving certain goals related to definite goods (one product) or a service (Parasuraman, 1997).

Customer value has also been the subject of Ph. Kotler's analysis. He defined it as a difference between the total customer value and the total customer costs. The total value is composed of a bundle of benefits anticipated by the customer, whereas the total cost is made up of a bundle of costs expected by the customer in connection with the evaluation, purchase, and consumption of a product or service (Kotler, 1997: 38). According to Ph. Kotler, the total customer value comprises the anticipated value of a product, service, personnel, and corporate image. The total cost, on the other hand, is composed of such costs as the money, time, energy, and psychical cost expected by the customer. In his definition, Ph. Kotler (1997: 38) emphasizes the fact that customer value is not delivered to the customer (as Ph. Kotler initially declared), but is expected by him/her.

Alongside the definitions of customer value discussed above, the marketing literature presents several others that, in great detail, refer to selected issues connected with the concept of customer value. All the definitions reflect the multifaceted character of studies conducted by scientists and marketing theorists doing research on the category. Although not all of them are considered successful, the overview of the definitions helps to understand the problems encountered by researchers. To provide some examples, B. Gale defines customer value as the quality perceived in the market in relation to the price of a given product (Gale, 1994). Value in industrial markets is, in turn, a perceived equivalence, expressed in monetary units, between a bundle of economic, technical, social, or service benefits gained by a customer's company and the price paid for the product, compared to the offers and prices of other possible deliverers (Anderson et al., 1993: 5). According to S. Slater and J. Narver (2000: 120), customer value appears when product-related benefits outweigh the costs over the life cycle of the product being consumed by the customer. For the institutional customer, the benefits materialize along with the growth of a unit profit or with an increase in the number of product units sold. The costs over the life cycle of a product being consumed by a customer comprise costs related to finding the product, the operational costs of the product, the disposal costs of the product, and the price of the product. Customer value is perceived as an emotional relationship between the customer and the producer as a result of consumer consumption of a product or a service that, in his/her opinion, provided him/her with added value (Butz and Goodstein, 1996: 63).

Bearing in mind the definitions and achievements in the theory of consumer behavior, consumer psychology, and marketing theory presented above, it can be concluded that customer value appears in the process of consumption of a purchased product. This value is developed through a consumer's subjective estimation of costs and benefits after product purchase and consumption. These costs and benefits are the only significant element in the assessment of the value obtained by the customer, and customer value itself represents a predominance of benefits over costs perceived by the customer. Based on this, one can venture a statement that customer value is an excess of subjectively perceived benefits over subjectively perceived costs related to the purchase and consumption of a given product.

Benefits gained by customers are connected with the needs they want to satisfy through some product purchase and product consumption. Individual customers seek benefits that can meet their consumption needs. Costs, in turn, have a financial dimension connected with the exchange of goods and money between the company (seller) and the customer (buyer). Besides the financial costs, there are costs that refer to time loss, inconvenience, extra efforts, negative emotions, and other costs for consumers.

In the discussion of customer value, a distinction should be made between the value that is expected and the value that is obtained by the customer. The **value expected** by the customer can be referred to as an excess of subjectively perceived and expected benefits compared to the costs relating to product purchase and consumption. In light of this definition, such a value constitutes the basis for customer market choices, and is closely related to the concept of utility in the theory of consumer choice. As for **value gained** by the customer, i.e., customer value, it can be defined as an excess of subjectively perceived customer benefits over subjectively perceived customer costs resulting from the product purchase and consumption. Such a definition of customer value corresponds to the notion of customer advantage in the theory of consumer choice and with added-value, introduced to the management literature by M. Porter.

With respect to the issues discussed above, the following **attributes of customer value** can be distinguished.

– Subjectivity: Customer-patient value is not dependent solely on the service itself, but also on a patient's individual needs to be satisfied by a medical service and on a patient's individual capability of covering the costs related to service purchase and service use.
– Situational character: The benefits and costs related to the purchase and use of a service are always conditional on the situation in which the service is bought; depending on the situation, the same patient may have a different perception of the benefits to be gained and the costs to be borne.
– Perceived value: This means that the assessment of patient value comprises only the benefits and costs that are perceived (recognized) by the patient, and not the benefits that were actually gained or the costs that were actually borne by him/her; the process of benefit and cost perception is connected not only with cognitive processes but also with emotional ones (Szymura-Tyc, 2005).

All the attributes of patient value do not allow direct measuring of the category. Although patient satisfaction can be used as a basic benchmark for customer value estimation, it should be remembered that satisfaction itself is not exclusively dependent on the value gained, but also the value expected by the patient. Even more so, satisfaction appears only when the effects of service purchase and use go beyond consumer expectations of these results.

Another important attribute of patient value concerns its dynamic character, which means that the value changes over time and embraces the whole process of service purchase and service use. In its endeavor to provide a patient with some value, a medical facility ought to focus on the whole life cycle of a service, including all costs and relevant benefits. Thus, patient value represents a complex set of benefits and costs perceived by the patient in the process of buying and using medical services. It is impossible to enumerate all the benefits and costs that are components of value for the patient because their number and variety correspond to the number of patient needs, expectations, and constraints. These needs, expectations, and constraints are subject to alterations because satisfaction of some needs opens the door to other, superior ones. Needs change or diversify, and new ones arise, thus necessitating the development of new medical services that can meet patients' changing needs and expectations and that can adapt to patients' varying constraints. Being aware of the fact that benefits and costs are the only determinants of the medical service value perceived by the patient, healthcare units tend to arrange miscellaneous activities that are designed to teach patients to appreciate the attributes of their services. In practical terms, a medical facility can create and model patients' needs and expectations with respect to the services offered and, ultimately, may affect the assessment of the final value gained by patients.

12.3 Value expected by customers on the European e-healthcare market

With reference to the views presented above, it was necessary to carry out studies that could allow researchers to identify the value that customers-patients expect from medical facilities and the services offered by them in the virtual environment in Europe.

In order to reach this goal, direct research was conducted on test groups of consumers representing five European countries. The study of patients' attitudes towards e-healthcare services in the German, British, Swedish, Belgium, and Polish markets was conducted by means of a survey of a group of 1,000 respondents in each country in 2013. The completion rate of the questionnaires was 54 percent, but after verification of the responses, 47 percent of the questionnaires were approved for further analysis. The choice of the countries was deliberate and based on different organizational models of the healthcare systems in the selected countries.

Study results showed that the value expected by patients in the virtual medical services market are similar or even identical across all European countries being studied. Differences emerge only in the significance of particular values for patients from the various countries. It should be emphasized that these differences result not only from the organizational model of the healthcare services market in a given country but also from the country's cultural characteristics as described by Hofstede (2009). Consequently, value related to safety is highly expected by patients from all the countries, except for Great Britain. Apart from safety of e-healthcare services, Germans, Swedes, Belgians, and Poles expect to have faster access to medical information as well as to obtain more comprehensive and accessible information via electronic channels. It is noteworthy that the countries being studied represent cultures where, according to the concept proposed by Hofstede, the Uncertainty Avoidance Index is high and people tend to avoid risk. The element of suspicion towards the new and unknown is deeply rooted in these cultures and a general safety orientation prevails. In Great Britain, however, the Uncertainty Avoidance Index equals 35, as the culture of this country is oriented toward risk acceptance and, consequently, contributes to innovations such as e-healthcare services.

Among other values expected by patients with respect to the provision of **e-healthcare services**, one can distinguish better quality of patient service as a result of intense competition between healthcare facilities and a wider range of accessible medical services. Individualization of services presents another value that is highly expected and appreciated, especially by patients in Sweden, Great Britain, and Belgium. In these countries, the Individualism Index is the highest of all the countries. In individualistic countries, people take care of themselves and want to be distinguished from others. In Germany and Poland as well as in countries with a collective-orientation, this value is also of great significance; yet it is not as highly deemed as in Sweden, Great Britain, and Belgium. It is worth noting that a great number of Polish patients expect value of an economic character, particularly lower prices for healthcare services and free-of-charge e-healthcare services. The considerable importance of economic value with respect to e-healthcare services declared by Polish patients reveals that the level of wealth among Poles is still low (Maciejewski, 2003). Additionally, compared to other countries, Polish patients more often point to the necessity of faster provision of services, which unveils some shortages and malfunctions of the transforming healthcare system in Poland.

Tab 12.1: Value expected by patients in the e-healthcare services market in Europe

Factors	Germany	Great Britain	Sweden	Belgium	Poland
Safety	53.4	13.2	59.5	54.9	52.3
Comprehensive information	47.5	18.4	48.9	60.1	36.5
Faster information access	38.6	21.3	32.9	31.3	30.4
Wider offer	29.2	30.8	32.2	28.7	25.5
Service Individualization	28.7	52.1	58.3	48.4	15.1
Better service quality	27.0	40.7	45.9	42.6	27.1
Free-of-charge services	17.0	8.2	8.1	11.4	35.7
Lower prices	16.3	11.7	9.3	10.8	46.2
Channel diversification	11.7	8.4	12.2	5.4	19.8
Faster service access	8.5	9.1	6.3	4.5	34.8
Others	3.7	2.6	1.8	2.6	4.3

12.4 Model of customers' attitudes towards e-healthcare services

As mentioned earlier in the text, customer-patient value is a very complex and diverse category; as a result, it is difficult to identify all its aspects and elements. In order to better address the issue of value for the patient, it is necessary to refer to models that describe the phenomenon. One of the most common model approaches to value found in literary sources is the consumption value model elaborated by J. N. Sheth, B. I. Newman, and B. L. Gross (Sheth et al., 1991: 157). The authors of the model try to describe value from the perspective of the value declared, respected, or preferred by buyers (customer value). The model refers to the theory of consumer choice and points to five types of value contained in products offered on the market.

The Sheth–Newman–Gross consumption value model was developed in order to explain why the consumer makes choices on the market. It consists of several components and presents a range of specific measures defining factors that determine consumer behavior. The model by Sheth–Newman-Gross focuses on estimating the consumption value, which explains why the consumer chooses between purchasing a certain product or withdrawing from it (using or not using a definite item); why the consumer prefers one type of product over another one; and, finally, why the consumer chooses one particular brand and rejects another. The model can be applied to making choices on a full range of products (consumers of consumer durables, services, or industrial goods) (Sheth et al., 1991: 167).

The model by Sheth-Newman-Gross is based on three central principles:
- consumer choice is a function of little amount of consumer values;
- the specific value of consumption differentiates the effort put into each particular situation; and
- the values that constitute the core of the model are functional, social, emotional, cognitive, and conditional values (Smyczek and Sowa, 2005: 138).

The functional value of a consumer choice is perceived as the functional, utilitarian, or psychological utility obtained through the attributes of the choice (e.g., positive or negative attributes). The functional value is strictly related to the theory of rationality, which is expressed in the popular phrase of 'the man acting rationally'. The center of the functional value is occupied by such attributes as durability, reliability, and price. This can be exemplified by a car purchase decision, which should be based on the price and the promise of economy during the life of the car.

The social value of a consumer choice occurs as a consequence of the relationship that exists between one or more specific social groups and a consumer choice. Consumer choice produces the social value through correspondence with positive or negative stereotypes of demographic, socio-economic, and cultural-ethnic groups (including benchmark groups). Thus, choices are made both with respect to products of daily use (e.g., bicycles, shoes) and 'socially engaged' goods (e.g. presents, products used for entertainment).

The emotional value of a choice reveals the utility of some goods with regard to their ability to stimulate consumer emotions and feelings. Consumer choice provides the consumer with emotional values when it is related to some specific feelings and when it evokes or sustains these feelings. Products often have some emotional connotations (e.g., excitement while watching one's favorite sports team or a thrill experienced while driving a new car).

The cognitive value of a choice displays the utility that is connected with the ability to satisfy curiosity or provide some novelty and/or satisfaction derived from the need for knowledge. A cognitive value is provided particularly by new purchases and experiences, although even a slight 'change in arrangement' (e.g., change in ice cream flavor) can provide the consumer with cognitive value.

The conditional value of consumer choice shows that the latter is the result of a definite situation or circumstance surrounding the consumer. Consequently, the purchase of some products is related to some specific period or event (e.g., a birthday present). Some goods generate a certain atmosphere or provide local benefits (e.g., a suntan lotion); some are connected with a once-in-a-lifetime opportunity (e.g., purchase of the first car); and, finally, some are used only in emergency situations (e.g., a visit to the dentist on Sunday evening).

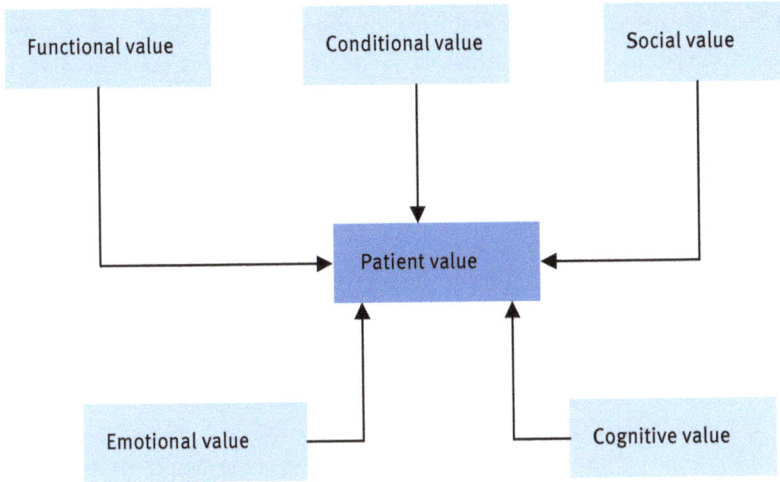

Fig. 12.1: Model of five customer-patient values
Source: Adopted from Sheth et al. (1991: 162)

The Sheth–Neman–Gross model is attractive not only due to its composition but also, above all, due to its manner of measuring (Sheth et al., 1991: 159) the five values in different consumer choice situations. Thus, the model presents, in a complex way, the types of value perceived by customers, whereby it is possible to demonstrate different kinds of value and to better explain the value expected by consumers. That is the reason the direct research conducted on the e-healthcare services market utilized the values (functional, social, emotional, cognitive, and conditional value) indicated by Sheth –Newman–Gross in their model of consumption value.

The factors describing value for patients in the e-healthcare services market in Europe and used for the customer attitudes for the e-healthcare services model construction were identified by means of exploratory factor analysis. First, an attempt was made to determine a set of variables that separately describe value defined by patients from the countries in the study, i.e., Germany, Great Britain, Sweden, Poland, and Belgium. The Likert scale responses for fifteen variables were used to identify variables that clustered together, which define the different kinds of value expected in the e-health services market. During the next stage of the factor analysis procedure, the variables used in the study were checked in terms of the existence of definite relationships among them. It is worth adding that if the correlations between the variables are low, they are rather unlikely to form strong and easy-to-interpret common factors.

In order to demonstrate that the choice of the factor analysis model as a method of data analysis was correct, the Kaiser-Meyer-Olkin (Walasiak, 2005) index was used. The KMO for the fifteen analyzed variables equaled 0.790, which was relatively high. This result, however, did not guarantee the distinction of some definite factors (or a factor). Therefore, it was necessary to calculate the adequacy of the selection of each separate variable by referring to the MSA_h index, which allows exclusion of some variables before the analysis. Low MSA_h values suggest that h variable correlations cannot be explained through other variables and, therefore, should be excluded from further research (Gorniak, 2000: 150).

Measures of sampling adequacy indicated that the variables, (4) fashion as a social value for the patient, (6) politeness as an emotional value, and (10) modernity as a cognitive value for the patient in the e-healthcare services market, have MSA_h index below 0.5, which excluded them from the analysis. Consequently, the rest of the analysis comprised twelve variables that achieved very high KMO (0.872) and MSA_h (over 0.8) indexes.

In order to determine the number of factors to be used in the remaining analysis, the method of scree plot was employed. This method is based on a scree plot where eigenvalues for definite factors are marked. According to the scree criterion, it is vital to preserve factors that form 'the slope' and to ignore the ones that build 'the scree', i.e., whose combined eigenvalues form almost a horizontal line. The analysis of variables defining the values for patients show that the 'scree' phenomenon appears at the third or fourth factor, which makes the choice of factors for further analysis problematic. In the literature on the subject, scientific opinions are divided: some researchers recommend keeping all factors in the 'slope', including the one that opens 'the scree'; others advise that this factor be ignored (Lehmann et al., 1998: 610).

Determination of the final number of factors to be used in the further analysis was performed through calculation of eigenvalues and the variance percentage explaining other components. The eigenvalue criterion marks the lower limit for the number of factors that are common in the correlation matrix for the population, which means that the number of factors is always equal to or higher than the number defined by the criterion. According to the eigenvalue criterion requiring an explanation percent higher than single digits, the remaining analysis should include factors that explain 68.47 percent of the variance capacity common for all variables. Application of the principal component method with quartimax rotation made it possible to determine factor loads for particular variables.

Using the analysis, it was possible to establish three factors that determine the attitudes of patients in the European market of e-healthcare services.

(1) The first factor is described by variables that give information about the circumstances that contribute to (or better the condition of) the use of e-healthcare services, namely: (11) current development of medical services, (12) risk management skills, (13) patient's health condition, and (14) attractive price offer from healthcare services available via electronic channels, as well as (15) patient's adequate knowledge, referred to as **conditional attitudes of the patient.**

(2) The second factor reveals variables that provide information on patients' expectations of medical facilities delivering e-healthcare services: (1) safety, (2) free-of charge medical services, (3) accessible medical information, and (7) a wider of-

fer of healthcare services, as well as (10) modernity, a factor called the **functional attitudes of the patient.**

(3) The third factor is described by variables that result from willingness to satisfy curiosity or to obtain some knowledge. These are (8) the use of definite e-healthcare services under the influence of some promotional activities and (9) expectations of sound and comprehensive medical information to be provided by a healthcare facility, called the **cognitive attitudes of the patient.**

All things considered, one can venture a statement that patient value regarding the European e-healthcare services market is affected by three factors, i.e., conditional, functional, and cognitive ones (Figure 11.2). Because of the specific character of the healthcare services market as well as of the virtual environment itself, emotional value does not play a major role in patients' market choices. Also social value, as indicated by research results, is not of great importance in this market. Patients willingly obtain information from informal sources, but final decisions about the use of certain e-healthcare services are made individually.

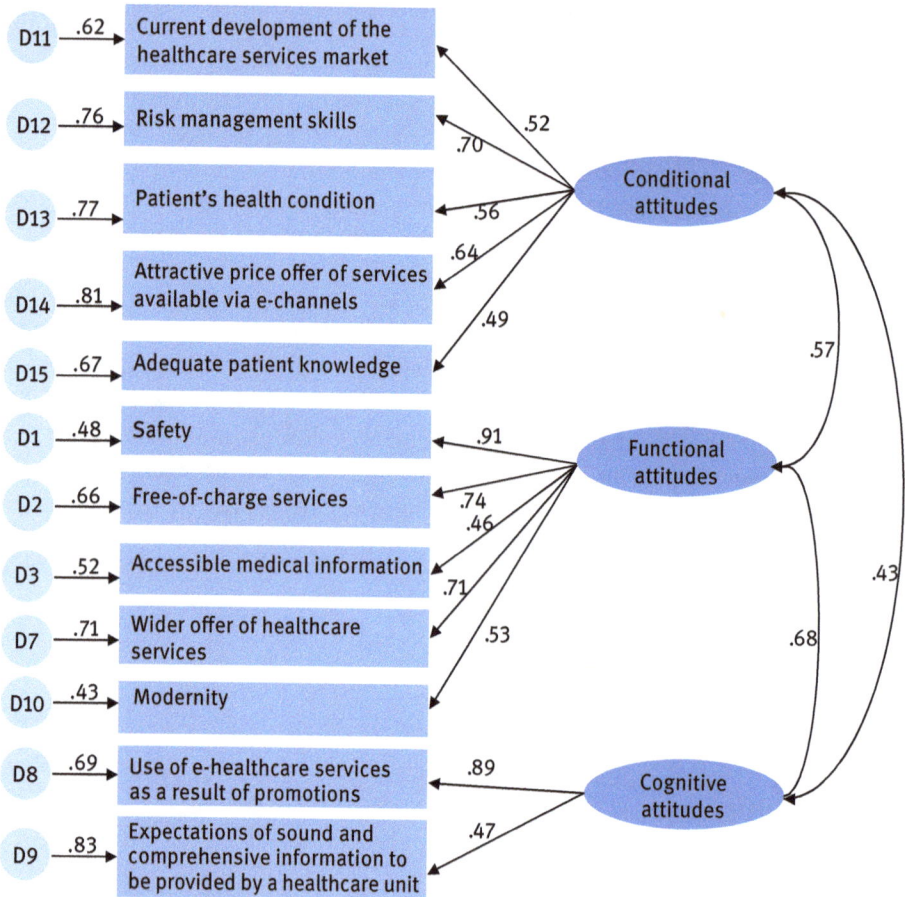

$\chi^2 = 249.21$; $df = 64$; level of significance $\alpha = 0.000$; $\chi^2 / df = 3.89$; $GFI = 0.89$; $AGFI = 0.87$; $NFI = 0.84$; $CFI = 0.81$; $RMSEA = 0.034$; Hoelter $0.05 = 272$.

Fig. 12.2: Model of customer-patient value in the European market of e-healthcare services

Conclusions

Bearing in mind the analysis presented above, it can be concluded that patients in the European e-healthcare services market demonstrate positive attitudes towards virtualization of services in this market. However, their expectations focus mainly on communication and service provision; on value connected with individualization of patient services; and on economic factors, the latter being more typical of economies undergoing transformation. Inclusion of this understanding of value in the strategy of medical facilities will allow for assessment of satisfaction and estimation of patient value in the European e-healthcare services market.

The elaborated model provides a complex description of consumer attitudes towards e-healthcare services with respect to cognitive theories. The model offers a wide range of applications; and, in the first place, it should help researchers and market participants comprehend the complex elements of patients' attitudes and consider patients' decision-making processes from another perspective (different from the one assumed in the subject literature). Moreover, the model takes into consideration that virtualization of the healthcare services market is a vital factor determining patients' behavior.

Thus, a conclusion can be drawn that the identified model of value for patients serves not only scientific, but, above all, practical functions (descriptive-explanatory). The model allows simple identification and explanation of market gaps between patients' expectations of the virtual environment and representatives of medical facilities responsible for provision of value.

References

Anderson, J. Jain, D. and Chintagunta, P. 1993. *Customer Value Assessment in Business Markets: A State-of Practice Study*, Journal of Business Marketing, Vol. 1, No 1

Butz, H. and Goodstein, L. 1996. *Measuring Customer Value: Gaining the Strategic Advantage*, Organizational Dynamics, Vol. 24, No 3

Drucker, P. 1954. T*he Practice of Management*, Harper, New York

Furtak, R. 2003. Marketing partnerski na rynku usług, PWE, Warszawa

Fuson, W.M. 1943. Attitudes: A note on the concept and its research context, American Sociological Review, Vol. 7.

Gale, B. 1994. *Managing Customer Value*, The Free Press, New York

Górniak, J. 2000. *My i nasze pieniądze*, Aureus, Kraków

Howard, J. and Sheth, N. 1969 *The Theory of Buyer Behaviour*, John Wiley and Sons, New York

Jachnis, A and Terelak, J. 1998. *Psychologia konsumenta i reklamy*, Branta, Bydgoszcz

Kamerschen, D., McKenzie, R. and Nardinelli, C. 1991. *Ekonomia*, Fundacja Gospodarcza NSZZ "Solidarność", Gdańsk

Kotler, Ph. 1997. *Marketing Management. Analysis, Planning, Implementation and Control*, Prentice-Hall International Inc., New Jersey 1997

Kotler, Ph. and Levy, S. 1969. *Broadening the Concept of Marketing*, Journal of Marketing Vol. 33, No 1

Lehmann, D.R., Gupta, S. and Steckel, J.H. 1998. *Marketing Research*, Addison-Wesley, Massachusetts

Maciejewski, G. 2003. *Poziom zamożności polskich gospodarstw domowych*, WSZiNS w Tychach, Tychy

Mądrzycki, T. 1970. *Psychologiczne prawidłowości kształtowania się postaw*, PZWS, Warszawa

Mika, S. 1982. *Psychologia społeczna*. Warszawa: PWN.

Mika, S. 1998. *Psychologia społeczna dla nauczycieli*, Warszawa: Wydawnictwo Akademickie Żak

Murray, H.A. and Morgan, C.D., 1945. A clinical study of sentiments, General Psychological Monographs, Vol. 32.

Parasuraman, A. 1997. *Reflections on Gaining Competitive Advantage through Customer Value*, Journal of the Academy of Marketing Science, Vol. 25, No 2

Porter, M. 1985. Competitive Advantage. Creating and Sustaining Superior Performance, The Free Press, New York

Ravald, A. and Gronroos, Ch. 1996. *The Value Concept and Relationship Marketing*, European Journal of Marketing Vol. 30, No 2

Rudnicki, L. 1996. Zachowania konsumentów na rynku, AE, Kraków

Sheth, J.N., Newman, B.I. and Gross, B.L. 1991. *Consumption Values and Market Choice. Theory and Applications*, Journal of Business Research

Slater, S. and Narver, J. 2000. *Intelligence Generation and superior Customer Value*, Journal of the Academy of Marketing Science, Vol. 28, No 1

Smyczek, S. and Sowa, I. 2005. *Konsument na rynku – zachowania, modele, aplikacje*, Difin, Warszawa

Światowy, G. 1998. Postawy konsumentów w procesie przemian rynkowych polskiej gospodarki, in: Konsument- Przedsiębiorstwo- Przestrzeń", AE, Katowice

Szymura-Tyc, M. 2003. *Budowa przewagi konkurencyjnej przedsiębiorstw*, Ekonomika i Organizacja Przedsiębiorstw No 1

Szymura-Tyc, M. 2005. *Marketing we współczesnych procesach tworzenia wartości dla klienta i przedsiębiorstwa*, AE, Katowice

Woodruff, R. 1997. *Customer Value: The Next Source for competitive Advantage*, Journal of the Academy of Marketing Science, Vol. 25, No 2

Zeithaml, V. 1988. *Consumer Perception of Price, Quality and Value: a Means-End Model and Synthesis of Evidence*, Journal of Marketing vol. 52, No 3

Marcin Tutaj

13 Efficiency Control of Building Relationships with Customers by using Social Media

Abstract In 2006, *Time* magazine noticed the importance of social media – granting the title 'Man of the Year' to all users of such sites (Levinson, 2010: 26). Data from September 2012 show, in turn, that in one of the most popular social networking sites, Facebook, 243 million users from Europe are registered (Internet World Stats, 2012). This extensive potential was observed by organizations creating their pages in such websites as Facebook, LinkedIn, Twitter, and YouTube. For effective use of these websites in building relationships with customers, it is necessary to assess the activities that have been conducted. This chapter presents basic parameters that should be taken into account when conducting activities on such websites.

Keywords: Healthcare, Social media, Efficiency control

13.1 Introduction

According to Michael Thomas, nowadays, the most valuable asset of each business has become its **relationships** (relations) with clients. By that we mean not groups of clients or market segments but individual clients, each of whom has different requirements and needs (1994: 6). In the process of building close relationships, four main conditions must be met:
- evoking trust,
- mutual agreement of the parties,
- an efficiently operating communication system, and
- customization of relationships.

Trust between partners in the exchange is treated as a function of opinions about their activity (reliability, honesty) and the use of certain ethical standards. Trust increases the value of a relationship and thus stimulates the tendency of customers to become involved in relations with the supplier. On the other hand, the basis for construction and control of relationships is effective **communication**. The system of such communication assists in learning about the needs and expectations of the parties to the relationship as well as adapting to these needs and expectations (Bilińska-Reformat, 2009: 108).

In this context, the Internet has gained particular importance. Clearly, the virtual space of communication creates areas where market entities can independently create and shape mutual relations. At this point, it should be emphasized that, when an intangible sphere starts to dominate, the most valuable technologies are those that expand, enhance, improve, and develop any kind of intangible relations (Kelly, 2001: 156).

Among the communication channels available on the Internet, the most interesting, from the point of view of conducting effective communication, establishing contacts, and building relationships, are the **social media**. Their attractiveness for users (both organizations and individuals) is mostly due to the possibility of easily implementing at least three activities: participation, sharing, and cooperation (Kaplan and Haenlein, 2010: 61–62).

In the case of websites of this type, we deal with building communities and establishing relationships with single users, which is reflected in the number of persons 'liking' a fanpage on Facebook or tracking entries, e.g., 'followers' on the Twitter website. Social media enable conducting a continuous dialogue of users with other users – individual people and organizations. The most frequent symptom of these activities is the function of assessing the posted publications – e.g., the 'Like' button on Facebook, '+1' tag in Google+, and graphic buttons 'thumbs up' or 'thumbs down' on YouTube. Greater importance, however, for developing relationships can be attributed to comments – they are the main activity of users on the Internet forums; blogs, e.g., Blogger; and micro-blogs, e.g., Twitter. The organizations that decide to begin conducting activities on **social networking sites (SNS)** must monitor these parameters. On the one hand, this is a considerable amount of information that has to be analyzed, while, on the other hand, it is an excellent opportunity to conduct a direct dialogue with clients, learning about their needs and sometimes preventing the occurrence of crisis situations.

13.2 Relationships as the value for organizations

Acknowledgment of relationships with a customer as the most valuable asset in business results from changes that took place in marketing in the first half of the 1990s. It was observed then that previous marketing using the effects of production scale (mass marketing) and marketing using various criteria for division of consumers (marketing based on market segments) no longer fulfilled their role. Thus, the next stage of development of marketing activities has become the marketing of relationships, whose basic characteristics include, among others, two-direction dialogue and long-term cooperation between a company and its individual consumer (Dyche, 2002: 40).

The primary purpose of the marketing of relationships is to create economically, technically, and socially strong bonds between parties, which leads to an increase in mutual trust and, at the same time, reduction of transaction costs (Pizło, 2008: 92).

From the point of view of the need for building relations in the **healthcare** industry, the specific character of the relationship occurring between the patient and the service provider (a medical unit, doctor), which is determined in many ways, has great importance. The following should be considered to be the most crucial (Matysiewicz and Smyczek, 2012: 80–81):

- strong dependence on unpredictable external factors,
- uncertainty concerning the result of the service process (treatment),
- asymmetry in access of the client to information,
- impact of the client on the course and result of the service process, and
- the phenomenon of stress usually experienced by the client during the exchange process.

The factors above may in turn be applicable to the mechanisms that are activated at passing from the plane of one-time transactions to the plane of long-term relationships, namely (Matysiewicz and Smyczek, 2012: 81):

- the mechanism of reducing a patient's uncertainty as to the result of the concluded transaction;
- the mechanism of growth in the efficiency of interaction between a facility, doctor, and patient; and
- the mechanism of satisfying social needs present at the emotional level.

Analyzing the issue of relations in more detail, five types of relationships taking place in the buyer (recipient)- seller (provider) line can be distinguished (Kotler et al., 2002: 531–534):

- basic – occurring when the vendor does not conduct any after-sale activities, focusing only on sales (conducting the transaction) of goods to the consumer;
- reactive – taking place when the seller, after the product sale, encourages the client to contact the company and creates the need to collect information on the consumer (asking questions, expressing doubts, etc.);
- responsible – performed by the organization when the seller contacts the client soon after the purchase to assess whether the product meets the buyer's (consumer's) expectations; at that time, the seller seeks information about the product (e.g.; on additional characteristics sought by the consumer, opinion about the product – particularly critical examples);
- proactive – occurring when the manufacturer's employee contacts the consumer and informs him/her during the conversation about additional, possible methods of use of a product or new offers of the company; and
- partner – consisting in maintaining permanent bonds with the consumer in order to seek methods of better delivery of the expected value for the buyer.

In the case of the entities in the healthcare industry, particular attention should be paid to building reactive and partner relationships that are characterized by encouraging a dialogue on a long-term basis and common striving for improvement of the services provided. In this way, the mechanisms associated with reducing uncertainty, increasing efficiency in interactions, and fulfilling social needs in patients

can be activated. Regardless of the system of solutions in the healthcare of particular countries, the actions of the healthcare sector entities aimed at building and
developing relations with patients should be a strategic area of operations for them.

13.3 Importance of social media in building relationships

Social media consist of a number of websites that vary among themselves, first of
all, in the kind and way of publishing content and the available functions as regards
interactions among users. Social media include such websites as (Kaplan and
Haenlein, 2010: 64) these:

- blogs (the so-called Internet diaries, created alone or with the use of websites,
  e.g., Blogger, Blogspot),
- social networking sites (SNS) (e.g., Facebook, LinkedIn, Bebo),
- virtual worlds (e.g., Second Life),
- projects co-created by users (e.g., Wikipedia),
- content websites (e.g., YouTube), and
- virtual worlds of games (e.g., World of Warcraft).

Differences in the published contents and available functions result in the fact that
different social media sites are applied differently in marketing activities
(Castronovo and Huang, 2012: 123).

Tab. 13.1: Examples of applications of selected social media
*Source: Adapted from Castronovo C., Huang L., 2012. Social Media in an Alternative Marketing
Communication Model. Journal of Marketing Development and Competitiveness, 6(1), 123*

Types of social media	Examples of applications
blogs (eg., Blogger, Blogspot)	– sharing opinions and recommendations. – building relations. – increasing loyalty.
microblogs (eg., Twitter)	– engaging consumers. – developing dialogue with users.
social networking sites (eg., Facebook, LinkedIn, Google+)	– Internet advertising. – developing communities on the Internet. – reaching certain communities. – joining the community of professionals.
content websites (eg., YouTube, DailyMotion, Vimeo)	– using video materials to increase dissemination of content on the Internet.

Social networking sites are particularly important among social media. They allow
users and organizations to reflect the networks of contacts and relationships they

have in the real world in virtual space. The main change, however, consists in social networking sites having the possibility, thanks to their functions, to increase the gaining and maintaining (developing) of relationships with contacts they already possess ('Friends') (Boyd and Ellison, 2007: 211).

At the end of 2009, Manhattan Research, a company dealing with market research and consulting in the pharmaceutical and healthcare industry on a global scale, conducted research on how doctors from Germany, Spain, France, Italy, and the UK use the Internet. Additionally, similar information about patients as Internet users was collected. According to the research, using social media is a growing trend in Europe; more than two-thirds of doctors are interested in joining social networking sites. On the other hand, patients usually use social media to exchange experiences as well as opinions about the products and services provided by the national health service (ManhattanRESEARCH, 2010: 1).

The publication of the Internet World Stats site since September 2012 shows that Facebook is the most well-known social media site in Europe. Knowledge of this site is declared by almost 100 percent of Internet users. Facebook has 243 million registered users in Europe, and this is the highest number of users of this website in the world (Internet World Stats, 2012).

Tab. 13.2: Number of Facebook users with breakdown into the regions of the world
Source: Adapted from Internet World Stats, 2012. Homepage – Facebook World Stats. Retrieved October 01, 2013 from: http://www.internetworldstats.com/facebook.htm.

Region	Millions of Subscribers
Europe	243.2
Asia	236.0
North America	184.2
South America	134.6
Africa	48.3
Central America/Mexico	47.0
Middle East	22.8
Oceania/Australia	14.6

On the other hand, the results of research among the patients of fourteen European countries (Austria, Belgium, Germany, Denmark, Estonia, Finland, France, Italy, Netherlands, Sweden, Slovenia, Slovakia, Spain, and the UK), announced in 2012, confirm that patients from Europe use the Internet, first of all, to search for information, use electronic mail (e-mail), and conduct activities on social networking sites (Citizens and ICT for Health in 14 EU Countries, 2012: 17).

Table 13.3: Purposes of using the Internet by patients from fourteen European countries
Source: Adapted from Citizens and ICT for Health in 14 EU countries, 2012. Brussels: European Commission.

	Every day or almost every day	At least once a week (but not every day)	At least once a month (but not every week)	Less than once a month	Never
use a search engine to find information	68%	24%	6%	2%	1%
send e-mails with attached files (documents, pictures, etc.)	41%	33%	16%	8%	3%
use a social networking site	39%	19%	10%	10%	22%
instant messaging, chat websites	23%	18%	12%	15%	32%
do home banking	20%	37%	18%	7%	18%
use the Internet through your mobile phone	19%	13%	9%	10%	49%
online gaming and/or playing game console	18%	18%	13%	15%	36%
post messages to chat rooms, newsgroups, or an online discussion forum	15%	17%	15%	19%	34%
use online software	14%	17%	19%	22%	28%
use websites to share pictures, videos, movies, etc.	12%	16%	16%	19%	36%
use the Internet to make telephone calls	9%	13%	12%	16%	52%
purchase goods or services online/online shopping (e.g., travel and holiday, clothes, books, tickets, films, music, …)	7%	21%	38%	28%	7%
use peer-to-peer file sharing for exchanging movies, music, etc.	6%	9%	10%	14%	60%
keep a blog (also known as weblog)	5%	7%	9%	11%	68%
create a web page	4%	6%	7%	16%	67%

The attractiveness of social media results from the expansion of their communication possibilities. The users have more and more possibilities of posting various multimedia materials – pictures, videos, and sound files. Also important are the mechanisms of interactions, such as assessment of information and video multimedia materials as well as sharing the content with other users of the site (Levinson, 2010: 18).

The popularity of social media, especially social networking sites, is different in different countries. According to the publication *The Economist*, Germans are most skeptical about using social networking sites. Thirty-seven percent of Internet users from this country use them. In Great Britain, Sweden, and Belgium, more than 50 percent of Internet users use them. In Latvia, Poland, Slovakia, and Cyprus, the number is 63 percent. The largest number of social networking site users is, on the other hand, among Hungarians – 80 percent (The Economist online, 2011).

Despite various attitudes in the society regarding this type of activity, it should be emphasized that social networking sites have become an important area of activity among Internet users. Additionally, the information made available by networking sites helps implement the idea of the marketing of relations in practice.

13.4 Control of effectiveness of activities building relationships

The intangible character of relationships results in the fact that organizations, in particular, look for methods of evaluating them as well as monitoring and controlling the effectiveness of the actions related to their establishment and development.

The stream of research associated with evaluation of relationships led to the development of classifications of relations, which are supposed to facilitate measurement of their value for both the client and the company. G. Urbanek proposes, for example, distinguishing of two types of relationships with a client (2005: 12): 1) relations in the sense of intangible assets that are the result of active relationship management by the company and 2) relations in general (such relations always come into being when a transaction between the company and the client takes place and are treated as part of goodwill). Thus, in order to speak about the relationship with the client as a part of the company's assets, the following two conditions must be met (Bilińska-Reformat K., 2009: 71):
- actual 'personal' relations must occur between the parties, and
- documentation regarding the relations (database) must exist.

Personal relations do not imply here family or friendly relationships, but mutual knowledge, allowing establishment of contacts by any party. For this purpose, a contact channel may be created, e.g., a helpline, a newsletter, or sending a folder (Bilińska-Reformat, 2009: 74).

Both of the conditions mentioned above are met in the case of using social networking sites. The users can contact the organization's page directly by connecting their profile with it on a social networking site. Any activity on the part of the organization and users is in turn accumulated in the site and made available for browsing.

The main parameter that may be used to evaluate the effects of activities on social networking sites is the number of 'Friends' (or 'Fans') or 'Followers'. These are individual users – sometimes organizations – who have connected their profile with a given site in a social networking site. Such a connection means that they express permission to receive information published on the site they 'Like'. The number of 'Friends' changes in time; usually it grows rapidly at the beginning of the organization's activities on a social networking site and achieves stabilization at a certain level. The size of communities is different for various organizations, e.g., Mc Donald's, at the end of July of 2012, had 21,911,010 'Friends' on Facebook and 10,496,341 on Google. In the healthcare industry, the National Health Service organization from the UK had 52,920 'Friends' on its website at the end of May 2013.

However, the most significant functions, from the point of view of building relationships between the organization and users, are the so-called social functions – mostly on social networking sites. They make it possible to assess particular information, comment on it, or make it available to other users of the site. For instance, in the case of the Facebook social networking site, users may use functions such as 'Like', 'Comment', and 'Share'. Use of any of these functions yields specific effects for the user and the organization. They have been described in more detail in Table 13.4.

It should be noted that the 'weight' of the functions mentioned above in building relationships with users varies. Using the 'Like' function does not require the users to show great commitment and, consequently, it affects the user-organization relations most poorly. Use of the 'Comment' function is very important from the point of view of building relations with the community already acquired by the organization because posting a comment requires the user to be involved in the preparation and publishing of an opinion. Additionally, maintaining the initiated discussion allows more users to join it. The 'Share' function makes it possible, on the one hand, to identify users who become 'the ambassadors' of the content published by the organization. On the other hand, publications of the organization published on private profiles of users make it possible to reach people who so far have not been interested in the organization's activity. This creates a chance to acquire them in the community of the organization.

To present an example of the effectiveness of building relationships by the entities of the healthcare system via the social networking sites, eleven entities responsible for organization and provision of services related to healthcare in five selected countries (Belgium, Germany, Poland, Sweden, and UK) were analyzed.

Tab. 13.4: Description of parameters for assessment of profitability of building relations on Facebook (SNS)
Source: Author's study

Parameter name	User	Organization
Like	– it allows the users to express their approval for the selected publication (entry). – a single user may use this function only once for a single entry. – the 'Friends' of the user receive information on liking the publication, which may encourage them to do the same. – it is also possible to cancel the approval expressed, using the 'I don't like' function.	– it enables basic evaluation of the quality of a publication (entry). – the more 'Likes', the greater the chance to promote the entry among users who have not encountered the organization so far.
Comment	– applied to express a written opinion concerning the selected publication. – it can be used many times, which makes it possible to develop a discussion between users. – the 'Friends' of the user are informed that he or she commented on particular entries. – the user is also notified about subsequent comments appearing under the entry. – additionally, the users can express their approval for single comments using the 'Like' function.	– it enables learning about specific opinions of users. – the organization may also post its comments–in the form of new threads or answers to the already posted opinions. – in turn, tracking 'Likes' of comments indicates the most popular opinions approved by users.
Share	– it allows the users to post, on their profile, publications from the organization's page. – the 'Friends' of the user may become familiar with the full entry, even if they are not connected with the organization's site.	– it gives the possibility of indirectly reaching, with full content publication, the users who have not been 'Friends' so far.

In the case of Germany, the entities were Der Verband der Ersatzkassen e. V. (vdek), Der AOK-Bundesverband, Der BKK Bundesverband, Dem IKK e.V., Die Knappschaft, Der Landwirtschaftlichen Sozialversicherung (LSV-SPV), and Der GKV-Spitzenverband. In the UK, the entity was the National Health Service (NHS); in Belgium, the entity was L'Institut national d'assurance maladie-invalidité (INAMI); in Sweden, the entity was the Swedish National Institute of Public Health; and in Poland, the entity was Narodowy Fundusz Zdrowia (NFZ).

It turned out that only the National Health Service in the UK has a Facebook site (https://www.facebook.com/NHSChoices) and conducts active operations there. Among the remaining organizations, a connection with community websites appears in four out of the seven entities in Germany. The organizations Der Verband der Ersatzkassen e. V., Der AOK-Bundesverband, Der BKK Bundesverband, and Der

GKV-Spitzenverband allow their users to publish entries from their web pages on such websites as Facebook, Google+, Xing, and Twitter. Such action, however, does not allow linking the user's profile on a social networking site with the organization. It also does not enable initiating direct contact.

The evaluation of the effectiveness of building relations with clients (patients) will thus be shown in the example of the National Health Service in the UK.

We will consider the period from May 1 to 31, 2013. During this period, the NHS posted, on its page on the FB website, twenty-one publications (entries) of various kinds: text information, multimedia materials, and links to external pages.

Table 13.5 presents the numbers corresponding to the proposed basic parameters for evaluation of the effectiveness of building relationships on Facebook. These are the totals for each kind of interaction for all entries posted by NHS in the period being examined.

Tab. 13.5: Statement of numbers for the parameters for the evaluation of the effectiveness of building relationships on Facebook for the National Healthcare Service (UK) for the period from May1 to 31, 2013
Source: Author's study

No.	Parameter name	Total
1.	number of 'Likes'	126
2.	number of 'Comments'	35
3.	number of 'Shares'	87

These publications brought about the activity level of 126 'Like' clicks, hence, on average, 6 'Likes' per entry. Under entries, there also appeared 35 'Comments' in total, which means, on average, more than 1 'Comment' (1.66) under a single entry was posted. On the other hand, taking into account the number of 'Sharing' entries, 4 'Sharing' actions took place on average for 1 entry.

From the point of view of developing reactive and partner relationships, which denote, in particular, a dialogue between the organization and a single user, the number of 'Likes' and 'Comments' to the entries of NHS can be considered sufficient. The number of 'Sharing' actions obtained is of great importance in establishing subsequent contacts and building a community around the NHS site on Facebook. The 'Share' function may be used by a single user only once for one entry. This means that 87 users regarded the content published by the NHS site interesting enough to include it on their private profile. This, in turn, resulted in a high probability of NHS reaching people who have not established relations with this organization so far. Thanks to the activities of the National Health Service on Facebook, from February 16, 2010, to May31, 2013, the number of users who joined the community of this organization amounted to 52,920.

Conclusions

The parameters presented concerned with measuring the effectiveness of building relationships on social media can be considered universal. On most social media websites, the functions of assessing, commenting, and sharing the content are available. Tracking these parameters makes it possible, at a basic level, to assess the size and the strength of relations occurring between an organization and the users. The parameters even have greater importance than the number of users – 'Friends' ('Followers') – related to the organization's page.

Along with the popularization of the use of social media in organizations, it is also possible to observe the development of tools enabling users' activity to be monitored in an advanced manner. An independent website 'Social Media Today', addressed to public relations, marketing, and advertising specialists, published a list of fifty tools for social media monitoring in May of 2013: http://socialmediatoday.com/pamdyer/1458746/50-top-tools-social-media-monitoring-analytics-and-management-2013.

This website contains links both to paid and free tools. Such applications make it possible to keep track of the effects of the activities of an organization on different social media as well as, in the case of selected tools, to manage the content published on different websites from one place.

The information presented in the publication concerning the activity of selected organizations from the health protection trade in social media show that most of them use these tools insufficiently to establish contacts and develop relationships with customers. From the point of view of relations marketing, it is important, however, that social media not be regarded as yet another mass communication channel but rather as a place for an organization to meet single users.

References

Bilińska-Reformat, K., 2009. *Relacje podmiotów rynkowych w warunkach zmian*. Warszawa: Wydawnictwo Placet.

Boyd, D.M. & Ellison, N.B., 2007. Social network sites: Definition, history, and scholarship. *Journal of Computer-Mediated Communication*, 13(1), 211.

Castronovo, C. & Huang, L., 2012. Social Media in an Alternative Marketing Communication Model. *Journal of Marketing Development and Competitiveness*, 6(1), 123.

Citizens and ICT for Health in 14 EU countries, 2012. Brussels: European Commission.

Dyche, J., 2002. *CRM. Relacje z klientami*. Gliwice: Wydawnictwo Helion.

Kaplan, A.M. & Haenlein, M., 2010. Users of the world, unite! The challenges and opportunities of social media. *Business Horizons*, 53(1), 65.

Kelly, K., 2001. *Nowe reguły nowej gospodarki*. Warszawa: WIG-Press.

Kotler, Ph., Armstrong, G., Saunders, J. & Wong, V., 2002. *Marketing. Podręcznik europejski*. Warszawa: Wydawnictwo PWE.

Levinson, P., 2010. *Nowe Nowe Media*. Kraków: Wydawnictwo WAM.

ManhattanRESEARCH, 2010. *Navigating the European Health Landscape*. Retrieved October 01, 2013 from: http://www.icmcc.org/pdf/2010_European_eHealth_Landscape.pdf.

Matysiewicz, J. & Smyczek, S., 2012. *Modele relacji jednostek medycznych z pacjentami w otoczeniu wirtualnym*. Warszawa: Wydawnictwo Placet.

Pizło, W., 2008. Marketing relacji – koncepcja i kierunki rozwoju. *Zeszyty Naukowe SGGW*, 69: 92.

Thomas, M., 1994. Przyszłość marketingu. *Marketing i Rynek*, 5, 6.

Urbanek, G., 2005. Wycena relacji z klientem. *Marketing i Rynek*, 12.

Internet World Stats, 2012. *Facebook World Stats*. Retrieved October 01, 2013 from: http://www.internetworldstats.com/facebook.htm.

The Economist online, 2011. *Where networking works*. Retrieved October 02, 2013 from: http://www.economist.com/blogs/dailychart/2011/07/europe%E2%80%99s-social-media-hotspots.

About the Authors

Beatrix Dietz has graduated from the University of Mannheim, Germany, where she also pursued her PhD at the chair of Professor Dr. Dr. h.c. mult. Christian Homburg. Currently, she is Professor of Marketing at the Berlin School of Economics and Law. Her research interests are healthcare-marketing and gender diversity. Prior to her academic career she worked – among others – as a marketing manager in the global business unit of Diabetes Care at Roche Diagnostics and as a team-leader at Pfizer.

Contact: Berlin School of Economics and Law, Department of Business and Economics, Badensche Strasse 52, 10825 Berlin, Germany

Mario Glowik is Professor of International Strategic Management at the Berlin School of Economics and Law in Germany. He holds a Doctorate in Business Administration from the Freie Universität Berlin in Germany and gained his habilitation (post-doctoral qualification) at the Vienna University of Economics and Business, Austria. His research is focused on the understanding and interpretation of global network configurations such as for example in healthcare, pharmaceutical and medical devices industries.

Contact: Berlin School of Economics and Law, Department of Business and Economics, Badensche Strasse 52, 10825 Berlin, Germany

Jagoda Gola is Ph.D. student at the University of Economics in Katowice, Poland. She graduated at the University at the Management faculty as well as at the Finance & Insurance faculty. Currently she works as a senior analyst at a consulting company providing concepts, among others, concerning financing and the efficient application of highly innovative technologies in different industries, including healthcare. She is specialized in investment projects profitability and feasibility studies. She has also published articles about consumer behavior and venture capital.

Contact: University of Economics in Katowice, Poland, Department of Consumption Research, 1 Maja Str. 50, Katowice, Poland

Marta Grybś is Ph.D. student in the Department of Consumption Research at the University of Economics in Katowice, Poland. Her scientific interests are focused around issues of modern trends in consumer behavior as well as integrated marketing communication and nonconventional advertising strategies. She developed her scientific experience inter alia through international projects where she gained valuable insights into global perspectives of healthcare markets and corresponding marketing communication.

Contact: University of Economics in Katowice, Poland, Department of Consumption Research, 1 Maja Str. 50, Katowice, Poland

Agnieszka Hat is Ph.D. student at the University of Economics in Katowice, Poland. Her research is focused on consumer behavior, particularly new consumer trends occurring in the contemporary world of medical and professional service markets. Her doctoral dissertation is devoted to the phenomenon of consumer ethnocentrism.

Contact: University of Economics in Katowice, Poland, Department of Consumption Research, 1 Maja Str. 50, Katowice, Poland

Agnieszka Marie is Ph.D. student at the Department of Consumer Research at the University of Economics in Katowice, Poland. She has earned a Master's degree both in Finance and Management. Her research is focused on consumer behavior in healthcare services markets. Agnieszka's doctoral dissertation is devoted to the phenomenon of the patient's dysfunctional behavior. As for her professional experience, she currently works as a specialist at PricewaterhouseCoopers Service Delivery Center Poland.

Contact: University of Economics in Katowice, Poland, Department of Consumption Research, 1 Maja Str. 50, Katowice, Poland

Justyna Matysiewicz is Assistant Professor at the University of Economics in Katowice, Poland. She holds a Doctorate in Economics. Her Ph.D. dissertation was related to concepts of structural conflicts in the company against its orientation changes. She has an extensive tertiary teaching and research experience. Her research is focused on management processes in healthcare service networks. She also conducts specialized training of medical staff.

Contact: University of Economics in Katowice, Poland, Department of Market Policy and Marketing Management, 1 Maja Str. 50, Katowice, Poland

Marcin Młodożeniec is founding director and co-owner of PRIME PR Agency. He is also Ph.D. student at the University of Economics in Katowice, Poland. Marcin is an enthusiast of engaging consumers in the world of brands and product innovation processes and author of publications related to the use of social media in business. Since 2004 he has planned and coordinated several marketing communications projects for companies doing business in healthcare, retail, and real estate as well as telecommunication industries.

Contact: University of Economics in Katowice, Poland, Department of Consumption Research, 1 Maja Str. 50, Katowice, Poland

Thuy Nguyen is a Manager at BIOTRONIK, one of the world's leading manufacturers of cardio- and endovascular medical devices. She gained her Master of Arts in Business Management from the Technical University of Applied Sciences in Wildau (Brandenburg, Germany). All her expertise in healthcare and medical devices she has gained during her employment at BIOTRONIK since 2008. Being responsible for an international physician training program, she is in permanent contact with different national and international hospitals for cardiology and acquired in-depth knowledge about the hospital structures, sales strategies of medical devices and the international medical device market.

Contact: BIOTRONIK, Woermannkehre 1, 12359 Berlin, Germany

Alexander J. Owczarek is Associate Professor at the Medical University of Silesia in Katowice, Poland. He holds a Doctorate in Electronics (digital biomedical signal processing) from the Silesian University of Technology and gained his habilitation (post-doctoral qualification) at the Medical University of Silesia in Katowice. His research is focused on biomedical data analysis relying on a broad range of statistical methods. Among others, he applies different types of classification trees and clustering algorithms, kernel and robust regression, structural equation modeling and time series analysis, and its use in cardiovascular epidemiology as well as in public health.

Contact: School of Pharmacy with the Division of Laboratory Medicine in Sosnowiec Medical University of Silesia, Katowice, Poland, Department of Instrumental Analysis, Division of Statistics, Ostrogórska Str. 30, Sosnowiec, Poland

Sławomir Smyczek is Full Professor and Vice-Rector for Internationalization and Marketing at the University of Economics in Katowice, Poland. He earned his Ph.D. from the same university. In 2010, the Polish Prime Minister awarded his habilitation (post-doctoral qualification) thesis as the best in Economics. He has an extensive international teaching and research experience. He also serves as consultant for institutions and international enterprises. His research is focused on consumer behavior, consumption models and relationship marketing such as for example in healthcare and pharmaceutical markets.

Contact: University of Economics in Katowice, Poland, Department of Consumption Research, 1 Maja Str. 50, Katowice, Poland

Artur Turek graduated from the Faculty of Pharmacy and Division of Laboratory Medicine at the Medical University of Silesia in Katowice. He obtained his Ph.D. in pharmaceutical sciences specializing in pharmaceutical biochemistry. His research deals with the modification of tissue-derived biomaterials, innovative drug configurations, as well as medicine consumption and consumer behavior in the pharmaceutical markets.

Contact: School of Pharmacy with the Division of Laboratory Medicine in Sosnowiec, Medical University of Silesia, Katowice, Poland, Chair and Department of Biopharmacy, Jedności Str. 8, Sosnowiec, Poland

Marcin Tutaj is a graduate of Silesian Higher School of Management and Upper Silesian Higher School of Economics in Katowice, Poland. He holds a degree in the field of Management and Marketing. Since 2003 he has been preparing and implementing communication strategies for companies and non-profit organizations as for example involved in healthcare. Marcin has participated in the development and implementation of various campaigns in the field of marketing communication using conventional and state-of-the-art social media tools. He works as a project consultant addressed to small and medium-sized enterprises.

Contact: University of Economics in Katowice, Poland, Department of Consumption Research, 1 Maja Str. 50, Katowice, Poland

Andreas Zaby teaches innovation & technology management, international management and entrepreneurial finance at the Berlin School of Economics and Law. He is also the Deputy President of this university. His research focuses on the management of high-technology firms, particularly from the biopharmaceutical industry. Prior to joining academia, Andreas worked as a strategy consultant in the healthcare practice of a leading US consulting company and, subsequently, as a CFO for a German-American biotechnology company. He holds an MBA (honors) from San Diego State University and a doctoral degree from the Friedrich-Schiller-University of Jena, Germany (summa cum laude).

Contact: Berlin School of Economics and Law, Department of Business and Economics, Badensche Strasse 52, 10825 Berlin, Germany

Index

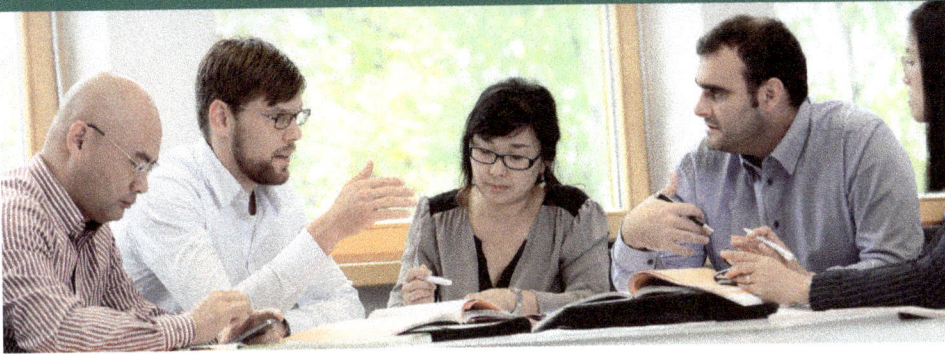

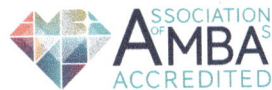

www.ingramcontent.com/pod-product-compliance
Lightning Source LLC
Chambersburg PA
CBHW050039220326

41599CB00041B/7210